Springer Tracts in Advanced Robotics 108

Editors

More information about this series at http://www.springer.com/series/5208

STAR (Springer Tracts in Advanced Robotics) has been promoted under the auspices of EURON (European Robotics Research Network)

Shane (S.Q.) Xie

Advanced Robotics for Medical Rehabilitation

Current State of the Art and Recent Advances

Springer

Shane (S.Q.) Xie
The Department of Mechanical Engineering
The University of Auckland
Auckland
New Zealand

ISSN 1610-7438 ISSN 1610-742X (electronic)
Springer Tracts in Advanced Robotics
ISBN 978-3-319-19895-8 ISBN 978-3-319-19896-5 (eBook)
DOI 10.1007/978-3-319-19896-5

Library of Congress Control Number: 2015950907

Springer Cham Heidelberg New York Dordrecht London

Printed on acid-free paper

Springer International Publishing AG Switzerland is part of Springer Science+Business Media
(www.springer.com)

Series Foreword

Robotics is undergoing a major transformation in scope and dimension. From a largely dominant industrial focus, robotics is rapidly expanding into human environments and vigorously engaged in its new challenges. Interacting with, assisting, serving and exploring with humans, the emerging robots will increasingly touch people and their lives.

Beyond its impact on physical robots, the body of knowledge robotics has produced is revealing a much wider range of applications reaching across diverse research areas and scientific disciplines, such as biomechanics, haptics, neurosciences, virtual simulation, animation, surgery and sensor networks, among others. In return, the challenges of the new emerging areas are proving an abundant source of stimulation and insights for the field of robotics. It is indeed at the intersection of disciplines that the most striking advances happen.

The *Springer Tracts in Advanced Robotics* (STAR) is devoted to bringing to the research community the latest advances in the robotic field on the basis of their significance and quality. Through a wide and timely dissemination of critical research developments in robotics, our objective with this series is to promote more exchanges and collaborations among the researchers in the community and contribute to further advancements in this rapidly growing field.

The monograph by Shane Xie presents the outcome of recent research results in the field of rehabilitation robotics, which is broadly surveyed. A number of novel methods are introduced including a physiological model of the masticatory system, a model of the human shoulder and elbow, a motion and interactive control of an exoskeleton for upper limb rehabilitation, a kinematic and computational model of human ankle, and an adaptive control of an ankle rehabilitation robot. Trends and opportunities for future advances in the design, modelling, control and development of medical robotic systems for rehabilitation are also discussed.

Most methods have been effectively implemented in experimental tests, and the source code of the robotic simulation and control is valuably provided. A fine addition to STAR!

Naples, Italy
September 2015

Bruno Siciliano
STAR Editor

Preface

Robots were used for rehabilitation purposes since the 1960s. Application of robots in rehabilitation was initially more focused on replacing lost functions in individuals with physical disabilities through the use of devices such as robotic orthoses, workstations, feeding devices and robotic wheelchairs. Over the last two decades, there has been an increasing amount of research into the use of robots in physical therapy. The goal of rehabilitation is to recuperate a patient from impairment or disability and improve mobility, functional ability and quality of life. This impairment can be the result of a stroke, a injury or a neurological disease.

Since robots are well suited for repetitive tasks and can be designed to have adequate force capabilities, their use in the execution of these exercises will be able to reduce the physical workload of therapists and can potentially allow the therapists to simultaneously oversee the treatment of multiple patients in a supervisory role. By using robotic devices, diagnosis and prognosis can be made more objectively with the help of quantitative data, and comparisons between different cases can also be made more easily. Several successful rehabilitation robots have undergone clinical trials and are currently being used in hospitals and clinics for neuromotor rehabilitation. However, the research and development of advanced robotics for medical rehabilitation are still at an early stage, and further research and development in this area are becoming more and more urgent.

This book systematically reviews the recent research and development of the innovative technologies for advanced robotics in medical rehabilitation. Through systematic overview of the existing systems and recent approaches of rehabilitation robots, interaction control and rehabilitation, the problems that emerged from recent approaches have been identified. To overcome these problems and to develop a series of novel advanced rehabilitation robotics, research and development of medical robotics for human impaired limbs have been carried out. These include the introduction of physiological masticatory model development, the modelling of human shoulder and elbow mechanisms, an exoskeleton development for upper limb rehabilitation, kinematic and computational model of human ankle, development of ankle rehabilitation robot and its adaptive control strategies. These research topics and findings constitute the main contents of this book.

The aim of this book is to provide a snapshot of our recent research outcomes and implementation studies in the field of advanced rehabilitation robotics. As the title suggests, Chap. 1 gives an overview of medical rehabilitation robotics. It briefly introduces the history and background of the medical robotics and this is followed by the discussion on the current issues involved in existing robotics and the motivation of our work presented in this book.

Chapter 2 presents the historical background of advanced robotics for medical rehabilitation. This chapter has highlighted the main motivations and objectives of this book through an overview of rehabilitation robots, interaction control and rehabilitation. The different types of rehabilitation devices developed in literatures were considered, with particular focus on their mechanical design, actuation methods and control schemes. Subsequently, studies relating to human limb kinematics and computational modelling of the ankle were also examined.

Targeting masticatory system modelling, Chap. 3 introduces the associated numerous complexities, and a new physiological model with two DOFs was developed for it. An in-depth study was performed on the mandibular muscles to properly characterise all accessible mandibular muscle EMG signals from which to base the physiological model. Based on the findings of the EMG signal study, the physiological model of the masticatory system was reconfigured and the concept of a hybrid model was introduced. The effectiveness of hybrid model was proven through experiments from multiple subjects and was analysed offline.

To further address the robotic system for upper limb, Chap. 4 proposes a kinematically redundant 4R spherical wrist model for shoulder and elbow joints, with its kinematics modelled by DH notation to solve the forward and inverse kinematic problems. This chapter also presents an EMG-driven physiological model of the elbow joint that was developed in the sagittal plane. In this chapter, the physiological model of the developed elbow joint model was coupled with linear envelope processing and experimentally validated with data from multiple subjects.

The design of an active upper limb exoskeleton prototype is presented in Chap. 5. A redundant 4R spherical wrist mechanism is proposed for a shoulder exoskeleton to solve the singularity and workspace limitations. The 4R mechanism has been optimised using multi-objective optimisation algorithm to achieve the entire human shoulder workspace while operating far away from singular configurations and without interfering with the user. Numerous important design factors were considered in this chapter in realising the final exoskeleton design to ensure that it can operate effectively alongside a human user's upper limb.

Chapter 6 further develops the motion and interactive control methods for upper limb exoskeleton. This chapter presents the minimum jerk trajectory planner, which is developed to generate smooth trajectories for the 5-DOF upper limb exoskeleton. This chapter also presents force-based control strategies that allow the exoskeleton to interact with and respond to the unpredictable behaviour of the user's limb. The concept of admittance and impedance in the interaction between two physical systems is discussed and applied to the exoskeleton system.

To model the human ankle joint, motion of the ankle–foot structure is discussed in Chap. 7. This chapter presents a computational ankle model developed to facilitate controller development of the ankle rehabilitation robot and provides a description of the ankle mechanical characteristics through considerations of forces applied along anatomical elements around the ankle joint, which include ligaments and muscle–tendon units. The dynamics of the ankle–foot structure and its surrounding ligaments and muscle–tendon units were formulated into a state space model to facilitate simulation of the robot. Finally, based on observations from preliminary testing, a modified recursive least squares algorithm was proposed and tested on experimental data.

Chapter 8 begins with an overview of the design requirements of an ankle rehabilitation robot. A suitable kinematic structure of the robot is then designed. Workspace, singularity and force analyses of mechanisms having this structure are then presented. This is followed by a description of the robot hardware and interface. Operation of the developed rehabilitation robot relies on implementation of a suitable interaction controller, and a force-based impedance control approach had been taken in this research. This chapter details the development of the multi-input multi-output (MIMO) actuator force controller devised in this work.

Chapter 9 further details the dynamic model of the parallel mechanism for ankle rehabilitation and presents variable impedance control approaches to achieve adaptive interaction control. In this chapter, the basic impedance control law is extended to yield a more advanced interaction control scheme for passive range of motion and active-assistive exercises. This chapter also explores the use of an assistance adaptation scheme to achieve the implementation of a control module to facilitate active user participation in the rehabilitation exercises.

Chapter 10 seeks to summarise the main outcomes and conclusions of this research, as well as highlight the contributions made in this book. This chapter also provides a discussion of future directions that can be explored to extend or advance the work presented in this book. The future trends in various aspects including the design, modelling and control of the advanced robotics for medical rehabilitation are discussed. This may be used to guide coming research, or act as a reference for institutions to design and develop new medical robotic systems.

This book also contains an Appendix that summarises some of the design and development of rehabilitation robotics. It provides the source code of the robotic simulation and control. These are excellent examples for users or developers.

I would like to take this opportunity to express my deep appreciation to those who have contributed to this book. The authors are also grateful to Wei Meng, Yun Ho Tsoi, James Pau and Ho Shing Lo for their assistance in compiling the book. It is our sincere hope that readers will find this book useful to their study and research.

Auckland, New Zealand
March 2015

Shane (S.Q.) Xie

Acknowledgments

The authors would like to acknowledge funding support from the Foundation for Research, Science and Technology of New Zealand, the Auckland Medical Research Foundation, the Lottery Healthcare Research Foundation and the University of Auckland.

Contents

Nomenclature

3D	Three-dimensional
Abduction	Drawing a limb away from the median sagittal plane (e.g. raising the shoulder)
Abduction/external rotation	Rotation of the foot on the transverse plane so that the big toe is moved away from the sagittal plane of the human body
AC	Activity coefficient
Adduction	Bringing a limb closer to the median sagittal plane (e.g. lowering the shoulder)
Adduction/internal rotation	Rotation of the foot on the transverse plane so that the big toe is moved closer towards the sagittal plane of the human body
Ankle/talocrural joint	The articulation between the tibia, fibula and talus
ANN	Artificial neural network
Anterior	In anatomy, nearer the forward end, or front of a human
AR	Autoregressive (coefficients)
Bilateral	Of both sides
CC	Correlation coefficient
CE	Contractile element
CMOS	Complementary metal–oxide–semiconductor
CMRR	Common-mode rejection ratio—ability of a device to reject common input signals (noise)
Concentric contraction	Condition where skeletal muscle shortens during a contraction (and overcomes external resistance)
Condition number	The ratio of the maximum to minimum singular values of a matrix
Contralateral	On the opposite side of the body
CPM	Continuous passive motion
DE	Differential evolution
DOF	Degree of freedom

Dorsiflexion	Rotation of the foot on the sagittal plane so that the toes are brought closer towards the shank
DSP	Digital signal processing
Eccentric contraction	Condition where skeletal muscle lengthens during a contraction (usually an already shortened muscle acting in a braking capacity)
EDF	Error dependency function
EEG	Electroencephalography—non-invasive measure of electrical brain activity taken from the surface of the scalp
EKF	Extended Kalman filter
Electromechanical delay	The time delay between the initiation of a muscle contraction and actual movement
EMA	Electromagnetic articulograph—device to track mandibular movement
EMG	Electromyography—non-invasive measure of electrical muscle activity taken from the skin surface
Euler angles	A sequence of angles used to define orientation of an object through consecutive rotations about the specified axes. For example, XYZ Euler angles give the X rotation about the x-axis, followed by a Y rotation about the resulting y-axis and then the Z rotation about the resulting z-axis
Eversion	Rotation of the foot so that the medial side of the foot is moved away from the sagittal plane of the human body
Exoskeleton	Powered anthropomorphic robotic device that moves in concert with a user
FFT	Fast Fourier transform
Frontal plane	The anatomical plane separating the body into front and back portions
GA	Genetic algorithm
GUI	Graphical user interface
HPF	High-pass filter
IMU	Inertial measurement unit
In vivo	Within a living environment
Inversion	Rotation of the foot so that the lateral side of the foot is moved closer to the sagittal plane of the human body
Ipsilateral	On the same side of the body
Isometric contraction	Muscle contraction during which muscle length is constant (only force increases)
Joint space	Generalised coordinates used to describe the motion or force quantities along the actuators of a robot
Lateral	Used to describe the side of a body part which is away from the sagittal plane of the human body

LE	Linear envelope—the result of linear envelope processing (LEP)
LEP	Linear envelope processing—filtering process that produces a smoothed signal, which is called a linear envelope
LMS	Least mean square
LPF	Low-pass filter
Manipulator Jacobian	A matrix describing the linear mapping between the joint space velocity and task space velocity
MAV	Mean absolute value—a time-domain feature of the EMG signal
MC	Movement coefficient
Medial	In anatomy, pertaining to the inside and closer to the midline
Medial	Used to describe the side of a body part which is facing towards the sagittal plane of the human body
MEM	Matrix element matching
MIMO	Multi-input multi-output
MMG	Mechanomyography—non-invasive measure of the surface oscillations of the skin during muscle contraction
MSE	Mean square error
MU	Motor unit—a motor neuron and all the muscle fibres it innervates
MUAP	Motor unit action potential—electrical impulse that stimulates contraction of a motor unit's muscle fibres
MVC	Maximum voluntary contraction—maximum contraction attainable without causing pain or discomfort
Myoelectric signal	Another name for the EMG signal
NI	Neuromuscular interface—all the hardware and software components involved in converting the raw EMG signals of a joint into an equivalent torque or displacement
Null space	A column-wise collection of the null vectors of a matrix
Null vector	A null vector of a matrix is a column vector of unit length whereby the matrix multiplication of this matrix and the null vector will result in a zero vector
PCB	Printed circuit board
PE	Parallel-elastic element
Plantarflexion	Rotation of the foot on the sagittal plane so that the toes are brought away from the shank
Posterior	In anatomy, nearer the back end, i.e. back of a human

Pronation	Rotational movement of the forearm that causes the palm to face downwards
Rank deficient	A matrix is considered to be rank deficient if it has zero as a singular value
RLS	Recursive least square
RMS	Root mean square—a time domain feature of the EMG signal
RMSE	Root mean square error—measure of average error between two sets of data collected over a set period of time
Robot singularity	A point in the robot workspace whereby the manipulator Jacobian becomes rank deficient
ROM	Range of motion
Sagittal plane	In anatomy, the vertical plane that passes from the front to rear of the body, dividing it into left and right halves
Sagittal plane	The anatomical plane separating the body into left and right portions
SDOF	Single degree of freedom
SE	Series elastic element
Shank	The portion of the lower limb between the knee and the ankle
Singular values	The values along the leading diagonal of the rectangular diagonal matrix resulting from the singular value decomposition of a matrix
Singular value decomposition (SVD)	A matrix factorisation that represents a rectangular matrix as the product of a unitary matrix, a rectangular diagonal matrix with non-negative real numbers along its diagonal and another unitary matrix
SISO	Single-input single-output
Subtalar joint	The articulation between the talus and calcaneus
Supination	Rotational movement of the forearm that causes that palm to face upwards
Task space	Generalised coordinates used to describe the motion or force quantities in the operational space of a robot
TMJ	Temporomandibular joint—connects the mandible to the maxilla at the base of the skull
TMJD	Temporomandibular joint disorder
Transverse plane	The anatomical plane separating the body into top and bottom portions

Chapter 1
Introduction

Robots can be considered as reprogrammable devices which can be used to complete certain tasks in an autonomous manner. While robots have long been used for automation of industrial processes, there is a growing trend where robotic devices are used to provide services for end users. An area where robots are believed to have a significant impact is healthcare. Accessibility to healthcare services is a vital component to improve the quality of life. This chapter provides background information on issues relating to this research, starting with the motivations behind the development of rehabilitation robots for physical therapy and successful examples of such systems.

1.1 Medical Background and Requirements

The goal of physical rehabilitation is primarily to recuperate a patient from impairment or disability and improve mobility, functional ability and quality of life. This impairment can be the result of a stroke, injury or a neurological disease. The most common cause of adult disability in developed countries is stroke [1]. Stroke is caused by an interruption of blood flow to the brain resulting in damage to brain cells and can be fatal. In New Zealand, an estimated 6000 stroke cases occur every year with approximately two-thirds of the victims surviving the stroke. The Stroke Foundation of New Zealand estimates that the number of stroke patients in New Zealand has reached 45,000 in 2011 [2]. As the population of the baby boom generation continues to age and life expectancy continues to improve, the number of elderly in the population is expected to increase in the next few decades [3]. As a result, stroke cases can be expected to increase as well.

Survivors of stroke commonly experience hemiplegia, the paralysis or loss of physical strength on one side of the body. Impairment of the upper limb can cause difficulties in performing basic day-to-day activities such as eating, dressing and hygiene tasks which can have a huge impact on the patient's life. Physical therapy (or physiotherapy) is the main treatment for these disabilities, a process that allows the stroke patient to relearn the best possible use of their limbs and regain independence. Current rehabilitation services utilise manual hands-on treatment

S.(S.Q.) Xie, *Advanced Robotics for Medical Rehabilitation*,
Springer Tracts in Advanced Robotics 108, DOI 10.1007/978-3-319-19896-5_1

provided by a physiotherapist. However, rehabilitation therapy can continue throughout most of a stroke patients' life [4] and is therefore labor-intensive and costly. As a result, current rehabilitation services are often unable to provide sufficient and timely treatment which hinders the rate of patient recovery.

Rehabilitation robots have the potential to overcome the limitations of conventional rehabilitation methods and can enable the development of new types of rehabilitation treatment. Compared to manual therapy, rehabilitation robots have the potential to provide intensive rehabilitation consistently for a longer duration [5] and are not affected by the skills and fatigue level of the therapist. Robots can treat patients without the presence of the therapist, enabling more frequent treatment and potentially reducing costs in the long term. In addition, it is possible for a rehabilitation robot to accurately measure quantitative data to evaluate the patient's condition. The use of specially designed virtual games with the robot can provide an entertaining therapy experience, promoting the patient to put in their own effort into the exercises [6].

Although a robot can provide many benefits, there are some processes in physiotherapy that may be difficult to achieve with a robot. For example, palpation is an important part of physiotherapy which involves the use of hands to examine the body. To achieve this with a robot, it may be necessary to cover the limb with actuators and sensors which is challenging and costly with current technology. The current goal in developing rehabilitation robots is to address some of the key issues that are limiting physiotherapy and enhance existing physiotherapy by providing physiotherapists with tools that utilise state-of-the-art technologies.

Current rehabilitation services in practice have the following limitations:

- Travelling difficulty: Patients are required to travel to rehabilitation clinics or medical centres to receive treatment. This is inconvenient, time-consuming and can be very challenging for an individual with physical disabilities. Rehabilitation robots can allow patients to receive treatment in more convenient locations such as at home or at work.
- Limited availability: Rehabilitation exercises involve manual hands-on treatment with the physiotherapist. This is tiring for both the patient and the physiotherapist and is difficult to perform continuously for extended periods of time. Therefore frequent treatment is preferable over long rehabilitation sessions. However, this is difficult to achieve due to the travelling difficulties and the limited availability of physiotherapists. Physiotherapists can only attend to a limited number of patients due to their physical involvement in rehabilitation sessions. Rehabilitation robots are not affected by fatigue and can operate for an unlimited duration of time.
- Subjectivity: Physiotherapists evaluate patient disability and recovery based on their own opinion. This can be inaccurate and lead to treatment that may not be optimal for the patient's condition. Furthermore, evaluations are inconsistent between different physiotherapists making it difficult to compare outcome results which reduce confidence in physiotherapy research. A rehabilitation

robot can be designed to provide an accurate objective measure of a patient's disability characteristics at specific joints and muscle groups in the body.

- Lack of patient motivation: Patients recover faster when they put in effort into their rehabilitation exercises [6]. Conventional rehabilitation methods tend to involve repetitive movements that are uninteresting and tedious. Since the patient is not enjoying the exercise, this will likely cause a reduction in the amount of voluntary effort put in by the patient. Rehabilitation robots can be used in conjunction with virtual games to give the patient a fun and engaging objective while performing rehabilitation exercises.
- Limited complexity of rehabilitation treatment: Physiotherapists are limited to providing rather basic treatment with currently available tools. It is difficult to provide a suitable amount of assistance only when required and to accurately manipulate multiple joints simultaneously without a complex multi-joint system. A rehabilitation robot can provide assistance only when needed and can be designed to move each joint independently to generate complex movements that resemble daily tasks.

1.2 Advanced Robotics for Medical Rehabilitation

1.2.1 Rehabilitation Robots

Robots were used for rehabilitation purposes since the 1960s [7]. Application of robots in rehabilitation was initially more focused on replacing lost functions in individuals with physical disabilities through the use of devices such as robotic orthoses, robotic workstations, feeding devices and robotic wheelchairs [8]. Over the last two decades however, there has been an increasing amount of research into the use of robots in physical therapy [9–12]. This section will discuss the main motivations behind this trend, notable robotic systems used for the rehabilitation of upper and lower limbs, as well as the some of the important features of these rehabilitation robots. In the context of this research, rehabilitation robots used for physical therapy purposes are considered as devices which utilises active feedback control to provide guidance, assistance or resistance to patients during their rehabilitation exercises.

Rehabilitation robots operate close to the human user and should be capable of controlling multiple human joints independently and simultaneously to emulate human tasks. This calls for a robot design that is ergonomic, safe and user friendly. Interaction forces between the human user and the robot should also be considered in controlling the robot in addition to position. The robot needs to not only be capable of moving the user's limb but also be capable of responding to force exerted by the user's limb as well. Furthermore, modulation of the interaction must be possible to allow for adjustments of the rehabilitation treatment to suit the patient's disability characteristics. These requirements introduce a number of challenges into the design and control of robots for rehabilitation:

- Kinematic compatibility: The robot must conform to the anatomy of the human limb in order to maintain kinematic compatibility during motion. The physical human–robot interfaces must only move the limb segment in paths achievable by the human limb.
- Design optimization: The robot design parameters need to be optimised to obtain a compact and efficient robot that can achieve the range of motion and forces required in rehabilitation without interfering with the user's body.
- Actuators: The desired actuator attributes for a rehabilitation robot are high power-to-weight ratio, high bandwidth and low noise.
- Control challenges: Position control for robots has typically involved either moving to a target position as fast as possible or moving with a constant velocity. In comparison, the movements of a rehabilitation robot should be smoother and have a velocity trajectory similar to that of normal human movement.
- Adaptive force control: The robot needs to be capable of interacting and responding to movements generated by the user. Different types of rehabilitation exercises will require different types of interaction. Furthermore, adjustments to the difficulty or amount of assistance provided during exercises are also required to accommodate users with different levels of disability.

1.2.2 Motivation for Rehabilitation Robots

One of the main motivations behind the adoption of robots in physical therapy is the potential improvement in productivity [13, 14]. Physical therapy normally requires manual manipulation of the patient's affected limb, and these manipulations can be rather repetitive and labor-intensive [15, 16]. Consequently, such rehabilitation exercises can easily lead to the onset of fatigue in the therapist, thus limiting the duration and intensity of the therapy session. Since robots are well-suited for repetitive tasks and can be designed to have adequate force capabilities, their use in the execution of these exercises will be able to reduce the physical workload of therapists, and can potentially allow the therapists to simultaneously oversee the treatment of multiple patients in a supervisory role [13, 15]. Additionally, by removing the physically demanding component of a therapist's workload, application of robots in rehabilitation also has the potential of reducing the likelihood of repetitive stress injuries amongst physical therapists.

The use of robots in physical therapy also offers further advantages due to their high repeatability and ability to collect vast amount of quantitative data when equipped with appropriate sensors. As therapists mainly operate based on their "feel", their evaluation of the patient's condition can be rather subjective. By using robotic devices, diagnosis and prognosis can be made more objectively with the help of quantitative data, and comparisons between different cases can also be made more easily [15, 17]. The high repeatability of the robotic devices also allows therapy to be applied more consistently and will help to identify the effectiveness of the treatment. As a result, in addition to the delivery of physical therapy, robots can also contribute to rehabilitation research.

Research has advocated that active participation of the patient in physical therapy is important in enhancing its effectiveness [18, 19]. This means that the patient will have to be motivated to carry out the required rehabilitation exercises. Robotic systems can provide a rich graphical user interface which can be designed to capture the attention of the patient. Many existing rehabilitation robots for the upper limb have administered robotic therapy in the form of "video games" [20, 21], where the required trajectory or end point of motion is displayed on a monitor and the patient is required to follow the target. This has made the rehabilitation exercises more goal-oriented and makes the exercises more engaging, thus giving the patients added motivation to complete the required exercises.

Several successful rehabilitation robots have undergone clinical trials and are currently being used in hospitals and clinics for neuromotor rehabilitation. Results from these clinical trials are predominantly positive, suggesting that the use of intensive robotic therapy on stroke patients has the effect of reducing the level of impairment and improving the mobility of the affected limb [22].

1.2.3 Examples of Rehabilitation Robots

Existing robots designed for physical therapy are commonly involved with neuromotor training of patients suffering from neurological disorders [22]. Robots used in this capacity are generally required to manipulate the patient's affected limb by guiding it along certain motion trajectories. For the rehabilitation of upper limbs, the MIT-MANUS is one of the more successful devices which had been clinically tested [13, 23]. The basic module of this robot is capable of guiding the patient's arm in 2-DOF motion on the horizontal plane, thus targeting motion in the shoulder and elbow joints. Additional modules were also developed to allow motion along the vertical direction, as well as motion of the wrist. The robotic manipulator used in this system was designed to have a low inertia and high backdrivability, making it inherently compliant and safe to operate. The rehabilitation exercises are carried out with the aid of a graphical user interface which provides visual feedback to the patient to indicate the location of their hand. The robot is controlled using a reference force field which gives the relationship between the desired patient–robot interaction force and the position of the patient's hand. Additionally, this force field is also designed to evolve with the performance of the patient in previous runs of the exercises in order to set the difficulty at a level that is challenging but yet manageable.

In terms of lower limb rehabilitation, the Lokomat® is a commercially available treadmill-based gait rehabilitation system [24]. This robotic system operates by suspending the patient over the treadmill to provide body weight support. A robotic orthosis is worn by the patient to guide the patient's lower limb through the gait cycle. Various control strategies had been devised to allow variation of the actual lower limb trajectory from the predefined reference trajectory to permit a certain degree of gait customisation for different patients [16, 18, 25, 26]. Additionally, it employs an assistance as required philosophy whereby the robotic orthosis will only provide assistive force if the patient fails to carry out the required gait pattern. Another rehabilitation robot used for gait training is the adaptive foot orthosis. This robot has a smaller scale compared to the Lokomat and takes the form of a wearable device driven by a series elastic actuator (an electric linear actuator placed in series with an elastic element). This orthosis can modify the stiffness at the ankle joint through different phase of the gait cycle. Additionally, it can also adapt its damping parameters to minimise the occurrence of drop foot gait [27].

Even though neuromotor task training is by far the biggest application area in therapeutic robots, devices were also developed for rehabilitation of musculoskeletal injuries. These robots share many similar requirements as those used for neuromotor rehabilitation. In fact, apart from the capability for passive and assisted motion of the affected limb, such robots also need to be able to provide resistive and proprioceptive training. A more detailed discussion on robots designed for rehabilitation is presented in Chap. 2.

1.2.4 Common Features of Rehabilitation Robots

It can be seen that the examples of rehabilitation robots presented above share several common traits. The obvious feature found in all these robots is the emphasis on the user's safety. As the patient is tightly coupled to the rehabilitation robot during its operation, it is vital that the patient–robot interaction forces or torques be maintained at safe levels to prevent any injuries. This therefore requires the robotic devices to have some degree of compliance or in other words, be backdrivable. Inherent backdrivability can be realised by using a low actuator transmission ratio or by decoupling the actuator mass from its end point through use of elastic elements. These are achieved by the MIT-MANUS and the adaptive foot orthosis, respectively, as described in the previous section. Alternatively, force feedback control can also be used to reduce the apparent actuator mass and improve the backdrivability of actuators [28, 29].

Physical characteristics such as size, shape, mass, joint kinematics, motion range and joint dynamics can vary considerably between individuals. Additionally, the level and severity of injuries are also likely to be different across different patients. Robots designed for rehabilitation must therefore be adjustable or adaptable so that they can cater for a larger population with different rehabilitative needs. Extrinsic characteristics such as size and shape are related to the ergonomics of the device and can generally be accommodated through incorporation of an adjustment mechanism or by replacing certain components in the device. On the other hand, variations in mass, joint kinematics and joint stiffness, will alter the mechanical properties of the robot's operating environment, and can dictate whether safe operation of the rehabilitation robot is possible. For example, closed loop system stability is influenced by joint dynamics, while joint kinematics determines directions of admissible motion. If these characteristics are not taken into consideration in the robot controller, the robot may become unstable or it may apply excessive forces in non-compliant directions, thus presenting a dangerous scenario for the patient. As a result, it is crucial that rehabilitation robots have the capability to operate safely in a range of environments. This can be achieved through use of robust or adaptive control strategies. Adaptive control strategies are also important in allowing the robot to cater for patients with different capabilities in performing the rehabilitation programme due to the specific extent of their injuries.

Another common feature among rehabilitation robots is the need to control the physical interaction between the patient and the robot. This means that both the motion of the robot and the contact forces applied to the patient must be regulated. Motion regulation is generally required when guiding the patient's limb along paths which are representative of reaching tasks for the upper limb or trajectories which corresponds to normal gait pattern for the limb. The requirement to control forces and torques on the other hand can arise from concerns of the patient's safety or from the need to apply resistive effort for strength training exercises.

1.3 Critical Issues in Rehabilitation

1.3.1 Upper Limb Rehabilitation

Initial rehabilitation robots developed for the human upper limb were end-effector robots that use one physical interface to manipulate the limb, typically at hand or forearm. End-effector robots can only move the user's limb in a very limited workspace and cannot independently control each upper limb joint. Owing to their lack of kinematic compatibility with the human user, developments soon shifted to exoskeleton robots [30, 31]. Exoskeleton robots have a similar kinematic structure to the human limb and are designed to operate alongside the user's limb. An example of end-effector robot is shown in Fig. 1.1.

1.3.2 Ankle Rehabilitation

The human ankle is one of the most complex structures in the human musculoskeletal system and plays an important role in maintaining body balance during ambulation [32]. A pictorial view of the various bones and ligaments found at the foot and ankle are shown in Fig. 1.2. In general use, the term "ankle" is used to

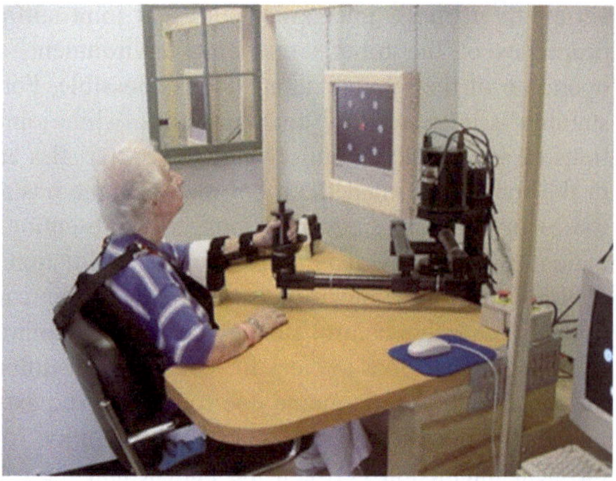

Fig. 1.1 The MIT-MANUS end-effector rehabilitation robot [9]

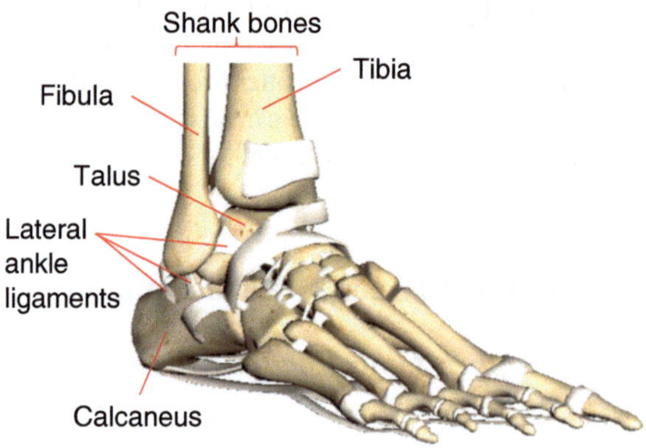

Fig. 1.2 Bones and ligaments at the human foot and ankle

describe the structure which encompasses both the ankle and subtalar joints, where the ankle (or talocrural) joint is the articulation between three bones of the lower limb, namely tibia, fibula and talus. The subtalar joint on the other hand, is formed by the interface between talus and calcaneus and is located beneath the ankle joint.

Owing to its location, the human ankle is frequently subjected to large loads which can reach up to several times the body weight. The exposure to such large loads also means a higher likelihood of injuries. In fact, the ankle is the most common site of sprain injuries in the human body, with over 23,000 cases per day in the United States. In New Zealand, approximately 82,000 new claims related to ankle injuries were made to the Accident Compensation Corporation (ACC) in the year 2000/2001, costing an estimated 19 million NZD and making ankle related claims the fourth biggest cost for ACC [33].

Ankle sprains are injuries which involve the overstretching or tearing of ligaments around the ankle and are often sustained during sporting or physical activities. Ankle sprains can be classified into several grades, ranging from mild overstretching to complete disruption of ankle ligaments. Depending on the severity of the sprain, the time required for recovery can range from 12 days to more than 6 weeks [34]. Researchers have reported that a significant number (>40 %) of severe ankle sprains can develop into chronic ankle instability [35], which makes the ankle more susceptible to further injuries. Chronic ankle instability is thought to be caused by a combination of mechanical and functional instability at the ankle. Mechanical instability is used to refer to changes of the ankle anatomy which makes it more prone to future injuries, while functional instability refers to changes which give rise to insufficiencies in the ankle neuromuscular system, such as impaired proprioception, muscle weakness and reduced neuromuscular control.

The general rehabilitation programme for ankle sprains is carried out in stages as shown in Fig. 1.3. The initial stage of treatment right after injury is considered the acute phase of rehabilitation and is focused on reducing effusion and swelling at the affected to promote healing of the injured tissues. A reduction in effusion can be achieved with elevation, application of ice and compression. The affected ankle is also often immobilised. However, as prolonged immobilisation of the ankle can lead to reduced range of motion (ROM) and muscular atrophy, the next phase of ankle rehabilitation typically involve ROM and muscle strengthening exercises. With reduced effusion, the rehabilitation enters into the subacute phase where active and passive ROM exercises are normally carried out within the pain-free range of the patient to improve the range of motion and reduce muscular atrophy. Research has also suggested that this has the ability to stimulate healing of torn ligaments [35].

The rehabilitative phase is achieved once pain-free weight bearing gait is possible. During this phase, ROM exercises are continued together with the commencement of muscle stretching and resistive exercises [35]. The resistance level of these strengthening exercises should be increased as the patient progresses with recovery. Muscle stretching is important to assist the recovery of joint ROM while resistance training is used to improve the strength of muscles surrounding the ankle to prevent future injuries [36]. Finally, proprioceptive and balancing exercises should be carried out towards the end of the rehabilitation programme (functional phase) to enhance the patients' sense of joint position, thus giving them better foot and ankle coordination and improving their ability to respond to sudden perturbations at the ankle [35].

As can be seen from the previous discussion, muscular strength and good proprioception are vital in preventing functional instability in the ankle. Emphasis must therefore be placed on these areas and an extensive rehabilitation programme is

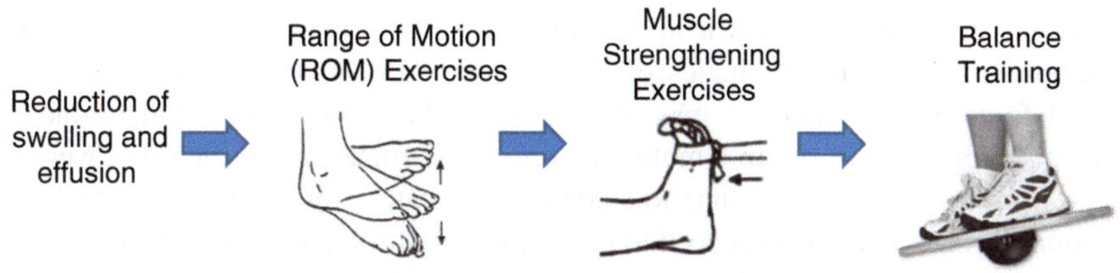

Fig. 1.3 The typical ankle rehabilitation programme for ankle sprains

needed to minimise the likelihood of recurrent injuries. The repetitive and tedious nature of such exercises therefore makes robotic devices an attractive alternative to manual manipulation. However, the great variability observed between different patients due to either their level of injury or their ankle characteristics such as joint limits and stiffness also means that any robotic device employed in this area must be adaptive to allow it to cater for the requirements of specific patients.

1.3.3 Interaction Control

Traditionally, many robotic devices are position-controlled and various mature control techniques had been developed for the design of position controllers. However, when robots are deployed in applications that require significant physical interaction with the external environment, pure position control is no longer adequate [37]. This is because the design of the position controller is normally done by considering the dynamics of the robot alone and treating externally applied forces/torques as disturbances. However, when the robot comes into contact with an external environment, the assumed robot model may no longer be valid and the robot will therefore deviate from its intended behaviour. Furthermore, as large controller gains are normally used in position controllers to minimise position-tracking errors, interaction with a stiff environment will result in large position errors which can in turn lead to force build up at the contact interface. This is of course unacceptable for robots which interact closely with humans as it is likely to cause injuries to the user. Clearly, a control strategy which takes more than just position into consideration is needed for the control of rehabilitation robots. Interaction control is an approach which aims to regulate both the forces and the motion of a robot which is in contact with an external environment. Two groups of interaction control schemes are commonly used. They are hybrid force-position control and impedance control [34, 38].

Hybrid force-position control [39] is a control strategy which splits the task space into two complementary subspaces using a selection matrix. A position control strategy is then applied in one of the subspaces and a force control in the other. Normally, directions where constraint-free motion is permissible are position-controlled while force control is applied in the constrained directions. This will allow accurate realisation of the desired force and motion when the kinematic constraints in the environment are known with little or no uncertainty. While such constraints may be well known in an industrial setting, there can be considerable variations in the joint kinematics of different individuals. This would mean that hybrid force-position control may still result in large interaction forces due to imprecise definition of the free motion directions. Furthermore, if the robot were to move from a constraint-free state to a constrained state, a switch in the control law is required since all directions need to be position-controlled prior to contact and the hybrid position-force control should only be active after contact has been made.

Impedance control is another type of interaction control scheme which aims to maintain a prescribed relationship between force and motion of the robot. This relationship is termed the mechanical impedance and is defined as the dynamic ratio of the error in applied forces to the velocity error of the robot end effector. Consequently, unlike the hybrid position-force controller, no switching of control law is required for impedance control [38].

Selection of the target manipulator impedance is an important issue in impedance control as it establishes the physical behaviour of the controlled manipulator. For a single-input-single-output system, it can be seen that an infinite impedance will result in pure position control while a zero impedance will lead to pure force control. From this observation, impedance control can be designed to give a similar performance as hybrid position-force control by selecting larger impedance values in directions of free motion and smaller impedance values in constrained directions. While the selection of target impedances can be achieved through experimental trial and error, more systematic approaches can also be taken. Researchers have suggested that the choice of impedance parameters should be based on optimisation of certain objective functions. For instance, the target impedance can be chosen to be proportional to the environmental admittance to minimise a weighted sum of position error and actuator force [40].

It is evident from the above discussion that impedance control is a more robust interaction control scheme than hybrid force-position control. It is therefore not surprising that a large proportion of rehabilitation devices have employed some form of impedance control to deal with the variability found among patients [41–44]. However, a more robust nature of impedance control does not mean that knowledge of the operating environmental is no longer important. Information of the environmental dynamic characteristics can be used to alter robot behaviour in such a manner that the robot performance can be enhanced. The ability to adapt the impedance controller according to changes in environmental conditions is therefore a desired feature in rehabilitation robots.

Several adaptive impedance controllers were developed to allow adaptation to variability in the robot dynamics [45–47]. This is due to the fact that a computed torque control approach is often used in position-based impedance controllers to allow the desired impedance to be realised with higher accuracy. As this control approach relies on accurate compensation of the robot dynamics, uncertainties in the robot dynamic parameters will degrade the controller performance. This issue is particularly important for fast moving robots where the robot dynamic terms are large due to high accelerations and velocities. Serial robots are also more severely affected, as they generally have larger link inertias. However, if the manipulator is designed in such a way that the robot inertia is low, robot performance may not be severely affected by the lack of such dynamic compensation terms. In fact, impedance control can be successfully implemented using merely proportional derivative position control in some applications. With this in mind, computational resources can potentially be allocated for adaptation of environmental parameters instead of robot parameters if the robot dynamic terms are relatively small in magnitude (in comparison with the interaction forces/moments) and when the application involves motion of lower velocity and acceleration.

1.4 Summary

This chapter has highlighted the main motivations and objectives of this book through an overview of rehabilitation robots, interaction control and rehabilitation. The main incentives for the use of robotic devices in physical therapy can be summarised as: their ability to reduce physical workload of therapists; the possibility to log relevant data for more objective diagnosis and prognosis; and their potential in making rehabilitation exercises more engaging experience via interactive user interfaces. A study on several successful rehabilitation robots have highlighted that backdrivability, interaction control and adaptability are important elements in rehabilitation robots. Limitations of conventional rehabilitation methods are identified and robotic devices are suggested as a potential solution. The key challenges in the design and control of rehabilitation robots are highlighted.

References

1. G.A. Donnan, M. Fisher, M. Macleod, S.M. Davis, Stroke. The Lancet **371**, 1612–1623 (2008)
2. Annual Report 2009. Stroke Foundation of New Zealand Inc. (2010)
3. M. Khawaja, N. Thomson, Population ageing in New Zealand (2000)
4. R.W. Teasell, L. Kalra, What's New in stroke rehabilitation. Stroke **35**, 383–385 (2004)
5. V.S. Huang, J.W. Krakauer, Robotic neurorehabilitation: A computational motor learning perspective. J. NeuroEng. Rehabil, **6** (2009)
6. K. Laver, S. George, J. Ratcliffe, M. Crotty, Virtual reality stroke rehabilitation—hype or hope? Aust. Occup. Ther. J. **58**, 215–219 (2011)
7. W.S. Harwin, T. Rahman, R.A. Foulds, A review of design issues in rehabilitation robotics with reference to North American research. IEEE Trans. Rehabil. Eng. **3**, 3–13 (1995)
8. N. Tejima, Rehabilitation robotics: a review. Adv. Robot. **14**, 551–564 (2000)
9. H.I. Krebs, J.J. Palazzolo, L. Dipietro, M. Ferraro, J. Krol, K. Rannekleiv, B.T. Volpe, N. Hogan, Rehabilitation robotics: performance-based progressive robot-assisted therapy. Auton. Robots **15**, 7–20 (2003)
10. S. Hesse, H. Schmidt, C. Werner, A. Bardeleben, Upper and lower extremity robotic devices for rehabilitation and for studying motor control. Curr. Opin. Neurol. **16**, 705–710 (2003)
11. H.I. Krebs, B.T. Volpe, M.L. Aisen, W. Hening, A. Adamovich, H. Poizner, K. Subrahmanyan, N. Hogan, Robotic applications in neuromotor rehabilitation. Robotica **21**, 3–11 (2003)
12. M. Girone, G. Burdea, M. Bouzit, V. Popescu, J.E. Deutsch, Stewart platform-based system for ankle telerehabilitation. Auton. Robots **10**, 203–212 (2001)
13. H.I. Krebs, B.T. Volpe, M.L. Aisen, N. Hogan, Increasing productivity and quality of care: Robot-aided neuro-rehabilitation. J. Rehabil. Res. Dev. **37**, 639–652 (2000)

14. J.A. Saglia, N.G. Tsagarakis, J.S. Dai, D.G. Caldwell, Control strategies for ankle rehabilitation using a high performance ankle exerciser, in IEEE International Conference on Robotics and Automation (2010), pp. 2221–2227
15. R. Riener, M. Frey, M. Bernhardt, T. Nef, G. Colombo, Human-centered rehabilitation robotics, in IEEE International Conference on Rehabilitation Robotics (2005), pp. 319–322
16. A. Duschau-Wicke, J. Von Zitzewitz, A. Caprez, L. Lunenburger, R. Riener, Path control: a method for patient-cooperative robot-aided gait rehabilitation. IEEE Trans. Neural Syst. Rehabil. Eng. **18**, 38–48 (2010)
17. A. Roy, H.I. Krebs, S.L. Patterson, T.N. Judkins, I.K. Larry, R.M. Macko, N. Hogan, Measurement of human ankle stiffness using the anklebot, in International Conference on Rehabilitation Robotics (2007), pp. 356–363
18. H. Vallery, A. Duschau-Wicke, R. Riener, Generalized elasticities improve patient-cooperative control of rehabilitation robots, in 2009 IEEE International Conference on Rehabilitation Robotics, ICORR 2009 (2009), pp. 535–541
19. L. Marchal-Crespo, D.J. Reinkensmeyer, Review of control strategies for robotic movement training after neurologic injury. J. NeuroEng. Rehabil. **6** (2009)
20. T. Nef, M. Mihelj, R. Riener, ARMin: a robot for patient-cooperative arm therapy. Med. Biol. Eng. Compu. **45**, 887–900 (2007)
21. J.E. Deutsch, J. Latonio, G. Burdea, R. Boian, Post-stroke rehabilitation with the Rutgers Ankle System: a case study. Presence **10**, 416–430 (2001)
22. D.J. Reinkensmeyer, J.L. Emken, S.C. Cramer, Robotics, motor learning, and neurologic recovery. Annu. Rev. Biomed. Eng. **6**, 497–525 (2004)
23. H.I. Krebs, D. Williams, J. Celestino, S.K. Charles, D. Lynch, N. Hogan, Robot-aided neurorehabilitation: a robot for wrist rehabilitation. IEEE Trans. Neural Syst. Rehabil. Eng. **15**, 327–335 (2007)
24. Hocoma, http://www.hocoma.com/en/products/lokomat/
25. R. Riener, L. Lunenburger, S. Jezernik, M. Anderschitz, G. Colombo, V. Dietz, Patient-cooperative strategies for robot aided treadmill training: first experimental results. IEEE Trans. Neural Syst. Rehabil. Eng. **13**, 380–394 (2005)
26. S. Jezernik, G. Colombo, M. Morari, Automatic gait-pattern adaptation for rehabilitation with 4-dof robotic orthosis. IEEE Trans. Robot. Autom. **20**, 574–582 (2004)
27. J.A. Blaya, H. Herr, Adaptive control of a variable-impedance ankle-foot orthosis to assist drop-foot gait. IEEE Trans. Neural Syst. Rehabil. Eng. **12**, 24–31 (2004)
28. N. Hogan, Stable execution of contact tasks using impedance control, in IEEE International Conference on Robotics and Automation (1987), pp. 1047–1054
29. N. Hogan, S.P. Buerger, Impedance and interaction control, in *Robotics and Automation Handbook*, ed. by T. Kurfess (CRC Press, New York, 2005)
30. H.S. Lo, S.Q. Xie, Exoskeleton robots for upper-limb rehabilitation: state of the art and future prospects. Med. Eng. Phys. **34**, 261–268 (2012)
31. R.A.R.C. Gopura, K. Kiguchi, Mechanical designs of active upper-limb exoskeleton robots state-of-the-art and design difficulties, in IEEE International Conference on Rehabilitation Robotics (2009), pp. 178–187
32. M. Dettwyler, A. Stacoff, I.A. Kramers-de Quervain, E. Stussi, Modelling of the ankle joint complex. Reflections with regards to ankle prostheses. Foot Ankle Surg. **10**, 109–119 (2004)
33. Accident Compensation Corporation, New Zealand. http://www.acc.co.nz/for-providers/resources/WCMZ002647?ssSourceNodeId=4249&ssSourceSiteId=1494
34. G. Zeng, A. Hemami, An overview of robot force control. Robotica **15**, 473–482 (1997)
35. M.R. Safran, J.E. Zachazewski, R.S. Benedetti, A.R.I. Bartolozzi, R. Mandelbaum, Lateral ankle sprains: a comprehensive review Part 2: treatment and rehabilitation with an emphasis on the athlete. Med. Sci. Sports Exerc. **31**, S438–S447 (1999)
36. C.G. Mattacola, M.K. Dwyer, Rehabilitation of the ankle after acute sprain or chronic instability. J. Athletic Training **37**, 413–429 (2002)
37. B. Siciliano, L. Villani, *Robot force control* (Kluwer Academic Publishers, Boston, 1999)

38. T. Lefebvre, J. Xiao, H. Bruyninckx, G. Gersem, Active compliant motion: a survey. Adv. Robot. **19**, 479–499 (2005)
39. M.H. Raibert, J.J. Craig, Hybrid position/force control of manipulators. J. Dyn. Syst. Meas. Control Trans. ASME **103**, 126–133 (1981)
40. N. Hogan, Impedance control: an approach to manipulation: Parts I, II and III. J. Dyn. Syst. Meas. Contr. **107**, 17–24 (1985)
41. A. Roy, H.I. Krebs, D. Williams, C.T. Bever, L.W. Forrester, R.M. Macko, N. Hogan, Robot-aided neurorehabilitation: a novel robot for ankle rehabilitation. IEEE Trans. Rob. **25**, 569–582 (2009)
42. J. Yoon, J. Ryu, K.-B. Lim, Reconfigurable ankle rehabilitation robot for various exercises. J. Rob. Syst. **22**, S15–S33 (2006)
43. J.A. Saglia, N.G. Tsagarakis, J.S. Dai, D.G. Caldwell, A high-performance redundantly actuated mechanism for ankle rehabilitation. Int. J. Rob. Res. **28**, 1216–1227 (2009)
44. M. Bernhardt, M. Frey, G. Colombo, T. Rahman, Hybrid force-position control yields cooperative behaviour of the rehabilitation robot LOKOMAT, in IEEE International Conference on Rehabilitation Robotics (2005), pp. 536–539
45. R. Colbaugh, H. Seraji, K. CGlass, Direct adaptive impedance control of robot manipulators. J. Rob. Syst. **10**, 217–248 (1993)
46. C.-C. Cheah, D. Wang, Learning impedance control for robotic manipulators. IEEE Trans. Robot. Autom. **14**, 452–465 (1998)
47. S.K. Singh, D.O. Popa, Analysis of some fundamental problems in adaptive control of force and impedance behavior: theory and experiments. IEEE Trans. Robot. Autom. **11**, 912–921 (1995)

Chapter 2
Literature Review

A comprehensive literature review on rehabilitation robots is carried out to identify the key issues. The main design requirements and development complications are identified and the various approaches used in past robots are reviewed. It begins with a survey of existing human rehabilitation devices designed for use in human assistance and treatment. An overview of the kinematic and computational biomechanical models of the human limb is also provided. This is followed by a review of the state of the art of interaction control strategies, with primary focus on its application in rehabilitation robots. Finally, the reviewed materials are assimilated in a discussion that highlights issues in rehabilitation robots that require further development, and are hence the subject of investigation for this research.

2.1 Medical Needs and Existing Rehabilitation Devices

2.1.1 Upper Limb Rehabilitation Robots

Early research on rehabilitation robots for the human upper limb was based on end-effector robots. End-effector rehabilitation robots hold the patient's hand or forearm at one point and generate interaction forces at this sole interface as shown in Fig. 2.1a. The kinematic structure of these end-effector robots are based on industrial robots and the kinematics of the human limb are not considered in their design. This type of robot is simpler, easier to fabricate and can be used for patients with different arm lengths. However, determining the posture of the upper limb can be difficult with only one interface, especially if the interface is at the patient's hand. This is because the upper arm and forearm are unconstrained and are free to move about the pivots at the shoulder and hand. Controlling the torque at specific upper limb joints is also not possible, resulting in uncontrolled load transfer between upper limb joints. As a consequence, generating isolated movement at a single upper limb joint is difficult since movement of the end effector can cause a combination of movements at the wrist, elbow and shoulder joints. In addition, the range of motion that end-effector robots can generate for the upper limb tends to be limited therefore only a limited set of rehabilitation movements can be produced by

S.(S.Q.) Xie, *Advanced Robotics for Medical Rehabilitation*,
Springer Tracts in Advanced Robotics 108, DOI 10.1007/978-3-319-19896-5_2

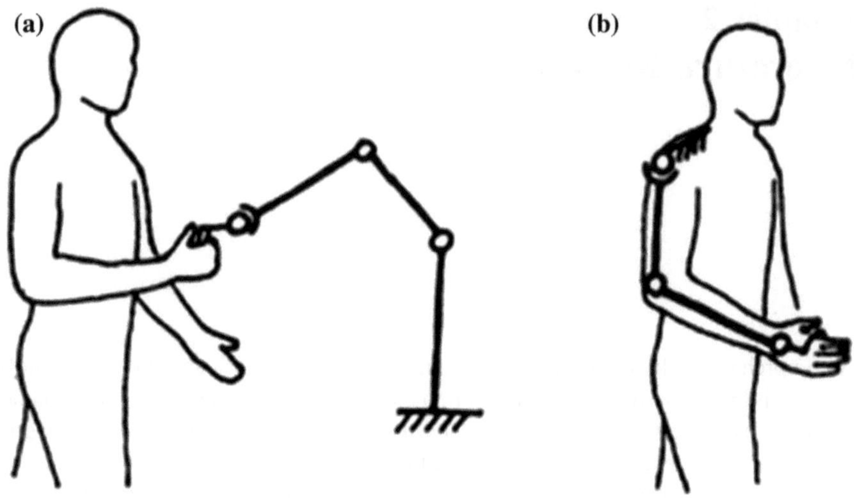

Fig. 2.1 Kinematics of a an end-effector robot and b an exoskeleton robot [10]

these robots. Examples of end-effector rehabilitation robots include the MIT-MANUS [1, 2], the MIME [3] and the GENTLE/s [4]. Extensive clinical testing has been done on these devices to evaluate their effectiveness as rehabilitative devices [5–9]. The results indicate reduced motor impairment of the upper limb for patients who received robotic therapy. The positive results justify research on the more sophisticated exoskeleton robots as rehabilitation devices.

Exoskeletons have a structure that resembles the human upper limb, having robot joint axes that match the upper limb joint axes as shown in Fig. 2.1b. Exoskeletons are designed to operate alongside the human upper limb, and therefore can be attached to the upper limb at multiple locations. Although this can make it more difficult for the robot to adapt to different arm lengths, multiple interfaces allow the exoskeleton to fully determine the upper limb posture and apply controlled torques to each upper limb joint independently. It is possible for exoskeletons to target specific muscles for training by generating a calculated combination of torques at certain joints. In addition, a larger range of motion is possible compared to end-effector robots which enable a wider variety of movements to be used in rehabilitation exercises.

The majority of past upper limb exoskeletons focus on movements for the 3-DOF spherical rotation of the shoulder joint and 1-DOF of the elbow. A lower number of exoskeletons have included movements for the 3-DOF wrist joint and even fewer have included movements for the 2-DOF translations of the shoulder joint. One exoskeleton studied during this literature review has also included 1-DOF for grasping movement of the hand. From this, it can be seen that the upper limb DOF that has larger influence on the hand's position have been the focus of upper limb exoskeletons. Rehabilitation of these movements is of the highest priority since they are the most important in controlling the position of the hand.

The ARMin III (Fig. 2.2a) [11], MGA [12] (Fig. 2.2b) and IntelliArm [13] exoskeletons have implemented an actuated DOF for shoulder elevation & depression. The MEDARM has included actuation for both shoulder elevation and depression, and retraction and protraction, allowing 5-DOF of actuated movement at the shoulder complex [14]. Other groups have opted to use passive DOF for these translation movements [13, 15, 16]. Passive DOF allows the joint to move freely but eliminates the ability to generate actuation forces at the joint.

There are a number of commercially available rehabilitation devices for the upper limb. One of the more sophisticated rehabilitation devices available are the Armeo products (Hocoma AG, Switzerland) [17]. These include the 7-DOF ArmeoPower active exoskeleton, ArmeoSpring passive exoskeleton and ArmeoBoom sling suspension system. The ArmeoPower is based on the ARMin III exoskeleton [11]. Examples of other commercial devices include the mPower arm brace (Myomo, Inc., Cambridge, MA) [18], a 1-DOF portable arm brace which uses electromyography (EMG) signals measured from the biceps and triceps muscles to generate assistive torques for elbow flexion and extension, and the Hand Mentor (Kinetic Muscles, Inc., Tempe AZ) [19], a 1-DOF wearable device for the rehabilitation of the wrist and fingers which provides force, position and EMG feedback and is actuated by an air muscle. The Robot Suit HAL-5 (Cyberdyne Inc., Japan) is a full-body exoskeleton for the disabled which uses measured EMG signals from the user to generate assistive torques. Examples of commercial end-effector rehabilitation robots include the InMotion robots (Interactive Motion Technologies, Inc., Boston, MA) [20], Biodex System 4 dynamometer (Biodex Medical Systems, Inc., New York) [21], HUMAC NORM (SCMi, Stoughton, MA) [22] and CON-TRES MJ (CMV AG, Switzerland) [23].

2.1.2 Ankle Rehabilitation Robots

Robotic devices had been developed for the rehabilitation of the human ankle. Although the main rehabilitation problem considered in this research is that of sprained ankle rehabilitation, devices used for gait rehabilitation for neurological disorders are also considered in this discussion for completeness. Ankle rehabilitation devices can be classified into two categories in terms of the mobility of the device during operation. These are wearable robots and robotic platforms with stationary bases. Wearable ankle robots typically take the form of a robotic orthosis or exoskeleton (Fig. 2.3) and are used to correct the user's gait pattern. Robotic platforms (Fig. 2.4) on the other hand, manipulate the user's foot using their end-effectors and are generally developed to facilitate the treatment of ankle sprains.

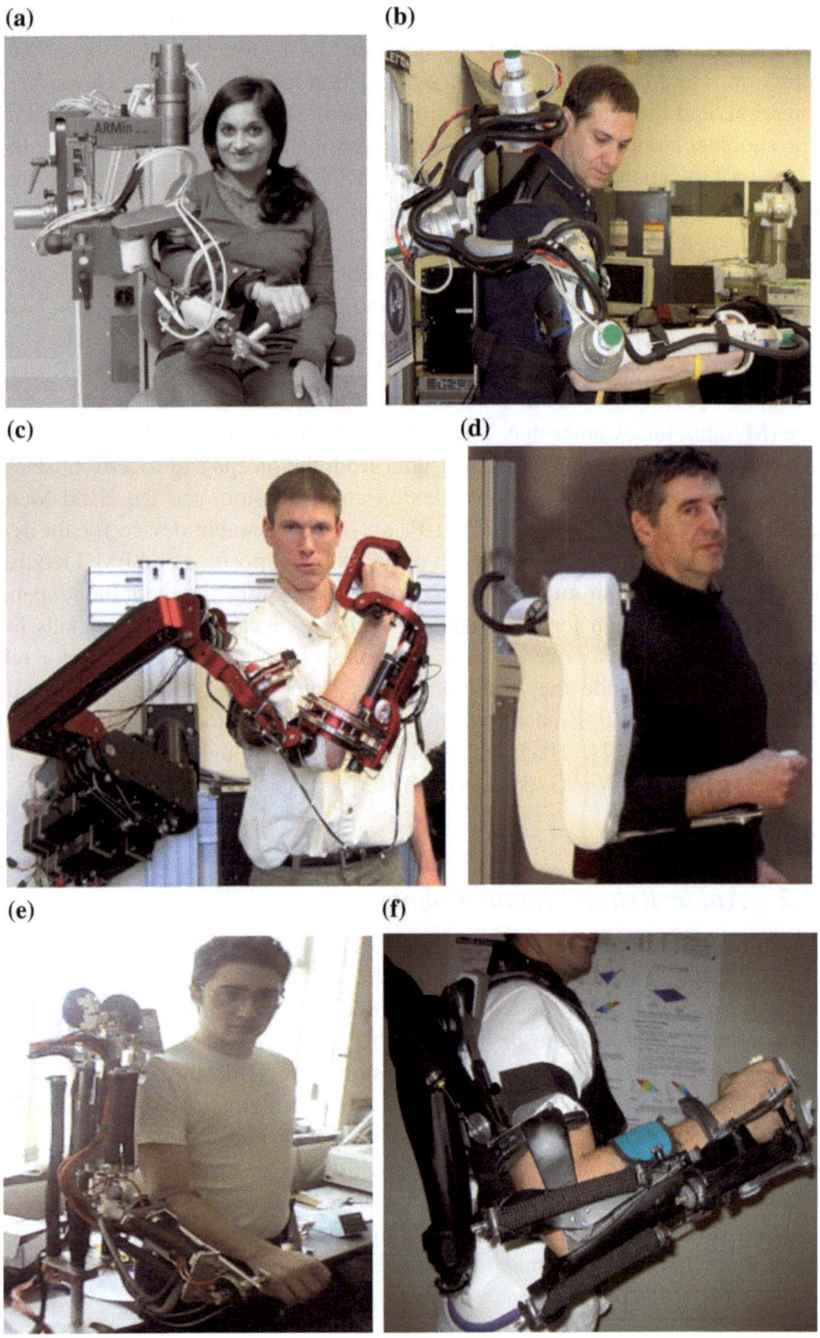

Fig. 2.2 Past upper limb exoskeletons. **a** ARMin III [11]. **b** MGA [12]. **c** CADEN-7 [24]. **d** ABLE [25]. **e** SRE [26, 27]. **f** RUPERT IV [28]

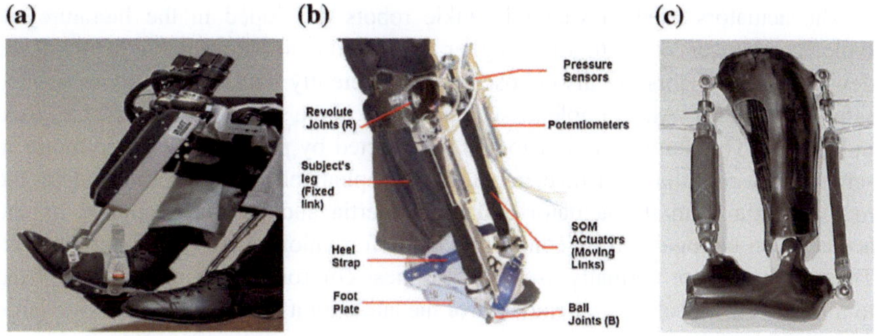

Fig. 2.3 Examples of wearable ankle rehabilitation robots. **a** The anklebot developed in [29]. **b** The robotic gait trainer developed in [30]. **c** The pneumatically powered ankle-foot orthosis developed in [31]. Images reproduced from [29–31]

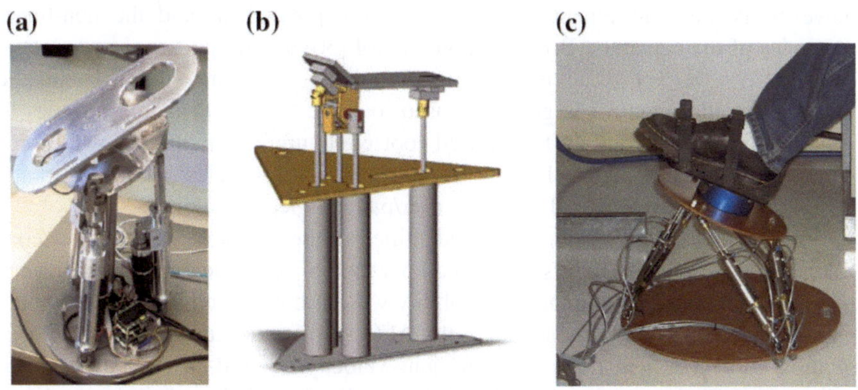

Fig. 2.4 Examples of platform-based ankle rehabilitation robots. **a** The ankle exerciser in [32]. **b** The reconfigurable ankle rehabilitation robot in [33]. **c** The Rutgers Ankle rehabilitation interface. Images reproduced from [32–34]

2.1.2.1 Wearable Ankle Rehabilitation Robots

To enable their use in gait rehabilitation, robotic devices developed for preventing foot drop must be wearable. It must also be controlled to limit the downward rotation of the foot during certain phase of gait. It is therefore not surprising that many robots used in this capacity take the form of actuated orthoses or exoskeletons. While some of these devices provide actuated motion in only 1-DOF to influence foot plantarflexion and dorsiflexion [35–38], others also include the possibility of controlled or passive inversion and eversion movements [9, 39, 40]. The internal-external rotation of the foot, however, is rarely controlled as it is assumed to be a negligible component of gait.

The actuators used in wearable ankle robots developed in the literature are typically of lower inertia to allow higher mobility due to the wearable nature of the device. The actuators are also chosen to be inherently backdrivable to ensure the safety of the user. An example of such actuators is the series elastic actuators used in [35, 38]. This family of actuators is constructed by placing an electric motor in series with a compliant elastic element. The compliant element therefore isolates the motor inertia from the actuator end point inertia and the force applied by the actuator can be regulated by controlling the deformation of the compliant element. These actuators are normally used with stiffness control and are in general utilised to influence the mechanical behaviour of the ankle joint rather than to provide large assistive moments.

Pneumatic muscle is another type of actuator commonly used in wearable ankle robots due to its high power-to-weight ratio and inherent compliance. It is typically used in systems with higher moment capacity, thus allowing these devices to provide a greater level of assistance during the user's gait. The disadvantage, however, is the requirement of a source of compressed air and the non-linear dynamics of the actuators. Both position control [30] and proportional myoelectric control [31, 36, 37] strategies had been applied on systems using pneumatic muscles. Position control is generally used to drive the length of the muscles to values which correspond to the desired foot configuration/orientation while proportional myoelectric control activates the pneumatic muscles according to the myoelectric signals measured from the user/patient's leg muscles.

Some notable features can also be identified in the wearable ankle robots considered in this review. The first is the incorporation of some element of intelligence into these devices. For example, adaptability was introduced in [35] to improve the performance of the AFO by adjusting the AFO stiffness to reduce the occurrences of drop foot gait, while the previous gait velocity is used in [38] to generate references for subsequent gait cycles. Additionally, knowledge of the general gait pattern had also been incorporated in higher level control schemes which coordinate the switching of AFO behaviour according to the current phase of gait.

Another important feature worth noting can be found in the mechanical designs of [9, 30, 40], where the AFOs were designed to be under-actuated when not attached to the user/patient. The advantage of this is that it will not be necessary to align the AFO's kinematic constraints to those of the human ankle, thus allowing the device to cater for a wider range of users and reducing set-up time. Furthermore, with an appropriate design, the device will be able to provide control or support in the important degree of freedom while at the same time acting passively in the remaining directions. This therefore helps to maintain natural movement of the ankle-foot structure and ensures that no unnecessary constraints are imposed on the user's ankle-foot complex.

2.1.2.2 Platform-Based Ankle Rehabilitation Robots

A range of platform-based devices had also been developed by researchers for the purpose of sprained ankle rehabilitation [41, 42]. They are therefore designed to carry out various ankle rehabilitation exercises such as motion therapy and muscle strength training. Motion therapy can be divided into passive, active-assist and active exercises, each requiring a different level of participation from the patient, ranging from no active effort in the passive exercises to full user-driven motion in active exercises. Strength training requires the robot to apply a resistive load to impede the user's movement to improve muscle strength.

One of the key differences between these platform-based devices and the wearable devices discussed previously is that the platform-based devices have a fixed base and thus cannot be used during gait training. Given the rather limited range of motion at the ankle-foot complex, parallel mechanisms are typically used for multiple DOF systems to reduce the size of the robot. With the exception of the Stewart platform-based device proposed in [43] which is capable of 6-DOF motion, most researchers have opted for designs which offer 2- or 3-DOF in rotational motion, where robot movements in the yaw direction (internal-external rotation) are typically constrained on 2-DOF devices. Most of the lower DOF devices also include a central strut in the robot's kinematic structure to provide the kinematic constraint required to restrict the movement of the end effector so that it is purely rotational [41, 44].

Different actuators had been used in platform-based ankle rehabilitation robots. The Stewart platform-based device in [43] and the reconfigurable ankle rehabilitation platform in [33] have utilised pneumatic cylinders to provide actuation, while electric motors were used in devices developed in [41, 45, 46]. A custom-designed electric actuator was proposed in [32, 48] to improve actuator backdrivability, whereby a cable-driven pulley system is used to convert the rotational motion of a DC motor to linear motion of the actuator rod.

A variety of control schemes had been implemented on these platform-based ankle rehabilitation robots. One approach involves the use of either pure force or pure position control for the execution of different exercises [43]. For instance, position control of the platform is typically used for passive range of motion ankle exercises where the user's foot is guided by the robot along the prescribed rehabilitation trajectory, or for isometric exercises where the orientation of the robot is kept constant while the user exerts a particular moment on the robot. Force control on the hand is used to maintain a desired level of interaction torque between the user and the robot during resistive or assistive exercises. Impedance/admittance control strategies had also been implemented, usually through a position-based approach whereby the robot's reference trajectory is modified based on the desired robot impedance and the measured interaction forces/moments [32, 33, 47, 48]. Such control schemes are also generally used with a computed torque/inverse dynamics based position controller to allow accurate tracking of the desired reference trajectories. While the basic interaction control schemes had been implemented on existing platform-based ankle rehabilitation robots, little emphasis had been placed on the realisation of adaptive control in such devices to allow adjustment of the robot behaviour due to variation in the user's joint characteristics and capability.

2.1.3 Rehabilitation Robots for Masticatory System

There is no specific medical condition called "jaw motion disorder". For the scope of this book, jaw motion disorder will be used to describe a deviation from ideal or normal function of the masticatory system, due to a single factor or combination of pathologies that affect mandibular movement. The causes of this dysfunctional movement can be from temporomandibular joint disorder (TMJD), which is an affliction of the TMJ, or paralysis or weakening of mandibular muscle.

TMJD is also known as myofascial pain dysfunction or Costen's syndrome and it is mostly caused by habitual behaviours that place excessive wear on the TMJ, trauma, disease or wear from aging [49, 50]. It is estimated that at any one time in the USA, 10 million people suffer from TMJD, making it a major health problem [51]. The symptoms and effects of TMJD are numerous and affect other areas in the craniofacial region as well as the mandible itself. Symptoms such as headaches, ear pain, dizziness, fullness of the ear (where the ear feels clogged) and tinnitus (ringing in the ear) can all be caused by TMJD. More intuitively, TMJD also causes muscle pain, pain within the TMJ and grinding, crunching or popping sounds [49]. Pain in the facial muscles and jaw joints can also be extended to the neck or shoulders. The most significant effect, however, is on the actual motion of the mandible. TMJD reduces the range of motion, causing the mandible to not fully open or to deviate to one side during opening. These unnatural movements feel awkward and affect the nature of occlusion [50].

Besides TMJD, the other significant contributing factor to jaw motion disorder is a loss in mandibular muscle function and this can be due to a weakened or paralysed muscle or group of muscles. The causes of detrimental mandibular muscle function are no different from those of other muscles within the body, and include muscular dystrophy (MD) [52], muscular atrophy [53] and stroke.

Most of the pathologies described in this section which contribute to jaw motion disorder can be treated with varying degrees of physical therapy. The therapy has to be tailored to a particular patient and should suit their specific needs. Passive motion therapy followed by active therapy can help strengthen and increase the movement range of muscle. However, existing aids are not sufficient at emulating all the motions that may be required for mastication and a more sophisticated device is required that accommodates the multiple DOFs of the mandible to restore mandibular function in rehabilitative processes.

2.2 Human Musculoskeletal Models

2.2.1 *Movements of Upper Limb*

Operating alongside the human upper limb, exoskeletons need to be capable of producing movements similar to those of the upper limb. The upper limb effectively has a total of 9-DOF from the shoulder to the wrist with the finger joints excluded as shown by q_1 to q_9 in Fig. 2.5 [54, 55]. This 9-DOF gives the upper limb exceptionally high manoeuverability and allows the hand to reach a very large workspace. The proximal joints of the upper limb are often considered a higher priority for rehabilitation as these joints have the largest influence on the hand's position and provide support for the rest of the limb.

The shoulder joint has 5-DOF, 3-rotational DOF which allow spherical rotation of the upper arm and 2-translational DOF which move the upper arm along the vertical axis and the anterior–posterior axis. The movements of each DOF are commonly described by a pair of terms, one for movement in the positive direction and one for the negative direction:

Shoulder flexion Rotation of the upper arm about the shoulder ICOR (instantaneous centre of rotation) out of the plane of the torso so that it points forwards.

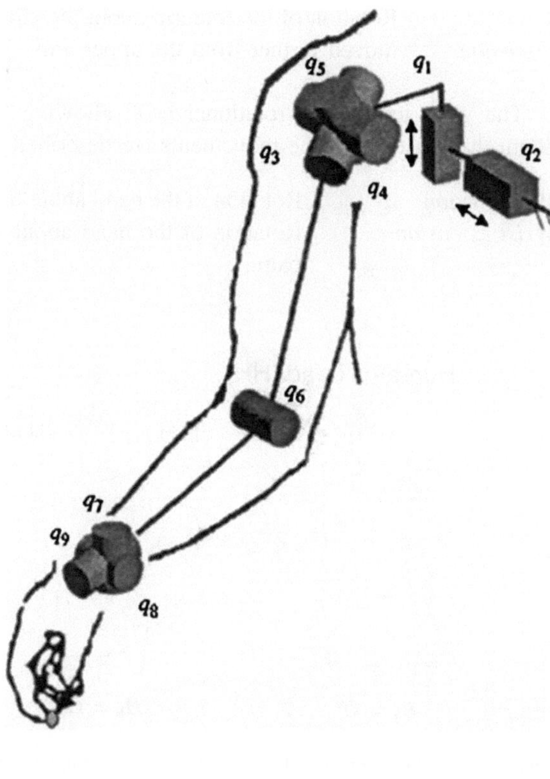

Fig. 2.5 9-DOF of the human upper limb [55]

Shoulder extension	Rotation of the upper arm about the shoulder ICOR out of the plane of the torso so that it points backwards.
Shoulder abduction	Rotation of the upper arm about the shoulder ICOR in the plane of the torso so that it is lifted upwards.
Shoulder adduction	Rotation of the upper arm about the shoulder ICOR in the plane of the torso so that it is dropped downwards.
Shoulder medial rotation	Axial rotation of the upper arm towards the torso.
Shoulder lateral rotation	Axial rotation of the upper arm away from the torso.
Shoulder elevation	Translation of the shoulder ICOR upwards.
Shoulder depression	Translation of the shoulder ICOR downwards.
Shoulder protraction	Translation of the shoulder ICOR forwards.
Shoulder retraction	Translation of the shoulder ICOR backwards.

An interesting phenomenon of the shoulder is that abduction of the upper arm above the horizontal plane will occur simultaneously with elevation as shown in Fig. 2.6 [56]. Without this elevation, abduction above the horizontal plane cannot be achieved.

The elbow joint has 1-rotational DOF which moves the forearm with the following movements:

Elbow flexion	Rotation of the forearm about the elbow joint so that the forearm is moved closer to the upper arm.
Elbow extension	Rotation of the forearm about the elbow joint so that the forearm is moved further from the upper arm.

The wrist joint has 3-rotational DOF allowing the hand to rotate spherically about the wrist joint. The movements are described as:

Wrist flexion	Rotation of the hand about the wrist joint towards the palm.
Wrist extension	Rotation of the hand about the wrist joint away from the palm.

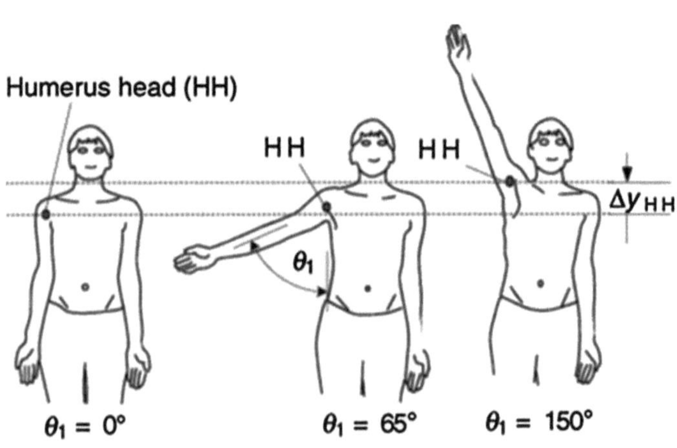

Fig. 2.6 Shoulder elevation during abduction of the upper arm [57]

Wrist radial deviation	Rotation of the hand about the wrist joint towards the thumb.
Wrist ulnar deviation	Rotation of the hand about the wrist joint away from the thumb.
Forearm pronation	Rotation of the hand about the axis of the forearm so that the palm faces backwards when the hand is pointing downwards.
Forearm supination	Rotation of the hand about the axis of the forearm so that the palm faces forwards when the hand is pointing downwards.

2.2.2 Model of Ankle Joint

Kinematics of the ankle-foot complex had been extensively studied in the literature. The simplest representation of ankle-foot motion is that of a hinge joint perpendicular to the sagittal plane. This description considers the entire foot as a rigid body that can rotate about the shank in the plantarflexion and dorsiflexion directions. This is a gross oversimplification of the ankle-foot motion as movements in other DOF are ignored. Additionally, early studies had found from examination of the talus bone surface geometry that the axis of rotation of the talus will vary with its orientation [58, 59]. The actual kinematics of the foot is therefore very complex as it is governed by the articulating surfaces between the different foot bones, as well as constraints imposed by ligaments, tendons and soft tissues. This was highlighted in various studies which investigated the movement patterns of foot bones in terms of 6-DOF motion in either in vitro or in vivo scenarios [60–63]. The general findings of these works were that the axes of rotations of the ankle and subtalar joints do vary rather considerably between different foot orientations and different individuals/specimens. Additionally, translational motions of the joint centres were also recorded, although it was found that these movements are typically within the range of one to two centimetres.

Information of ankle kinematics is essential in applications such as gait analysis, diagnosis of normal ankle-foot function and design of implants for total ankle replacement. However, the complex motion observed at the ankle makes it difficult to describe the complete ankle kinematics concisely with a mathematical model. Models of varying levels of complexity had been established for different applications. As discussed above, the simplest model used is that of a single hinge joint model (Fig. 2.7a). Furthermore, ankle-foot motion had been described as purely rotational using an effective spherical joint (Fig. 2.7b) [64], while the biaxial model which considers the foot motion to be equivalent to rotations about two hinge/revolute joints in series was also widely adopted in literature (Fig. 2.7c)

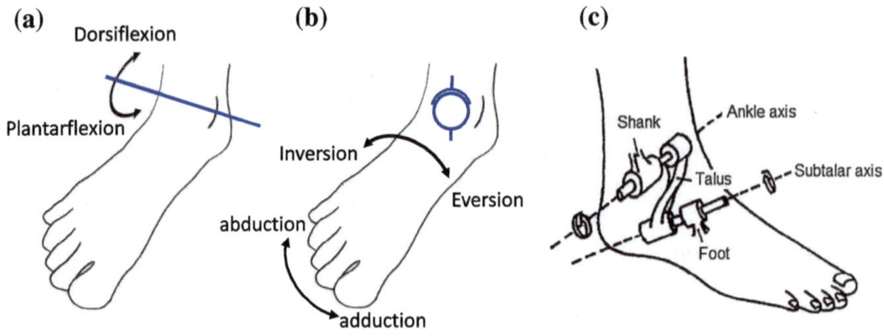

Fig. 2.7 Kinematic models used to describe ankle motion. **a** Hinge joint model. **b** Spherical joint model. **c** Biaxial joint model. Adapted from [65]

[64–69]. Additionally, recent studies had modelled the ankle-foot kinematics using four-bar linkages and spatial parallel mechanisms [63, 70].

Since large inter-subject variability is observed in ankle kinematics, a user-specific description of ankle kinematics should be used to adapt the robot behaviour to suit the current user. Most of the studies in literature that considers subject-specific ankle kinematics in full 6-DOF have utilised either motion tracking systems or medical imaging techniques [71, 72]. As these methods typically require offline processing, they are not suited for use in real-time systems. A simpler kinematic model with reduced degree of freedom which is amenable to online parameter identification is therefore more appropriate for this research. Additionally, since this representation of the ankle kinematics will also be incorporated in the dynamic model of the ankle-foot structure, the use of a straightforward model will reduce the computational complexity of the system, thus making its simulation more tractable. For the above reasons, the biaxial ankle model appears to be sensible choice and its parameter estimation will be further discussed.

Parameter identification for a biaxial kinematic model was investigated by van den Bogert in an in vivo manner using visual markers placed on the subject's foot [68]. The biaxial model considered has 12 parameters and these are determined through minimisation of the discrepancies between marker positions obtained from the assumed model and from measurements using the Levenberg–Marquardt algorithm. The resulting ankle and subtalar joint orientations using this method were found to be similar to corresponding values obtained from in vitro anatomical studies of the ankle. Good fit of the model in terms of the marker positions was also reported, with relatively small rigid body errors. Lewis et al. had also investigated the parameter identification of the biaxial ankle model on both biaxial mechanical linkage and cadaveric foot specimens [71]. The optimisation algorithm used is largely similar to that described by van den Bogert except that the ankle and subtalar joint displacements were estimated through optimisation using the Gauss–Newton algorithm. It was reported that the parameter identification of the biaxial mechanical linkages shows results that are largely consistent with the actual kinematic parameters of the structure. Considerable discrepancies, however, were observed between the ankle and subtalar joint orientations computed from the optimisation algorithm and the average helical axes obtained from successive measurements of the foot bone orientations. This had therefore led them to conclude that the biaxial ankle model with fixed revolute joints can only give a limited representation of the actual ankle-foot kinematics, and that an alternative model, perhaps one with configuration-dependent joint axes orientations, be explored. It should be noted that both the previous works discussed above on the identification of biaxial ankle kinematic model parameters were completed using offline optimisation techniques.

Studies in the biomechanical characteristics of the ankle go beyond the understanding the kinematic behaviour of the ankle. It seeks also to identify how the human ankle will react under certain loading conditions, as well as the loading distribution among different anatomical structures of the ankle-foot complex such as foot bones, ligaments, tendons and other soft tissues.

One of the core components of a computational ankle model is a description of the ankle-foot kinematics as it determines how the foot bones will move relative to one another, thus ultimately influencing the length of ligaments and muscle-tendon units, as well as deformation of other soft tissues. While the use of three-dimensional contact constraints [73–75] can lead to more realistic results, it can be computationally intensive and therefore limit the speed of simulations. In this aspect, the biaxial ankle kinematic model described previously appears to be able to provide a good balance between simplicity and the ability to provide a reasonably description of the ankle-foot motion.

Another important modelling decision is found in the treatment of bones and soft tissues. Some models treat the bones as rigid bodies and ignore effects caused by deformation of soft tissues [67, 73], while others apply finite element analysis on the bones and soft tissue in order to obtain the stress distribution across the articulating bone surfaces [74, 75]. Clearly, use of finite element analysis will improve the accuracy of the model at the expense of increased computational complexity.

Effects of ligaments on the ankle-foot biomechanics had also been considered in some models. Typically, they are treated as tension-only elastic elements whose lengths are dependent on the configurations of foot bones [73–75]. Some models, however, include the influence of ligaments on passive joint stiffness as a lumped effect, and describe it through application of non-linear resistive moment-displacement functions at the ankle and subtalar joints [76, 77]. Properties of muscles and tendons are also commonly included in computational models which require consideration of active muscular contractions [67, 76, 77], and these models typically employ a Hill-based muscle model and are often used for gait analysis. Models which involve explicit modelling of the ligaments and muscle-tendon units generally require the acquisition of bone geometry and ligament/tendon attachment locations by means of medical imaging, and this can add to the complexity of the model. However, as forces and strains along the ligaments/tendons can be extracted from such models, the added complexity can be justified for applications requiring greater insights into the loading on these anatomical elements.

2.2.3 Model of Masticatory System

The purpose of the human masticatory system is to perform the initial breakdown of food via chewing and prepare it for swallowing. It includes the bones and soft structures, such as muscles, ligaments and tendons of the face and mouth, that are involved in mastication. There are multiple complex mechanisms involved in this process, including the secretion of saliva, manipulation of the chewed food into a bolus with the tongue and the muscular control of the mandible that produces chewing motions, which is the focus of this and following parts. The main problem is that if the temporomandibular joint (TMJ) or mandibular muscles are weakened, the patient is unable to properly chew and process food. Current solutions include modifying the texture or consistency of the food for easier processing, or bypassing the masticatory system by tubular feeding through the oesophagus or abdomen. However, there are also efforts that are attempting to reduce the effects of physical symptoms through therapy and physical rehabilitation of the mandibular muscles. Similar to gait or upper limb rehabilitation, these exercises consist of repetitive exercises that are conducted with the assistance of a therapist, and can therefore also benefit from the advantages robotics and exoskeletons provided in those applications.

This section introduces the components of the masticatory system directly involved in the formation of chewing motions, including the skeletal structure, primary mandibular muscles and the temporomandibular joint. These components form a unique complex structure that is not replicated elsewhere in the human body and allows the mandible to be manipulated in three-dimensional space. A review of the available literature regarding masticatory robotics and the development of jaw exoskeletons for rehabilitation is also presented, which lead to the motivations behind this particular case study.

2.3 Control of Rehabilitation Robots

2.3.1 Motion/Force Control Strategies

The main goal of interaction control is to establish a certain relationship between force and motion, and this relationship is typically expressed as either a mechanical impedance or admittance. To realise these relationships, both force and motion of the robot have to be obtained from sensors and acted upon accordingly through application of suitable control laws. However, the most tightly controlled loop in a rehabilitation robot typically deals with only one of the two interaction variables, and these control loops are considered as low-level controllers in this review. These lower level control loops of the interaction controllers are generally implemented using conventional position (or force) control to ensure that the desired motion (or force) is applied to the robot. An outer loop is then applied to alter this desired motion (or force) depending on the measured force (or motion) so that the overall behaviour of the robot resembles that of a mechanical system exhibiting the desired impedance or admittance.

2.3.1.1 Inner Loop Position/Velocity Control

In additional to the commonly used proportional-integral-derivative (PID) controller, another popular strategy used in the implementation of a position-controlled inner loop is the computed torque control [78]. This method is an established method for position tracking of robotic manipulators and operates by linearizing the robot dynamics through application of feedback terms which aim to cancel the non-linear terms in the robot dynamic equations. An additional proportional derivative (PD) term acting on the position error is also applied to facilitate tracking of the reference position. The computed torque control scheme therefore requires a good knowledge of the robot dynamics as well as the ability to measure actuator velocities. In applications where the robot velocity is low, the velocity-dependent terms can be neglected and gravity compensation alone can be used to reduce the computational complexity of this approach [79].

Variants of the computed torque control laws had been used in interaction control of rehabilitation robots [80, 81]. In robots with inner position control loops, the observed interaction forces are used to compute reference accelerations according to the desired impedance relationship. These reference accelerations are then fed to the inner motion control loop to realise the prescribed interaction behaviour.

2.3.1.2 Inner Loop Force/Torque Control

Inner force or torque control loops can also be used to provide the required interaction behaviour. In this alternative approach, the motion of the robot is used to generate the force/torque reference. Similar to the case of motion control, the simplest force controller can be obtained through the use of PID-type controllers. More advanced control strategies such as disturbance observers [82, 83] had also been used to reject disturbances stemming from frictional forces and modelled dynamics. It should be noted that computed torque control used in robot motion control also ultimately requires some form of actuator level force/torque control. This is because it operates on the assumption that the desired torque is accurately delivered by the actuators.

Naturally, actuator force control can be carried out with the feedback of actuator forces. The main challenge associated with the implementation of control laws requiring force feedback, however, is system stability. Since compliant force sensors are typically required to measure the actuator force, it contributes to additional position feedback [84]. As a result, large sensor stiffness will lead to a large, effective position feedback gain, thus creating severely under-damped systems which could become unstable when higher order modelled dynamics are taken into account. Force sensors that are too soft on the other hand will result in inaccurate position measurements due to additional unmonitored force sensor deformations.

Researchers have proposed that the passivity of the controlled system must be preserved if stability were to be maintained during interaction with arbitrary passive environments [85, 86]. This imposes an upper limit on the force feedback gain that can be used depending on how the actuator mass is distributed when the actuator's first resonance is considered in the actuator model. Since the main contribution of increasing the force feedback gain is shown to be a reduction in the apparent actuator inertia, the above limitation also restricts the extent to which this inertia can be reduced. Recent work, however, had proposed the use of environmental information to relax the passivity criterion to permit performance improvements of the actuator [87, 88]. The authors have imposed bounds on the expected human arm impedance and utilised it to numerically compute force feedback gains that satisfy the robust stability criterion based on the small gain theorem.

An alternative strategy in the regulation of actuator force involves the use of a force sensor-less control scheme. Instead of measuring the actuator force/torque through force/torque sensors, this method uses a disturbance observer based approach [89] to estimate the reaction torque/force from current and motion variables. This was shown in [90] to reduce the oscillations found in the resulting force response. Such a control strategy, however, requires the measurement of actuator velocity and a good knowledge of model parameters such as actuator inertia, damping and friction. Torque control was also achieved in [91] through the use of a position disturbance observer in the control of a rotary series elastic actuator, which consisted of a highly geared motor coupled in series with a torsional spring. In this approach, torque control is realised by accurately controlling the deformation within the torsional spring.

While a considerable amount of research had been made in force/torque control, manipulator force control is still mainly achieved by independent control of individual actuators, where the torque/force of each actuator is regulated in its own feedback loop. It is therefore worthwhile to investigate whether force control performance can be improved when the robot actuators are treated collectively as a multi-input, multi-output system.

2.3.2 EMG Signals Based Control

Muscle tissue can be divided into two main types based on their fundamental structure: striated muscle and smooth muscle [92]. Striated muscle is involved with conscious movement and its basic structure consists of thick and thin filaments that slide against each other to produce movement [93]. Skeletal muscle is a type of striated muscle that is usually attached to a bone on each end by tendons. Upon voluntary activation, the muscles contract and shorten pulling on the tendons, and the resulting tension causes the bones to move relative to each other.

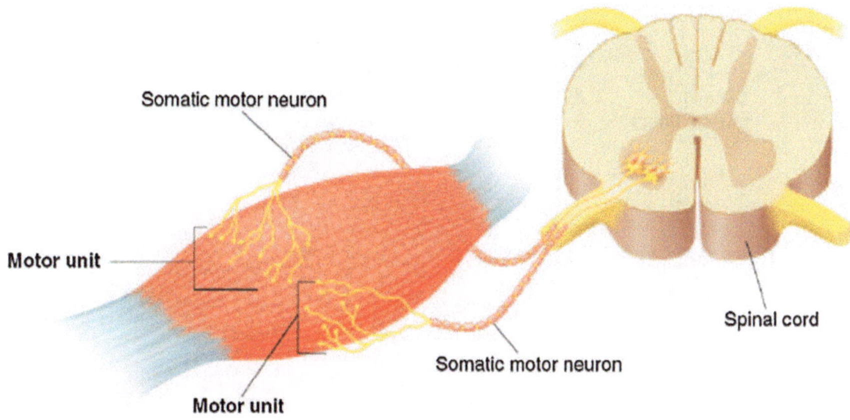

Fig. 2.8 The motor unit [94]

Each skeletal muscle cell is essentially a muscle fibre and two stages of bundling of muscle fibres result in the formation of skeletal muscle tissue. Somatic motor neurons externally stimulate the muscle cells to cause contractions. The cell body of a motor neuron is located in the grey matter of the spinal cord and its axon (main branch) splits into a number of collateral branches (motor neuron fibres) before being distributed about the muscle fibres as nerve fibre branches. Each branch innervates or activates a single muscle fibre, and the somatic motor neuron, together with all the muscle fibres it innervates, is collectively known as a motor, as shown in Fig. 2.8. For more details of muscle structure and function, see [94].

The control signals of skeletal muscle are called action potentials and these are electrical impulses that originate in the brain. The signals propagate through the central and peripheral nervous systems and are transmitted down the axons of motor neurons where they reach a specialised synapse called the neuromuscular junction, where the action potentials cross the boundary from muscle motor neuron to muscle fibre, and stimulate contraction [95]. This is illustrated in Fig. 2.9. Note that the muscle fibres of a single motor unit are not necessarily adjacent to each other and are instead interspersed throughout the muscle.

To take advantage of the benefits, the EMG signal can provide to interfacing, the term "neuromuscular interface" (NI) has been coined to describe a new type of self-contained module with a specific role. This role is to obtain and process EMG signals into a predicted joint torque or position of the joint or limb of interest. The NI includes all the hardware and software components that would be required to perform this procedure. The part an NI plays in the grander scheme of a complete control system and its more detailed constituents is shown in Fig. 2.10. The input to the interface are the EMG signals of the target joint, and the output is the user-intended torque or position of the associated limb, which can then be used by a controller or similar component to operate an exoskeleton. The focus on the development of a dedicated module to serve as the interface means that the NI can

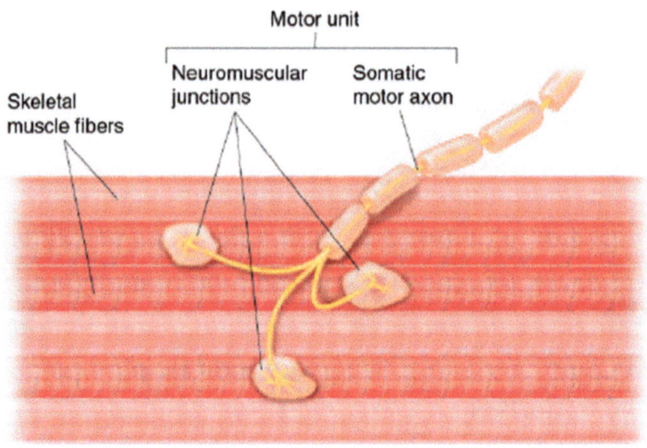

Fig. 2.9 The neuromuscular junction [94]

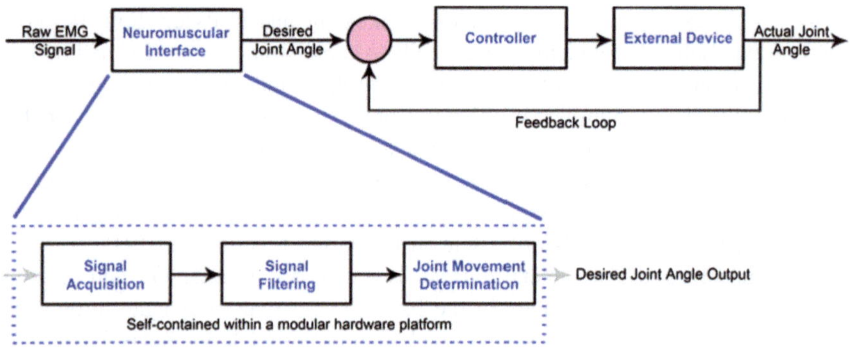

Fig. 2.10 The concept of a neuromuscular interface

be included in an unlimited number of applications both within and outside the health industry. The concentration on such a specific module for interfacing is unprecedented, with interfacing methods commonly a secondary consideration as a component of an overall system that includes controller, actuator and sensor design, and implementation. The output of the NI will only need to be post-processed further depending on the purpose, and the input signal should be able to drive exoskeletons, prostheses, mobility devices, communication tools, industrial equipment and any other relevant applications.

The realisation of an NI depends on and requires the development of several key areas of importance. Challenges in areas such as the EMG signal filtering process, conversion and interpretation of the signals into an equivalent joint torque or position and the specialised hardware development of the interface; all need to be addressed before an NI can become robust, reliable and practical enough for real-world applications. As mentioned previously, one of the main limitations of current exoskeleton devices is the lack of an adequate interface for information exchange between the user and the device. This is the current-limiting technology, which will continue to hold back exoskeleton development despite any advances in power supply, actuator or sensor technologies.

Most of the interfacing methods and approaches presented and discussed use commercial EMG or biosignal acquisition systems that have been specifically designed for clinical or research purposes. The conversion of an interface into a re-usable module includes the specialised hardware necessary to acquire EMG signals and the non-existence of such hardware is a key problem that is preventing EMG interfaces from becoming practical. Custom hardware interfaces are required to maximise performance while reducing unnecessary bulk and reviews of examples of wearable hardware systems can be found in [96, 97]. These hardware systems are targeted more towards patient or individualised monitoring applications, rather than interfacing and control, but they share similar design considerations, such as durability, portability, power consumption requirements, cost and aesthetics.

The realisation of EMG interfaces on hardware is an important consideration because the transfer from a laboratory environment to a real-world embedded system will inevitably have lower quality hardware components (to save cost) and have to account for additional sources of noise and disturbances. There is also an emphasis on reducing power consumption and volume to ensure that electrodes and corresponding processing circuitry and systems are as unobtrusive to the user as possible [98]. Progress in this area has been relatively lacklustre with only a few minor developments. This is partly because interfacing methods have their own fundamental problems and are barely on the cusp of being robust or practical enough to make it beyond the research or laboratory stage.

2.3.3 Interaction Controllers for Rehabilitation Robots

2.3.3.1 Basic Interaction Controllers

One of the most basic forms of interaction controllers can be found in simple impedance control, which essentially applies the torque command in an open loop manner without any force feedback. This torque command, however, is determined based on the desired impedance relationship and the discrepancies between the desired and actual robot motion. Owing to the lack of force feedback, this interaction control approach has poorer disturbance rejection but does not suffer from the stability issues discussed previously. It is therefore suitable for the use with devices with low inherent inertia and low friction. Force feedback control can also be used in impedance control schemes to allow reduction of the apparent robot inertia and improve the force tracking ability of the robot. However, the force feedback gain and hence the performance improvement are again limited due to stability constraints. Natural admittance control can be used to regulate the end point admittance of a robotic manipulator. It does so by using both force and velocity feedback in the same control loop. It was proposed that the mechanical admittance used in this approach be selected in such a way that the apparent end point mass of the controlled system is identical to that of the actual physical system to maintain passivity. Stiffness and damping characteristics, however, can be chosen as desired. Additionally, the velocity feedback gain is chosen to be large so that effects of disturbance forces such as friction can be reduced.

2.3.3.2 Higher Level Interaction Control

In addition to the basic interaction control strategies described above, higher level interaction control schemes had also been investigated in rehabilitation robots, with many such schemes focusing on improving the safety and incorporating adaptability in the rehabilitation robots. These higher level controllers are also generally designed with a particular type of rehabilitation exercise in mind.

Safety and adaptability in rehabilitation robots are somewhat related. For instance, different patients will have different joint or limb kinematics. It is therefore unreasonable to have the robot strictly enforce one set of rehabilitation trajectories for all patients as it may result in application of large forces and thus lead to discomfort/injuries. In fact, impedance control in itself can be viewed as having a built-in adaptive mechanism as it permits positional deviation from a virtual reference when external forces are encountered. Some higher level interaction controllers extend on this and provide greater freedom to the user to dictate the actual path taken in rehabilitation. However, the extent of this freedom must also be bounded to ensure that the required exercises are still being carried out.

In order to achieve adaptability of this nature, some controllers for lower limb rehabilitation define a particular region or tunnel around the reference trajectory within which the interaction forces between the robot and user are minimised [99, 100]. This is typically achieved through feed forward compensation of the robot inertial and gravitational forces. It is also possible to reduce the time dependency nature of the reference trajectory by identifying the reference point using a nearest neighbour approach [99]. Various strategies for the adaptation of rehabilitation trajectory had also been considered in [101] for a position-controlled gait rehabilitation robot. Some of these strategies were aimed at reducing the active patient torques through modification of the reference gait trajectory while another utilises impedance control to allow deviation from the reference trajectory. The recorded deviation due to impedance control is then incorporated into the reference trajectory of the next gait cycle.

An alternative approach taken in [102] to provide adaptability in upper limb rehabilitation is to avoid the prescription of reference trajectories in the Cartesian space, and instead define the virtual trajectory in terms of Euclidean distance to the desired end point. In other words assistance is given to the user through impedance control when the distance between the current position and the end position exceeds that desired for the particular time instant. In [103], a moving potential field is used to define the level of forces applied to move the user's limb to the current reference position. This potential field, however, is selected in such a way that it will not impede the user's movement should the current arm position be closer to the target destination compared to the current reference. This means that the controller is designed so that it would not penalise users when they are performing better than required.

One other way to improve safety is to use a smaller manipulator impedance to allow larger deviations from the reference trajectory. An obvious shortcoming associated with this approach is that certain positions in the limb or joint range of motion will not be reached as insufficient forces are available for guidance. A method to overcome this problem is to apply a reference force on top of the force command generated from impedance control. This will provide adequate forces to move the affected limb or joint while also allowing for greater flexibility in terms of the limb or joint position. In [104], this reference force is generated from a series of radial basis functions whose weights are adaptively tuned to compensate the inertial and gravitational forces of the robot and user.

Another aspect of adaptability can be described as the ability of the robot to cater for the physical capability of the patients. Various researchers have proposed that robots used in neuromotor training should encourage the patient to actively participate in the rehabilitation exercises by providing assistance or intervention only when it is needed [103, 105, 106]. It was also observed that given the opportunity, the user will decrease their effort and rely on the robot's assistance to complete the rehabilitation exercises [107]. Robots used in rehabilitation must therefore also be able to adjust the task difficulty or level of assistance it provides to the user according to some performance indicator. A common approach is to reduce the level of assistance over time. This can be done by reducing the assistive forces by decreasing the impedance or feed forward force parameters as in [102, 104]. Clearly, a mechanism must also be put in place to halt the decay in assistance should the performance of the patient deteriorate, and this is typically accomplished via the addition of a term which increases the reference force or impedance parameter based on variables derived from motion error. A fuzzy inference system has also been used in [80] to vary the robot behaviour between that of a minimal interaction force-controlled and impedance-controlled robot depending on the position-tracking errors. This means that when the user is moving as required, the robot will merely actuate to support its own gravitational and inertial forces. However, as the user fails to follow the required motion trajectories, the robot will provide assistance according to the prescribed impedance relationship.

2.4 Discussion

Recent technological advances have enabled the development of feasible exoskeleton robots. Modelling software has allowed exoskeletons to be tested in simulations before they are fabricated, allowing rapid prototype development. Biomechanics modelling allows the exoskeleton to mimic the dynamics of the human limb. Sensor technologies, control strategies and computing power have advanced to the extent where they are no longer major obstacles. However, actuator and power supply technologies still have limitations.

One of the fundamental limitations in past upper limb exoskeletons is the inability of the shoulder mechanism to achieve the entire human shoulder workspace with adequate performance. This is due to the singular configurations present in the 3R spherical wrist mechanism that are used in the shoulder complex of the exoskeletons. Operating at a singular configuration results in the loss of 1-DOF in the 3R mechanism and therefore the exoskeleton becomes unable to achieve the same movements as that of the 3-DOF human shoulder. Even operating near a singular configuration reduces the ability of the 3R mechanism to rotate about the affected DOF and requires the 3R mechanism to move at undesirably high velocities. Several recent upper limb exoskeletons have considered this problem and designed the exoskeleton so that the singular configurations occur at uncommon shoulder postures at the edge of the shoulder workspace. Although this change partially improves the performance of the exoskeleton, the singular configurations are still present in the shoulder workspace and operating near these configurations causes poor performance in the 3R mechanism.

Among the 9-DOF in the human upper limb, the 3-DOF spherical movement of the shoulder has the largest range of motion and has the most influence on the rest of the upper limb since it is the most proximal joint in the limb. Therefore, recovery of the shoulder joint is often more urgent than the other joints in the upper limb. The shoulder joint is also highly complex and is the most powerful joint in the upper limb making it the most difficult joint to provide rehabilitation for. Thus, designing an exoskeleton that is capable of implementing all movements of a normal human shoulder is highly challenging, but such capabilities can provide significant improvements to existing shoulder rehabilitation methods.

Clinical results are available for some of the early end-effector type robots which provide strong evidence that robotic rehabilitation has a beneficial effect on motor function. However, comparing clinical data is rather difficult as different groups use different devices, control strategies, intervention strategies and assessment criteria. There are many patient-specific parameters that can affect the outcomes of the treatment which may also need to be taken into consideration. There are currently insufficient guidelines and tools used in clinical evaluations of robotic rehabilitation, and to some degree in conventional rehabilitation, which is limiting the amount of quality data that can be acquired. Many assessment methods, such as the assessment of posture, are based on subjective impressions which make it difficult to justify the effectiveness of rehabilitation treatments. Future research will need to focus on developing and refining these guidelines and tools to ensure researchers to get as much reliable data as possible out of clinical evaluations. With better data, the effects of variations in the rehabilitation treatment and the patient's condition on motor and functional recovery can be better understood. This will enable the development of more effective rehabilitation exoskeletons and intervention strategies. Exoskeleton technologies have the potential to initiate new areas of research as well as support existing research work. New approaches to rehabilitation treatment and patient assessment may be discovered and a better understanding of the human neuromuscular system can be achieved.

One promising approach for patient treatment is the application of task-based exercises in rehabilitation. There is evidence that suggests task-based rehabilitation specifically designed to deal with lost abilities produce better results than resistance-strengthening exercises. However, realistic task-based exercises are difficult to achieve with manual rehabilitation methods. Exoskeletons have the ability to accurately control multiple joints at the same time, enabling them to produce more realistic task-based exercises for the patient. In addition, studies have found that rehabilitation is more effective when the patient exerts voluntary effort in intensive and frequent exercises, much like recreational exercises. Incorporating rehabilitation exercises into virtual games can make rehabilitation more enjoyable thus motivating the patient to put in effort and encouraging more exercise. In addition, the use of virtual reality enables more realistic task-based exercises to be performed. The concept of using virtual games to provide therapy exercises has already been applied in a number of exoskeletons. The next step is to design games based on rehabilitation principles and allow the games to be adjusted to better match the patient's level of motor deficiency.

It can be seen from the above review that rehabilitation robots had already been proposed in the literature, with wearable devices mainly aimed at gait rehabilitation and platform-based devices focusing more on treatment of ankle sprains. However, it should be noted that the Stewart platform-based ankle rehabilitation robot had also been applied in the area of stroke rehabilitation, thus indicating that it is worthwhile to develop a rehabilitation robot which can be potentially extended to cater for treatment of both ankle sprains and neurological disorders.

One major shortcoming in existing platform-based ankle rehabilitation devices with 2- to 3-DOF is that the rotation of the robot end effector is typically constrained about a point on the robot rather than allowing the user's lower limb to govern the end-effector motion as in the designs proposed. The consequence of this is that the motion of the user's foot will not be limited to movements between the shank and the foot during operation of the robot. Under such conditions, measurements of the robot end-effector orientation may no longer be the true ankle joint displacements, thus limiting the repeatability of the actual ankle-foot motion while also compromising the ability of the robot to act as a reliable evaluation/measurement tool. This issue is therefore addressed during the mechanical design of the ankle rehabilitation device developed in this research.

Additionally, even though existing platform-based ankle rehabilitation devices are already capable of basic interaction control and can perform various rehabilitation exercises, not much emphasis was placed on the adaptability of these devices. As the kinematics and impedance characteristics of the ankle can vary considerably between individuals, the controller for rehabilitation robots should ideally be able to detect these variations and adjust for it accordingly. An example of this is the reduction of robot impedance in regions of large stiffness to prevent exertion of excessive forces. It is therefore the intention of this research to incorporate adaptability into an ankle rehabilitation robot through online parameter estimation. A suitable interaction control scheme can then be developed to capitalise on the additional information available to improve the safety of the device. Furthermore, the assistance adaptation schemes available in robots designed for motor training were also considered in this research so that the developed device will be able not only to accommodate variations in the users' joint characteristics but also to adapt its behaviour to ensure that the level of assistance provided is based on the user's capability to carry out the required exercises. While the aim of this research is to create a system which is primarily targeted at rehabilitation of sprained ankles, development of an assistance adaptation scheme will also facilitate future extension of the developed system to cover neuromotor rehabilitation.

It is worth noting that many of the assistance adaptation schemes vary the assistive effort either directly or indirectly based on observation on the position-tracking errors, and the adaptation rules are typically formulated in ways which do not place much consideration on the possibility of constrained motion in the robot's task space. This is perhaps due to the predominant application of these algorithms in upper limb rehabilitation where the subject's arm can normally move within the workspace of interest in a constraint-free manner. This is, however, unlikely to be the case for ankle-foot movements due to the existence of coupled rotations which imposes constraints in the three-dimensional rotational space. Assistance adaptation rules which are more suitable for constrained motion are therefore investigated in this work.

It can be seen from the above discussion on ankle models that numerous computational ankle models had been developed to study foot pathology and biomechanics. However, to the best of the author's knowledge, none of these models were applied in the controller development of ankle rehabilitation devices. In addition to its use in controller simulation and in providing information on the configuration-dependent ankle characteristics such as ankle stiffness which can be used for parameter adaptation and stability analysis of the interaction controller, a suitable computational ankle model can also be used to approximate the forces along different ligaments or muscle-tendon units as well as reaction forces and moments encountered at the ankle and subtalar joints. It can therefore also serve as a tool to evaluate the performance of a controller or the effectiveness of a particular rehabilitation programme. It can be seen that a computational ankle model which provides all the functionalities above will greatly facilitate the overall goal of this research in the development of an adaptive ankle rehabilitation robot. Such a model is therefore developed in this research to facilitate both the design and the implementation of the adaptive control scheme.

Lastly, given the considerable variation in the ankle kinematics and the need to incorporate adaptability into the developed system, user-specific ankle kinematic parameters should ideally be available to facilitate adjustment of the controller parameters. It can be seen that while identification of the biaxial ankle kinematic model had been explored in the literature, such identification was carried out in an offline manner. However, due to the real-time requirements of this application, an online parameter identification algorithm is required. Consequently, the development of such an algorithm is also addressed in this research. Owing to the importance of computational tractability, it is proposed that a biaxial ankle model be used to describe the ankle kinematics in the identification algorithm. However, as it is commonly found in literature that orientations of the ankle and subtalar joint axes change with foot configuration, the conventional biaxial ankle model with constant axes orientations is also extended in this research to allow variation of these parameters with foot displacement so that a better fit between the model and measured foot orientations can be obtained.

2.5 Summary

This chapter presented a review of existing works relevant to this research. Numerous issues in the development of robots for rehabilitation have been identified and there is much room for improvement. Of particular concern is the inability of the robots to achieve the full range of motion of the joint's spherical movement with adequate performance. The different types of human rehabilitation devices developed in the literature were considered, with particular focus on their mechanical design, actuation methods and control schemes. Subsequently, studies relating to human joint kinematics and computational modelling were also examined. The state of the art of control strategies for rehabilitation robots was reviewed.

References

1. N. Hogan, H.I. Krebs, J. Charnnarong, P. Srikrishna, A. Sharon, MIT-MANUS: a workstation for manual therapy and training. I, in *IEEE International Workshop on Robot and Human Communication*, 1992, pp. 161–165
2. H.I. Krebs, J.J. Palazzolo, L. Dipietro, M. Ferraro, J. Krol, K. Rannekleiv, B.T. Volpe, N. Hogan, Rehabilitation robotics: performance-based progressive robot-assisted therapy. Auton. Robot. **15**, 7–20 (2003)
3. C.G. Burgar, P.S. Lum, P.C. Shor, H.F.M. Van Der Loos, Development of robots for rehabilitation therapy: The Palo Alto VA/Stanford experience. J. Rehabil. Res. Dev. **37**, 663–673 (2000)
4. R. Loureiro, F. Amirabdollahian, M. Topping, B. Driessen, W. Harwin, Upper limb robot mediated stroke therapy—GENTLE/s approach. Auton. Robot. **15**, 35–51 (2003)

5. P.S. Lum, C.G. Burgar, M. Van Der Loos, P.C. Shor, M. Majmundar, R. Yap, MIME robotic device for upper-limb neurorehabilitation in subacute stroke subjects: a follow-up study. J. Rehabil. Res. Dev. **43**, 631–642 (2006)
6. H.I. Krebs, N. Hogan, B.T. Volpe, M.L. Aisen, L. Edelstein, C. Diels, Overview of clinical trials with MIT-MANUS: a robot-aided neuro-rehabilitation facility. Technol. Health Care **7**, 419–423 (1999)
7. P.S. Lum, C.G. Burgar, P.C. Shor, M. Majmundar, M. Van der Loos, Robot-assisted movement training compared with conventional therapy techniques for the rehabilitation of upper-limb motor function after stroke. Arch. Phys. Med. Rehabil. **83**, 952–959 (2002)
8. P.S. Lum, C.G. Burgar, P.C. Shor, Evidence for improved muscle activation patterns after retraining of reaching movements with the MIME robotic system in subjects with post-stroke hemiparesis. IEEE Trans. Neural Syst. Rehabil. Eng. **12**, 186–194 (2004)
9. S. Coote, B. Murphy, W. Harwin, E. Stokes, The effect of the GENTLE/s robot-mediated therapy system on arm function after stroke. Clin. Rehabil. **22**, 395–405 (2008)
10. A. Frisoli, L. Borelli, A. Montagner, S. Marcheschi, C. Procopio, F. Salsedo, M. Bergamasco, M.C. Carboncini, M. Tolaini, B. Rossi, Arm rehabilitation with a robotic exoskeleleton in Virtual Reality, in *International Conference on Rehabilitation Robotics*, 2007, pp. 631–642
11. T. Nef, M. Guidali, R. Riener, ARMin III—arm therapy exoskeleton with an ergonomic shoulder actuation. Appl. Bion. Biomech. **6**, 127–142 (2009)
12. C. Carignan, J. Tang, S. Roderick, Development of an exoskeleton haptic interface for virtual task training, in *IEEE/RSJ International Conference on Intelligent Robots and Systems*, 2009, pp. 3697–3702
13. Y. Ren, H. S. Park, L.Q. Zhang, Developing a whole-arm exoskeleton robot with hand opening and closing mechanism for upper limb stroke rehabilitation, in *IEEE International Conference on Rehabilitation Robotics*, 2009, pp. 761–765
14. S.J. Ball, I.E. Brown, S.H. Scott, MEDARM: A rehabilitation robot with 5DOF at the shoulder complex, in *IEEE/ASME International Conference on Advanced Intelligent Mechatronics*, 2007
15. R.A.R.C. Gopura, K. Kiguchi, Y. Yi, SUEFUL-7: a 7DOF upper-limb exoskeleton robot with muscle-model-oriented EMG-based control, in *IEEE/RSJ International Conference on Intelligent Robots and Systems*, 2009, pp. 1126–1131
16. A.H.A. Stienen, E.E.G. Hekman, F.C.T. van der Helm, H. van der Kooij, Self-aligning exoskeleton axes through decoupling of joint rotations and translations. IEEE Trans. Rob. **25**, 628–633 (2009)
17. *Armeo Therapy Concept*. Available: http://www.hocoma.com/products/armeo/
18. *myomo*. Available: http://www.myomo.com/myomo-solutions-mpower-1000
19. *Hand Physical Therapy*. Available: http://www.kineticmuscles.com/hand-physical-therapy-hand-mentor.html
20. *Interactive Motion Technologies*. Available: http://interactive-motion.com/
21. *Biodex*. Available: http://www.biodex.com/
22. *HUMAC NORM*. Available: http://www.csmisolutions.com/products/isokinetic-extremity-systems/humac-norm
23. *CMV AG Con-Trex*. Available: http://www.con-trex.ch/index.php?option=com_content&task=blogcategory&id=21&Itemid=88
24. J.C. Perry, J. Rosen, S. Burns, Upper-limb powered exoskeleton design. IEEE/ASME Trans. Mechatron. **12**, 408–417 (2007)
25. P. Garrec, J.P. Friconneau, Y. Méasson, Y. Perrot, ABLE, an innovative transparent exoskeleton for the upper-limb, in *IEEE/RSJ International Conference on Intelligent Robots and Systems*, 2008, pp. 1483–1488
26. D.G. Caldwell, N.G. Tsagarakis, S. Kousidou, N. Costa, I. Sarakoglou, "Soft" exoskeletons for upper and lower body rehabilitation—design, control and testing. Int. J. Humanoid Rob. **4**, 549–573 (2007)

27. S. Kousidou, N. Tsagarakis, D.G. Caldwell, C. Smith, Assistive exoskeleton for task based physiotherapy in 3-dimensional space, in *1st IEEE/RAS-EMBS International Conference on Biomedical Robotics and Biomechatronics*, 2006, pp. 266–271
28. S. Balasubramanian, H.R. Wei, M. Perez, B. Shepard, E. Koeneman, J. Koeneman, J. He, Rupert: an exoskeleton robot for assisting rehabilitation of arm functions, in *2008 Virtual Rehabilitation, IWVR,*, 2008, pp. 163–167
29. A. Roy, H.I. Krebs, S.L. Patterson, T.N. Judkins, I.K. Larry, R.M. Macko, N. Hogan, Measurement of human ankle stiffness using the anklebot, in *International Conference on Rehabilitation Robotics*, 2007, pp. 356–363
30. K. Bharadwaj, T.G. Sugar, J.B. Koeneman, E.J. Koeneman, Design of a robotic gait trainer using spring over muscle actuators for ankle stroke rehabilitation. J. Biomech. Eng. **127**, 1009–1013 (2005)
31. D.P. Ferris, J.M. Czerniecki, B. Hannaford, An ankle-foot orthosis powered by artificial pneumatic muscles. J. Appl. Biomech. **21**, 189–197 (2005)
32. J.A. Saglia, N.G. Tsagarakis, J.S. Dai, D. G. Caldwell, Control strategies for ankle rehabilitation using a high performance ankle exerciser, in *IEEE International Conference on Robotics and Automation*, 2010, pp. 2221–2227
33. J. Yoon, J. Ryu, A novel reconfigurable ankle/foot rehabilitation robot, in *IEEE International Conference on Robotics and Automation*, Barcelona, Spain, 2005, pp. 2290–2295
34. Human-Machine Interface Laboratory, Rutgers University. http://www.caip.rutgers.edu/vrlab/projects/ankle/ankle.html
35. J.A. Blaya, H. Herr, Adaptive control of a variable-impedance ankle-foot orthosis to assist drop-foot gait. IEEE Trans. Neural Syst. Rehabil. Eng. **12**, 24–31 (2004)
36. G.S. Sawicki, D.P. Ferris, A pneumatically powered knee-ankle-foot orthosis (KAFO) with myoelectric activation and inhibition. J. NeuroEng. Rehabil. **6**(23) 2009
37. G.S. Sawicki, K.E. Gordon, D.P. Ferris, Powered lower limb orthoses: applications in motor adaptation and rehabilitation, in *2005 IEEE International Conference on Rehabilitation Robotics*, 2005, pp. 206–211
38. A.W. Boehler, K.W. Hollander, T.G. Sugar, D. Shin, Design, implementation and test results of a robust control method for a powered ankle foot orthosis (AFO), in *IEEE International Conference on Robotics and Automation*, 2008, pp. 2025–2030
39. A. Agrawal, S.K. Banala, S.K. Agrawal, S.A. Binder-Macleod, Design of a two degree-of-freedom ankle-foot orthosis for robotic rehabilitation, in *IEEE International Conference on Rehabilitation Robotics*, 2005, pp. 41–44
40. J.W. Wheeler, H.I. Krebs, N. Hogan, An ankle robot for a modular gait rehabilitation system, in *IEEE/RSJ International Conference on Intelligent Robots and Systems*, Sendai, Japan, 2004, pp. 1681–1684
41. G. Liu, J. Gao, H. Yue, X. Zhang, G. Lu, Design and kinematics simulation of parallel robots for ankle rehabilitation, in *IEEE International Conference on Mechatronics and Automation*, Luoyang, China, 2006, pp. 1109–1113
42. C.E. Syrseloudis, I.Z. Emiris, A parallel robot for ankle rehabilitation-evaluation and its design specifications, in *IEEE International Conference on BioInformatics and BioEngineering*, 2008
43. M. Girone, G. Burdea, M. Bouzit, V. Popescu, J.E. Deutsch, Stewart platform-based system for ankle telerehabilitation. Auton. Robot. **10**, 203–212 (2001)
44. J.S. Dai, T. Zhao, Sprained ankle physiotherapy based mechanism synthesis and stiffness analysis of a robotic rehabilitation device. Auton. Robot. **16**, 207–218 (2004)
45. C.-C.K. Lin, M.-S. Ju, S.-M. Chen, B.-W. Pan, A specialized robot for ankle rehabilitation and evaluation. J. Med. Biol. Eng. **28**, 79–86 (2008)
46. J.G. Sun, J.Y. Gao, J.H. Zhang, R.H. Tan, Teaching and playback control system for parallel robot for ankle joint rehabilitation, in *IEEE International Conference on Industrial Engineering and Engineering Management*, 2007, pp. 871–875
47. J. Yoon, J. Ryu, K.-B. Lim, Reconfigurable ankle rehabilitation robot for various exercises. J. Robot. Syst. **22**, S15–S33 (2006)

48. J.A. Saglia, N.G. Tsagarakis, J.S. Dai, D.G. Caldwell, A high-performance redundantly actuated mechanism for ankle rehabilitation. Int. J. Robot. Res. **28**, 1216–1227 (2009)
49. W.C. Shiel, Temporomandibular joint disorder (tmj). Retrieved 10 Jan 2010 from http://www.medicinenet.com/temporomandibular_joint_disorder/article.htm
50. W.C. Shiel, Temporomandibular joint (tmj) syndrome. Retrieved 10 Jan 2010 from http://www.emedicinehealth.com/temporomandibular_joint_tmj_syndrome/article_em.htm
51. D.M. Laskin, *Temporomandibular Joint Disorders* (SigmaMax Publishing, 2001), Chap. 79
52. NHS Choices, Muscular dystrophy. Retrieved 10 Jan 2010 from http://www.nhs.uk/Conditions/Muscular-dystrophy/Pages/Introduction.aspx
53. D.C. Dugdale, Muscle atrophy. Retrieved 10 Jan 2010 from http://www.umm.edu/ency/article/003188.htm
54. B. Tondu, Estimating shoulder-complex mobility. Appl. Bion. Biomech. **4**, 19–29 (2007)
55. J. Yang, K. Abdel-Malek, K. Nebel, Reach envelope of a 9-degree-of-freedom model of the upper extremity. Int. J. Robot. Autom. **20**, 240–259 (2005)
56. P.M. Ludewig, V. Phadke, J.P. Braman, D.R. Hassett, C.J. Cieminski, R.F. Laprade, Motion of the shoulder complex during multiplanar humeral elevation. J. Bone Jt. Surg.—Series A **91**, 378–389 (2009)
57. T. Nef, M. Guidali, R. Riener, ARMin III—arm therapy exoskeleton with an ergonomic shoulder actuation. Appl. Bion. Biomech. **6**, 127–142 (2009)
58. C.H. Barnett, J.R. Napier, The axis of rotation at the ankle joint in man; its influence upon the form of the talus and the mobility of the fibula. J. Anat. **86**, 1–9 (1952)
59. A. Lundberg, O.K. Svensson, G. Nemeth, G. Selvik, The axis of rotation of the ankle joint. J. Bone Jt. Surg.—Series B **71**, 94–99 (1989)
60. J.R. Engsberg, A biomechanical analysis of the talocalcaneal joint—in vitro. J. Biomech. **20**, 429–442 (1987)
61. D.M. Demarais, R.A. Bachschmidt, G.F. Harris, The instantaneous axis of rotation (IAOR) of the foot and ankle: a self-determining system with implications for rehabilitation medicine application. IEEE Trans. Neural Syst. Rehabil. Eng. **10**, 232–238 (2002)
62. N. Ying, W. Kim, Determining dual Euler angles of the ankle complex in vivo using "flock of birds" electromagnetic tracking device. J. Biomech. Eng. **127**, 98–107 (2005)
63. A. Leardini, J.J. O'Connor, F. Catani, S. Giannini, A geometric model of the human ankle joint. J. Biomech. **32**, 585–591 (1999)
64. J. Apkarian, S. Naumann, B. Cairns, A three-dimensional kinematic and dynamic model of the lower limb. J. Biomech. **22**, 143–155 (1989)
65. J. Dul, G.E. Johnson, A kinematic model of the human ankle. J. Biomed. Eng. **7**, 137–143 (1985)
66. S.H. Scott, D.A. Winter, Biomechanical model of the human foot: kinematics and kinetics during the stance phase of walking. J. Biomech. **26**, 1091–1104 (1993)
67. S.L. Delp, F.C. Anderson, A.S. Arnold, P. Loan, A. Habib, C.T. John, E. Guendelman, D.G. Thelen, OpenSim: open-source software to create and analyze dynamic simulations of movement. IEEE Trans. Biomed. Eng. **54**, 1940–1950 (2007)
68. A.J. van den Bogert, G.D. Smith, B.M. Nigg, In vivo determination of the anatomical axes of the ankle joint complex: an optimization approach. J. Biomech. **27**, 1477–1488 (1994)
69. V.T. Inman, *The Joints of the Ankle* (Williams and Wilkins, Baltimore, 1976)
70. R.D. Gregorio, V. Parenti-Castelli, J.J. O'Connor, A. Leardini, Mathematical models of passive motion at the human ankle joint by equivalent spatial parallel mechanisms. Med. Biol. Eng. Comput. **45**, 305–313 (2007)
71. G.S. Lewis, H.J. Sommer, S.J. Piazza, In vitro assessment of a motion-based optimization method for locating the talocrural and subtalar joint axes. J. Biomech. Eng. **128**, 596–603 (2006)
72. R.J. de Asla, L. Wan, H.E. Rubash, G. Li, Six dof in vivo kinematics of the ankle joint complex: application of a combined dual-orthogonal fluoroscopic and magnetic resonance imaging technique. J. Orthop. Res. **24**, 1019–1027 (2006)

73. P.C. Liacouras, J.S. Wayne, Computational modeling to predict mechanical function of joints: application to the lower leg with simulation of two cadaver studies. J. Biomech. Eng. **129**, 811–817 (2007)
74. J.T.-M. Cheung, M. Zhang, K.-N. An, Effects of plantar fascia stiffness on the biomechanical responses of the ankle-foot complex. Clin. Biomech. **19**, 839–846 (2004)
75. J.T.-M. Cheung, M. Zhang, A.K.-L. Leung, Y.-B. Fan, Three dimensional finite element analysis of the foot during standing—a material sensitivity study. J. Biomech. **38**, 1045–1054 (2005)
76. I.C. Wright, R.R. Neptune, A.J. Van den Bogert, B.M. Nigg, The influence of foot positioning on ankle sprains. J. Biomech. **33**, 513–519 (2000)
77. I.C. Wright, R.R. Neptune, A.J. Van den Bogert, B.M. Nigg, The effects of ankle compliance and flexibility on ankle sprains. Med. Sci. Sports Exerc. **32**, 260–265 (2000)
78. F.L. Lewis, D.M. Dawson, C.T. Abdallah, *Robot Manipulator Control*, 2nd edn. (Marcel Dekker, New York, 2004)
79. T. Nef, M. Mihelj, R. Riener, ARMin: a robot for patient-cooperative arm therapy. Med. Biol. Eng. Comput. **45**, 887–900 (2007)
80. A. Deneve, S. Moughamir, L. Afilal, J. Zaytoon, Control system design of a 3-DOF upper limbs rehabilitation robot. Comput. Methods Programs Biomed. **89**, 202–214 (2008)
81. D. Erol, N. Sarkar, Design and implementation of an assistive controller for rehabilitation robotic systems. Int. J. Adv. Rob. Syst. **4**, 271–278 (2007)
82. C.J. Kempf, S. Kobayashi, Disturbance observer and feedforward design for a high-speed direct-drive positioning table. IEEE Trans. Control Syst. Technol. **7**, 513–526 (1999)
83. Y. Wang, Z. Xiong, H. Ding, X. Zhu, Nonlinear friction compensation and disturbance observer for a high-speed motion platform, in *International Conference on Robotics and Automation*, New Ordleans, LA, 2004, pp. 4515–4520
84. C.H. An, J.M. Hollerbach, Dynamic stability issues in force control of manipulators, in *IEEE International Conference on Robotics and Automation*, 1987, pp. 890–896
85. J.E. Colgate, N. Hogan, Robust control of dynamically interacting systems. Int. J. Control **48**, 65–88 (1988)
86. J.E. Colgate, N. Hogan, An analysis of contact instability in terms of passive physical equivalents, in *IEEE International Conference on Robotics and Automation*, 1989, pp. 404–409
87. S.P. Buerger, N. Hogan, Relaxing passivity for human-robot interaction, in *IEEE/RSJ International Conference on Intelligent Robots and Systems*, 2006, pp. 4570–4575
88. S.P. Buerger, N. Hogan, Complementary stability and loop shaping for improved human–robot interaction. IEEE Trans. Rob. **23**, 232–244 (2007)
89. T. Murakami, F. Yu, K. Ohnishi, Torque sensorless control in multidegree-of-freedom manipulator. IEEE Trans. Ind. Electron. **40**, 259–265 (1993)
90. S. Katsura, Y. Matsumoto, K. Ohnishi, Analysis and experimental validation of force bandwidth for force control. IEEE Trans. Ind. Electron. **53**, 922–928 (2006)
91. K. Kong, M. Tomizuka, H. Moon, B. Hwang, D. Jeon, Mechanical design and impedance compensation of SUBAR (Sogang University's Biomedical Assist Robot), in *IEEE/ASME International Conference on Advanced Intelligent Mechatronics*, Xi'an, China, 2008, pp. 377–382
92. R. Raghu, Modelling surface electromyograms of the human masticatory system, Master's thesis, The University of Auckland, 2003
93. S.I. Fox, *Muscle: Mechanisms of Contraction and Neural Control*, 5th edn. (Wm. C. Brown Publishers, 1996), Chap. 12, pp. 306–341
94. S.I. Fox, *Muscle: Mechanisms of Contraction and Neural Control*, 8th edn. (McGraw-Hill Higher Education, 2003), Chap. 12, pp. 324–363
95. L. S¨ornmo, P. Laguna, *The Electromyogram* (Academic Press, 2005), Chap. 5, pp. 337–410
96. R.F. Yazicioglu, T. Torfs, P. Merken, J. Penders, V. Leonov, R. Puers, B. Gyselinckx, C.V. Hoof, Ultra-low-power biopotential interfaces and their applications in wearable and implantable systems. Microelectron. J. **40**(9), 1313–1321 (2009)

97. S. Patel, H. Park, P. Bonato, L. Chan, M. Rodgers, A review of wearable sensors and systems with application in rehabilitation. J. NeuroEng. Rehabil. **9**(21) 2012
98. A. Mohideen, S. Sidek, Development of emg circuit to study the relationship between flexor digitorum superficialis muscle activity and hand grip strength, in *4th International Conference on Mechatronics* (ICOM), Kualar Lumpur, pp. 1–7 May 2011
99. A. Duschau-Wicke, J. Von Zitzewitz, A. Caprez, L. Lunenburger, R. Riener, Path control: a method for patient-cooperative robot-aided gait rehabilitation. IEEE Trans. Neural Syst. Rehabil. Eng. **18**, 38–48 (2010)
100. H. Vallery, A. Duschau-Wicke, R. Riener, Generalized elasticities improve patient-cooperative control of rehabilitation robots, in *2009 IEEE International Conference on Rehabilitation Robotics, ICORR 2009*, 2009, pp. 535–541
101. S. Jezernik, G. Colombo, M. Morari, Automatic gait-pattern adaptation for rehabilitation with 4-dof robotic orthosis. IEEE Trans. Robot. Autom. **20**, 574–582 (2004)
102. M. Mihelj, T. Nef, R. Riener, A novel paradigm for patient-cooperative control of upper-limb rehabilitation robots. Adv. Robot. **21**, 843–867 (2007)
103. H.I. Krebs, J.J. Palazzolo, L. Dipietro, M. Ferraro, J. Krol, K. Rannekleiv, B.T. Volpe, N. Hogan, Rehabilitation robotics: performance-based progressive robot-assisted therapy. Auton. Robot. **15**, 7–20 (2003)
104. E.T. Wolbrecht, V. Chan, D.J. Reinkensmeyer, J.E. Bobrow, Optimizing compliant, model-based robotic assistance to promote neurorehabilitation. IEEE Trans. Neural Syst. Rehabil. Eng. **16**, 286–297 (2008)
105. D.J. Reinkensmeyer, J.L. Emken, S.C. Cramer, Robotics, motor learning, and neurologic recovery. Annu. Rev. Biomed. Eng. **6**, 497–525 (2004)
106. R. Riener, L. Lunenburger, S. Jezernik, M. Anderschitz, G. Colombo, V. Dietz, Patient-cooperative strategies for robot aided treadmill training: first experimental results. IEEE Trans. Neural Syst. Rehabil. Eng. **13**, 380–394 (2005)
107. L. Marchal-Crespo, D.J. Reinkensmeyer, Review of control strategies for robotic movement training after neurologic injury, J. NeuroEng. Rehabil. **6** (2009)

Chapter 3
Physiological Model of the Masticatory System

The purpose of the human masticatory system is to perform the initial breakdown of food via chewing and prepare it for swallowing. It includes the bones and soft structures, such as muscles, ligaments and tendons of the face and mouth, that are involved in mastication. There are multiple complex mechanisms involved in this process, including the secretion of saliva, manipulation of the chewed food into a bolus with the tongue and the muscular control of the mandible that produces chewing motions, which is the focus of this and following parts. This chapter introduced the masticatory system and its associated numerous complexities, and a new physiological model with two DOFs was developed for it.

3.1 Introduction to the Masticatory System

3.1.1 Skeletal Structure

The human masticatory system has a structure that is well developed and adapted for its primary functions of preparing food for swallowing and ingestion. The upper dentition is fixed to the base of the maxilla and is stationary (assuming no head motion) during jaw movement. The lower dentition is fixed to the mandible (or jawbone), which is a U-shaped bone shown in Fig. 3.1. This is a rigid structure that does not change in shape or form during the mastication process and in theory, if the geometry of the mandible is known, a single point's orientation and position can be used to reconstruct the position of the complete structure. The mandible is mobile and the driving force behind upper and lower dentition interactions, allowing teeth to move towards, across and against each other. The mandible is able to achieve a wide range of motions and does so by accommodating the attachments of a complex system of muscle tissues and ligaments [1].

The hyoid bone is another U-shaped bone situated in the neck between the chin and thyroid cartilage. It provides an attachment point for muscles that have their insertions at the floor of the mouth or beneath the mandible. The hyoid bone itself is not fixed, but suspended by muscles in the anterior, posterior and inferior directions. However, its service as an anchoring point for tongue movement, swallowing

S.(S.Q.) Xie, *Advanced Robotics for Medical Rehabilitation*,
Springer Tracts in Advanced Robotics 108, DOI 10.1007/978-3-319-19896-5_3

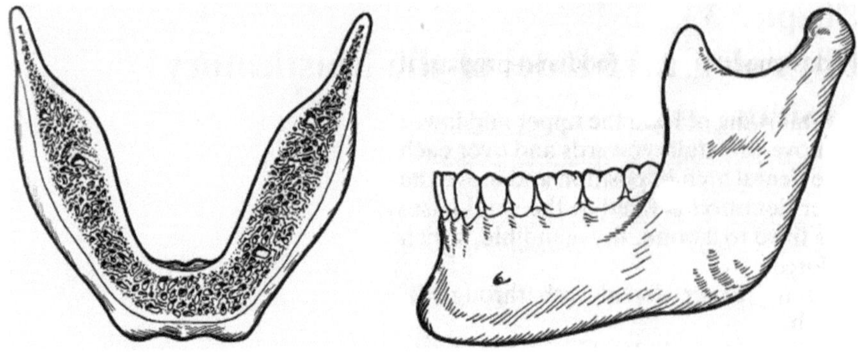

Fig. 3.1 The mandible (jaw). On the *left* is a sectioned image of the mandible when viewed from above and on the *right* is the lateral perspective [4]

and other mandibular movements suggests that relative to the mandible, it is quite stationary. If the maxilla and hyoid are assumed to be fixed in space, and the mandible is able to move freely between them except for where it is fixed to the maxilla at the temporomandibular joints (TMJs), then the interaction between the mandible and actuating muscles is similar to a parallel robot platform [2].

3.1.2 Mandibular Muscles

The masticatory system contains a large number of muscles, to the extent where it almost seems that there are more muscles than required to perform functional mandibular movements. From a mechanical perspective this may seem to be an inefficient arrangement, but the spatial limitations native to the masticatory system have to be considered. The confined space in the craniofacial region means that if the muscular system were to be in a mechanically optimal arrangement it would most likely interfere with the adjacent airways and digestive tract [3]. To compensate, the masticatory muscles are generally more complex than the skeletal muscle within other limbs. They have a multipennate structure, are complexly layered or are divided into active regions. The complexity addresses the non-ideal physical arrangement of the muscles and allows substantial differential contractile forces to be produced by the mandible.

The masseter is a bulky, rectangular muscle that is located on the lateral side of the mandible. It lies just beneath the surface of the skin and its cross section is wedge-shaped and bulky. The masseter can be divided into two parts in relation to their functional purposes: the superficial head and the deep head. Its origin is at the zygomatic arch of the skull and its insertion is at the lateral surface of the ramus (the ascending part of the mandible), as shown in Fig. 3.2. The muscle has a multipennate structure, where muscle fibres converge towards a central tendon on

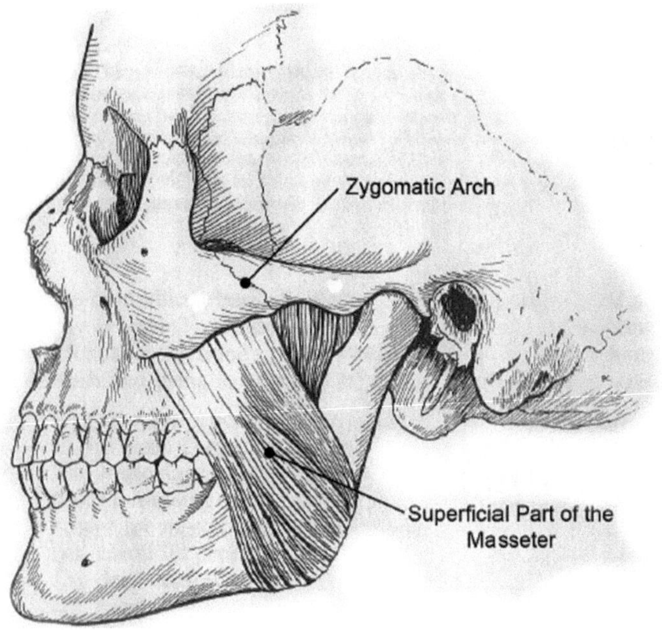

Fig. 3.2 The masseter muscle [4]

multiple sides, similar to a feather. This structure vastly increases muscle power and gives a broader range of directional pull.

In general, the masseter is used for the heavy crushing and grinding of food and primarily moves in the vertical direction. In addition to this, the masseters (on both sides of the jaw) are capable of exerting a range of forces in the anterior direction of the jaw and the deep head can produce retrusive movements (in the posterior direction) [4]. The superficial head of the masseter is the most likely contributor to surface EMG signal recordings and it is heavily involved in the mandible's ability to produce bite forces up to and in excess of 590 N (mean for males with standard deviation of 145.8 N [5].

The largest mandibular muscle, though not considered one of the power movers of the mandible, is the temporalis. Its origin is fan-shaped which results in it being very large and covers a wide area, as shown in Fig. 3.3. Converse to its origin, the attachment of the temporalis to the mandible is concentrated on a smaller area on the ramus. When viewed laterally, the temporalis can be separated into three regions: the anterior, middle and posterior, and it can be divided further into two layers, the superficial layer and the principal mass. The bulk of the muscle lies in the anterior region and the tendinous fibres are generally longer than those of the masseter. The problem with the fan-shaped arrangement of the temporalis is that only a few fibres will be aligned with the direction of movement at any one time,

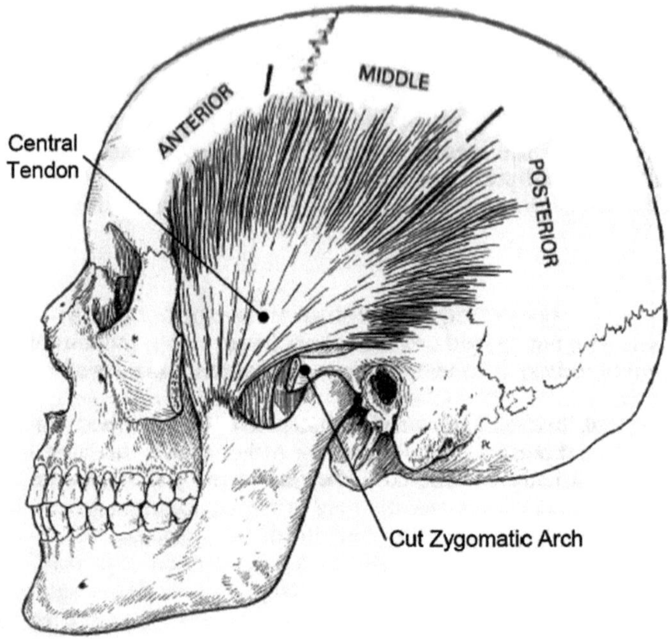

Fig. 3.3 The temporalis muscle [4]. Note that the anterior, middle and posterior sections are all part of the temporalis muscle

reducing maximum efficiency. However, this means that besides producing a vertical pull on the mandible, there is the possibility of other directions of movement in the sagittal and frontal planes. The temporalis acts primarily as an elevator and retractor, but due to the divergent arrangement of fibres, it also has the ability to contribute to the fine adjustment of the mandible antero-posteriorly, medio-laterally and vertically [4].

The digastric muscle has a unique structure and is formed from two belly-like masses of muscle tissue which are joined and separated by an intermediate tendon, as shown in Fig. 3.4. The anterior belly is smaller and is attached to the digastric fossa of the mandible while the posterior belly is attached to the mastoid notch of the temporal bone. The intermediate tendon is indirectly attached to the hyoid bone by a fascial tunnel, formed from a loop of cervical fascia. This structural arrangement is much like a pulley and allows the intermediate tendon to slide to and fro. The mechanism allows the digastric muscle to exert inferior and posterior traction and it is speculated that the two digastric muscles acting together, help to guide the mandible in a centred position as it approaches the intercuspal position during normal function. In these circumstances they act as antagonists to the action of the elevators and have the ability to guide the mandible laterally and medially, similar to the reins guiding a horse. The digastrics are the main depressors of the mandible and act as the antagonists to perform the controlled closure of the

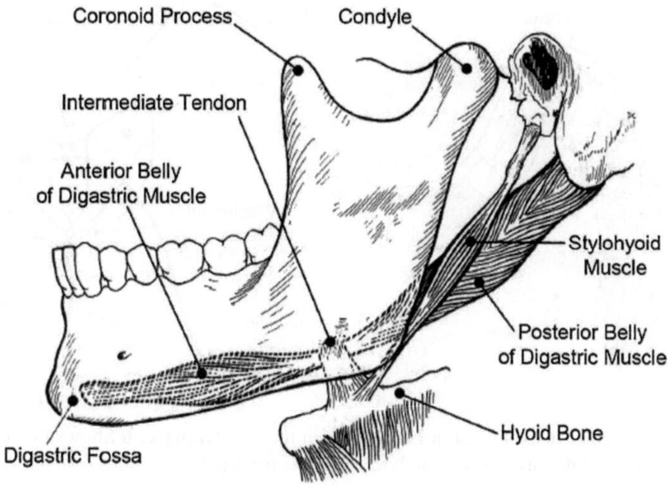

Fig. 3.4 The digastric muscle [4]

mandible. They are also active during positioning movements of the mandible in the transverse plane, including medial, lateral, protrusive and retrusive movements, and therefore appear to be the prime movers and antagonistic controllers in the horizontal plane [4].

3.1.3 The Temporomandibular Joint (TMJ)

In the craniofacial region there are 209 joints, 119 of which are synarthrodial (fibrous), 82 are special dental and eight are diarthrodial. The TMJ consists of a diarthrodial joint, which is a discontinuous arrangement and accommodates functional movements between bones [4].

Diarthrodial joints are subjected to shearing, abrasive and compressive forces and in order to withstand these forces they need to have strong and rigid articulating surfaces that maintain their shape. The ranges of movement of these joints are determined structurally and depend on how ligaments are attached, bone morphology, muscle activity and other structural restraints. The TMJ consists of a number of bony parts and soft tissue components. The bony parts include the condylar process of the mandible and the glenoid structures on the skull base. The condylar process can be seen in Fig. 3.4 and its function is to provide a supportive platform for the articular surface of the mandible. This is so that it can efficiently act as a pivot for three dimensional movement and as a fulcrum for third class leverage. It also provides suitable attachment points for the muscles which protract from the mandible. The glenoid structures are a group of several structural forms in the skull

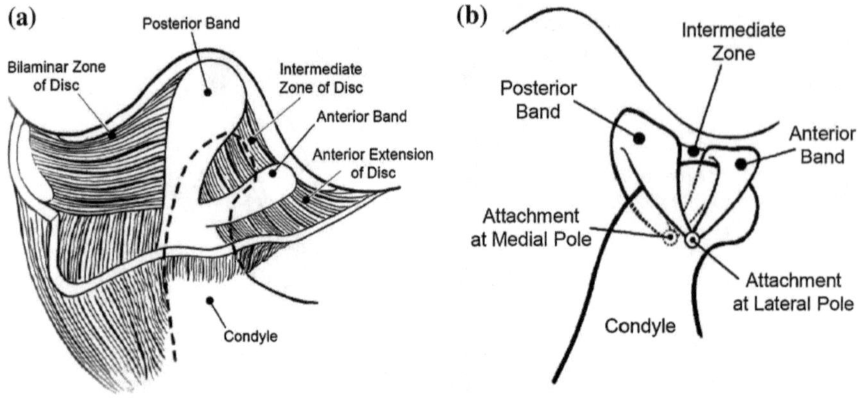

Fig. 3.5 The articular disc of TMJ. **a** Is the view in the sagittal plane. **b** Shows the details of the attachment points of the disc to the condyle. Adapted from [4]

base that approximately match the condylar process and also serve as guides for condylar movement [4].

The soft tissue components of the TMJ include the articular covering of the joint surfaces, the articular disc and muscle tissue, the joint capsule, ligaments, synovial membranes, blood vessels and nerves. The articular disc is a continuous structure that occupies the space between the bony and articular surfaces of the joint. It is shown in Fig. 3.5 and it has three distinct parts of varying thickness. The posterior band is the thickest and is separated from the anterior band by the intermediate zone of the disc which is quite thin. The anterior and posterior bands act together with lateral and medial thickenings of the disc to form a self-centring mechanical wedging arrangement that keeps the disc on the condyle [6].

The capsule of the TMJ is a loose, tapering, thin-walled cuff of white collagenous tissue that encloses the bony parts and the articular disc, and delineates two joint cavities [4]. In the inferior joint compartment created by the capsule of the TMJ, the condyles can rotate about a horizontal axis. This is part of the simple hinge movement of the mandible in the vertical plane and it occurs through the bilateral movement happening simultaneously at both TMJs. In the superior joint compartment, the condyle-disc assembly is a firmly bound and closely adapted mechanism that is able to slide in the joint compartment due to the slack nature of the joint capsule. This allows the condyle-disc assembly to perform a range of movements that include sliding along the articular eminence, pivoting and rotating around a vertical axis and sliding medio-laterally. Additionally, because the joint capsule is quite loose, different movements can occur simultaneously in the superior compartments of the right and left joints. This is shown in Fig. 3.6 and exemplified through lateral movement where the condyle-disc assembly on the side the mandible is moving towards, pivots. On the opposite side, from which the mandible

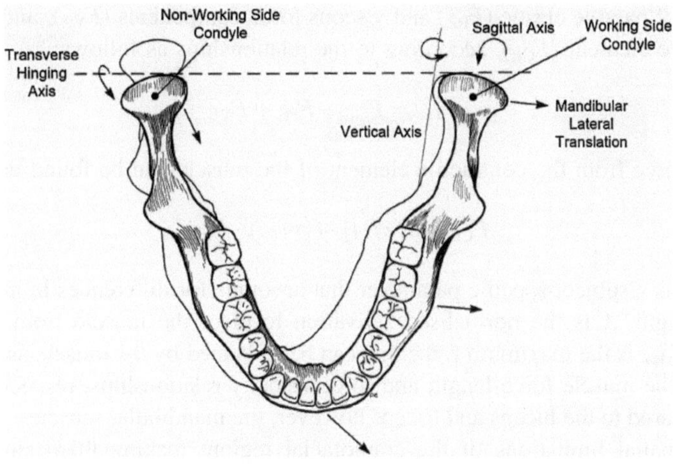

Fig. 3.6 Lateral movement of the mandible towards the subject's left. Adapted from [4]

is moving away, the condyle-disc assembly progresses antero-inferiorly and medially (which is a translatory movement). The pivoting and translation occurs in the superior joint compartments and at the same time, in the inferior joint compartments, a simple hinge movement of varying extent occurs [4].

3.2 Masticatory System Physiological Model Development

Exoskeleton development for the masticatory system is in its infancy with only a very recent transition from robotic chewing devices to exoskeletal pursuits [7]. The original purposes of these chewing robots were to study mandibular dynamics and control methods for dental training, jaw simulation, food texture and breakdown analysis, and speech therapy [8]. Modelling of the masticatory system has been done in a similar fashion with the intention of understanding the underlying biomechanical processes and forces [3, 9]. These models are able to include the key mandibular muscles because accessibility is not an issue and can therefore explore the full range of available movement.

3.2.1 Revised Musculotendon Model

The musculotendon models are re-applied and it is assumed that muscular structure does not significantly vary around the body—the main difference is the size while structural and compositional proportions remain similar. This model provides the embodiment of a Hill-type muscle model, derived from experimental data, and consists of passive elastic (F_{PE}) and viscous force components (F_{VE}), and an active contractile element (F_{CE}), according to the relationships as follows:

$$F_{Tot} = F_{CE} + F_{PE} + F_{VE} \tag{3.1}$$

The force from the contractile element of the muscle can be found using:

$$F_{CE} = R \cdot f(l) \cdot f(v) \cdot A \cdot F_{Max} \tag{3.2}$$

where R is a subject-specific parameter that accounts for differences in muscle size and strength, A is the normalised activation level of the muscle from the EMG signal, F_{Max} is the maximum force that can be produced by the muscle and $f(l)$ and $f(v)$ are the muscle force-length and force-velocity relationships, respectively.

Compared to the biceps and triceps however, the mandibular muscles are limited by the spatial limitations of the craniofacial region, making them smaller, and arranged differently to other joint systems. This provides different normalized and optimised length characteristics and the force-length relationship was adjusted from Eq. (3.3) to:

$$f(l) = 2.5 - ((l_n - 1)/0.75)^2, \quad l_n = l/l_{Opt} \tag{3.3}$$

where l_n is the normalized muscle length given by the current muscle length, l, and the optimum muscle length, l_{Opt}. The adjustment allowed more flexibility in the range of movement of the mandibular muscles to prevent model instabilities.

The effect is shown in Fig. 3.7, where it is apparent that the previous equation presented for the elbow joint would lead to a representation of the musculotendon behaviour that is incongruous with actual dynamic processes. Muscle lengths extending or decreasing beyond the x-axis intercepts would cause a negated output and cause the model to behave unexpectedly or become unstable. The direction of the forces produced by each musculotendon unit is along the axis that connects the

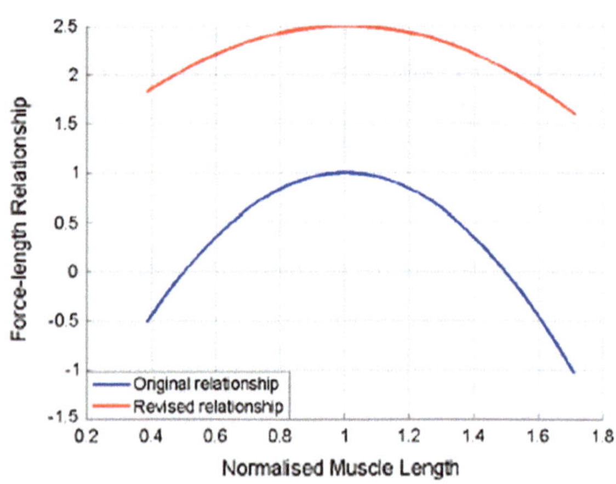

Fig. 3.7 Updated musculotendon force-length relationship. The *shallower curve* allows for a greater range of muscle length change

insertion and origin points of the musculotendon unit. Therefore, when considering three dimensional arrangements of the musculotendon units and the effect this has on the movement of a particular DOF, the total force needs to be broken down into its appropriate components.

3.2.2 *Jaw Musculoskeletal Model Derivation*

The preliminary structure of the model was first built in the biomechanical simulation software environment, ArtiSynth [10], because a pre-existing detailed model of the jaw and laryngeal structure had previously been developed, as shown in Fig. 3.8a. This first model had a single degree of freedom and two lumped actuating muscle groups classified as jaw elevators and jaw depressors acting on an 'L' shaped representation of the mandible as shown in Fig. 3.8b. The muscle groups had geometries and attachment points to the mandible that were determined from the masseter and digastric muscles, with origins at fixed points in space (equivalent to maxilla and hyoid bone anchorage positions). This provided the attachment locations of the muscle groups, and approximate muscle lengths and bone geometry were obtained from the literature [11].

The motion of the mandible at this stage is purely rotational and a polar coordinate system was used to define the muscle attachment locations and incisor point (jaw geometry) relative to the centre of rotation. Figure 3.9 shows this arrangement in the sagittal plane with the elevator and depressor muscle groups acting on a mandible representation with a hinge joint at the centre of rotation. The polar coordinate system provides a means of easily determining the movement of dynamic properties of interest such as the incisor point (indication of opening angle), muscle group lengths and insertion points.

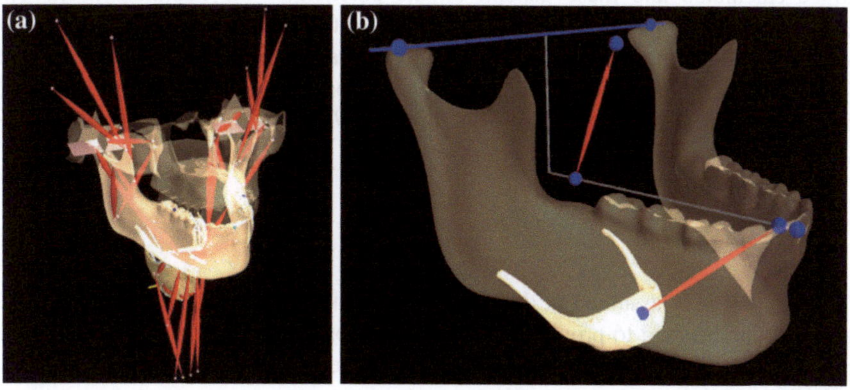

Fig. 3.8 Screenshots of ArtiSynth models. **a** Original model of the jaw and laryngeal structure. **b** Simplification of the masticatory system to a hinge joint

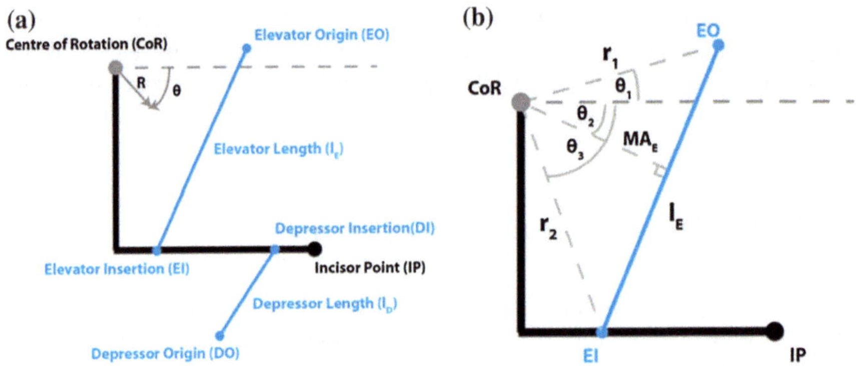

Fig. 3.9 Sagittal view of the musculoskeletal model. The model consists of the mandible and an antagonistic muscle group: elevator and depressor. **a** Labelling and coordinate system. **b** Elevator muscle group geometry

From the figure, it is apparent that because movements are only rotational, point locations only undergo rotational changes, and this is exemplified through the elevator muscle group. The insertion point on the mandible EI is the only point that moves as the origin EO remains fixed to the maxilla. The length of the elevator muscle group (l_{E}) can therefore be determined geometrically and is given by:

$$l_{\mathrm{E}} = \sqrt{r_1^2 + r_2^2 - 2 \cdot r_1 \cdot r_2 \cdot \cos(\theta_1 - \theta_2)} \tag{3.4}$$

where (r_1, θ_1) and (r_2, θ_2) are the polar co-ordinates to the elevator origin and insertion, respectively, as indicated in the figure. The length of the depressor muscle group can be found with a similar expression but the origin and insertion coordinates would represent those of the depressor points instead.

To determine total joint torque, the moment arms of the muscle groups still need to be calculated and these depend on the position of the mandible itself. The following is the derivation of the moment arm for the elevator muscle group ($\mathrm{MA_E}$), with labels illustrated in Fig. 3.10b. In general, if a line (l_a) passes through the pole (origin) of a polar coordinate system and is perpendicular to a line (l_b) with an intersection at point (r_o, θ_o) and the point (r, θ) lies on l_b, the equation for l_b is given by:

$$r = \frac{r_o}{\cos(\theta - \theta_o)} \tag{3.5}$$

Note that it is assumed l_b does not pass through the pole itself and this relationship can be used to provide two definitions for the muscle group length and its perpendicular line through the pole, which utilise the known origin and insertion coordinates of the elevator muscle group:

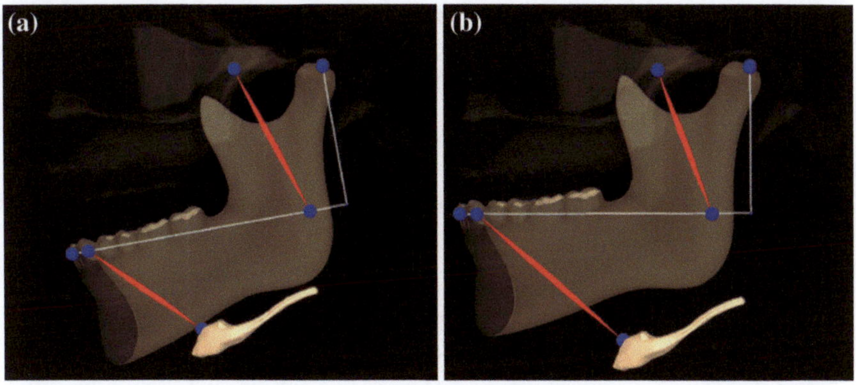

Fig. 3.10 Examples of jaw positions in the sagittal plane. Note the variation in muscle lengths and the fixed locations of the origin muscle attachment points. **a** Jaw open. **b** Jaw closed (occluded)

$$r_1 = \frac{\mathrm{MA_E}}{\cos(\theta_1 - \theta_3)} \tag{3.6}$$

$$r_2 = \frac{\mathrm{MA_E}}{\cos(\theta_2 - \theta_3)} \Rightarrow \mathrm{MA_E} = r_2 \cdot \cos(\theta_2 - \theta_3) \tag{3.7}$$

$$\mathrm{MA_E} = r_2 \cdot \cos\left(\theta_2 - \tan^{-1}\left(\frac{r_1 \cos\theta_1 - r_2 \cos\theta_2}{r_2 \sin\theta_2 - r_1 \sin\theta_1}\right)\right) \tag{3.8}$$

Movement of the mandible will affect angle θ_2 since the position of EO is fixed. The pure rotational movement also means that r_1 and r_2, once defined for an individual, remain constant throughout all movements. The moment arm for the depressor muscle group with origin and insertion points at DO and DI, respectively, and the moment arm $\mathrm{MA_D}$ can be derived in a similar fashion, but with the coordinates (r_1, θ_1), (r_2, θ_2) and (r_3, θ_3) representing DI, DO and $\mathrm{MA_D}$ respectively:

$$\mathrm{MA_D} = r_2 \cdot \cos\left(\theta_2 - \tan^{-1}\left(\frac{r_2 \cos\theta_2 - r_1 \cos\theta_1}{r_1 \sin\theta_1 - r_2 \sin\theta_2}\right)\right) \tag{3.9}$$

Up to this point, the weight of the mandible has not been considered, and it would be inappropriate to ignore its effect since movements are occurring in the sagittal plane. The difficulty, however, lies in determining the mass of the mandible and its attached muscles, and even approximating its centre of gravity is dependent on many factors. The passive activity of antagonistic muscles during movement contributes to moments of inertia and the suspension of the jaw by multiple muscles means that its mass is distributed. The inability to measure mass and inertial properties directly, or even estimate them with reasonable accuracy, means that values from the literature will have to be sought and combined with subject-specific parameters to account for variability and the inevitable inaccuracy. The weight can be assumed as acting at a single point and is attributed to the mass of the mandible and attached tissues that are part of the moving system. If the weight acts at the point $(r_{\mathrm{w}}, \theta_{\mathrm{w}})$, the resulting moment arm is:

$$\mathrm{MA_W} = r_{\mathrm{W}} \cdot \cos(\theta_{\mathrm{W}}) \tag{3.10}$$

Deriving the weight of the mandible from its approximated mass allows the determination of the resulting moment:

$$F_{\mathrm{W}} = m \cdot g \tag{3.11}$$

$$M_{\mathrm{W}} = F_{\mathrm{W}} \cdot \mathrm{MA_W} \tag{3.12}$$

$$\Rightarrow M_{\mathrm{W}} = K_{\mathrm{W}} mg \cdot r_{\mathrm{W}} \cdot \cos(\theta_{\mathrm{W}} + d) \tag{3.13}$$

where m is the approximate mass of the mandible, K_{W} is a subject-specific parameter to account for modelling inaccuracies, and d is the opening angle of the mandible which affects the position of the centre of gravity. The elevator, depressor and weight forces are enough to produce single DOF rotation motion in the sagittal plane. The ArtiSynth model in different stages of opening is shown in Fig. 3.10, and the lengthening and shortening of the muscle groups is apparent. The movement of the mandible will naturally be rotational but the trajectory of the incisor point does not necessarily have to follow a circular pattern. Additional passive degrees of freedom, such as a vertical translational component that is dependent on the opening angle of the mandible, could allow more realistic trajectories with a shallower arc to be produced by the model [12].

The model was developed to have two degree of freedom: open-close movement (about a hinge joint with fixed centre of rotation, denoted by CoR and about the x axis in Fig. 3.11) and lateral movements, where the mandible translates in the

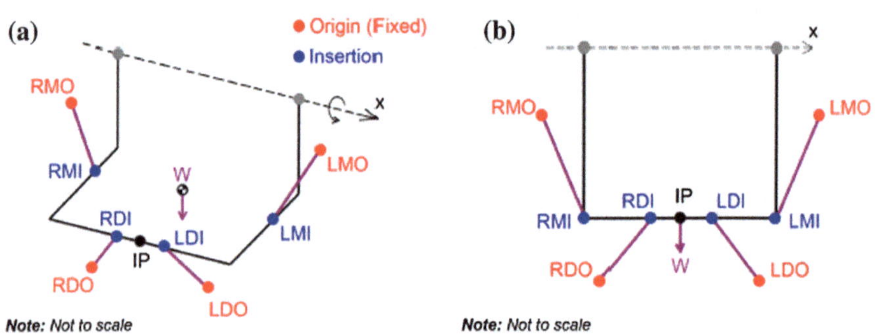

Fig. 3.11 2-DOF musculoskeletal model of the jaw. The 2-DOFs are given by rotation about and translation along the x axis. (R, θ, x) is the cylindrical coordinate system, W is the weight of the mandible, and the labels consist of combinations of: R right, L left, M masseter, D digastric, I muscle insertion and O muscle origin. EMG signals are therefore required from the bilateral masseters and digastrics. The view from the sagittal plane remains unchanged. **a** Top-left view. **b** Frontal view

horizontal direction (along the x axis in Fig. 3.11). The position of the mandible was measured by the movement of the incisor point (IP in the figure), in cylindrical co-ordinates (R, θ, x), which was the most convenient system to simultaneously output the predicted movements.

For force and torque calculations, the forces are broken down into their respective components relevant to the degree of freedom of motion being calculated. Both DOFs of movement, however depend on the lengths of the muscles and the definition of attachment points in cylindrical coordinates allows the model to be expanded easily to accommodate this (in the sagittal plane, the model looks unchanged and the x axis can be considered to only add depth). The total length of a muscle group is given by:

$$l_{\text{Muscle}} = \sqrt{r_1^2 + r_2^2 - 2r_1 r_2 \cdot \cos(\theta_1 - \theta_2) + (x_1^2 - x_2^2)} \tag{3.14}$$

where l_{Muscle} is the length of any muscle group given the coordinates of its origin (r_1, θ_1, x_1) and insertion (r_2, θ_2, x_2). The final implementation of the musculoskeletal model was in the MATLAB/Simulink environment where the mass and overall passive properties of the mandible were introduced to the model and were similar to the values used in the elbow model.

3.2.3 *Kinematic Model*

The concept of using kinematics in a rotational and translational capacity is applied here for the opening–closing and lateral movements, respectively. The total joint moment can be determined by combining the appropriate components of the forces calculated from the musculotendon models with the moment arms from the musculoskeletal model, and the horizontal components can be used to determine the forces contributing to lateral movement. For the opening and closing movement, the moments produced by each musculotendon unit is:

$$M_n = K_n \cdot \text{MA}_n \cdot F_n \tag{3.15}$$

where n = LM, RM, LD or RD, and the moment is given by the product of the force component in the sagittal plane determined from the musculotendon model, F_n, the moment arm determined from the musculoskeletal geometry, MA_n, and a subject-specific parameter to account for inaccuracies in the geometric model, K_n. The total joint moment can then be determined using:

$$M_{\text{Tot}} = M_{\text{LM}} + M_{\text{RM}} + M_{\text{LD}} + M_{\text{RD}} + M_{\text{W}} + M_{\text{Damp}} + O_z \tag{3.16}$$

where the total moment about the centre of rotation, M_{Tot}, is given by the sum of moments caused by the left masseter (LM), right masseter (RM), left digastric (LD), right digastric (RD), mandible weight (W), joint damping (Damp) and an offset value that determines resting position in the vertical direction, O_z. The kinematics of the joint can now be found with:

$$d(t+\Delta t) = d(t) + \omega(t) + \frac{M_{\mathrm{Tot}}}{2I}\Delta t^2 \tag{3.17}$$

$$\omega(t+\Delta t) = \omega(t) + \frac{M_{\mathrm{Tot}}}{I}\Delta t \tag{3.18}$$

where the new angular displacement (in the θ direction) of the mandible, $d(t+\Delta t)$, on the previous displacement $d(t)$, previous angular velocity $\omega(t)$, moment of inertia II, and sampling time Δt. Note that up to this point calculations have been implemented in polar coordinates so, to obtain the vertical displacement, $z(t)$, a geometric conversion is required that uses the $(R,\ \theta)$ coordinates of the incisor point: IP_R and IP_θ respectively. The vertical displacement of the mandible is necessary for comparisons with data from the literature and actual measurements of jaw movement because the concept of a rotational angle, while based on anatomical structure, is largely arbitrary when considering the distance between the approximated centre of rotation and incisor point. The vertical displacement is shown in Fig. 3.12, and given by:

$$z(t) = \mathrm{IP}_R \cdot \sin(\mathrm{IP}_\theta + d(t)) - \mathrm{IP}_R \cdot \sin(\mathrm{IP}_\theta) \tag{3.19}$$

The translational component of movement is found with similar relationships, but along the x axis. The horizontal force components of the muscles is found by determining the horizontal component of the muscle forces in the x direction, using the acute angle between the force vector and x axis, α. The vertical distance is given by:

$$y = r \cdot \sin(\theta) \tag{3.20}$$

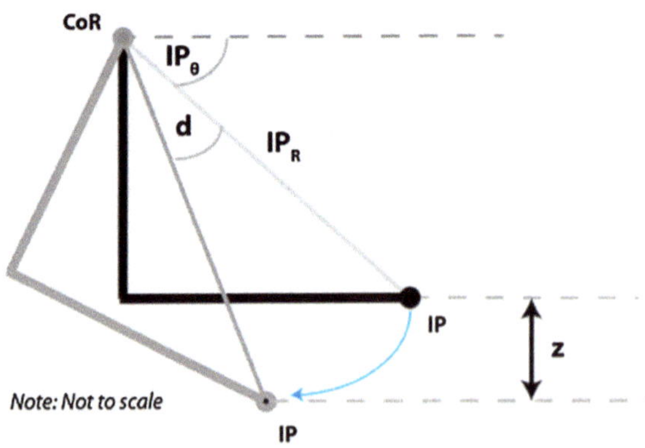

Fig. 3.12 Determination of vertical displacement, z

$$\alpha = \tan^{-1}\left(\frac{r_1 \sin\theta_1 - r_2 \sin\theta_2}{x_2 - x_1}\right) \tag{3.21}$$

$$F_x = F \cdot \cos(\alpha) \tag{3.22}$$

where 1 and 2 are subscripts for insertion and origin cylindrical coordinates, and F_x is the lateral component of total musculotendon force, F. Once all the horizontal force components are known, the total force in the lateral direction can be determined and linear kinematics applied to find the horizontal displacement and velocity:

$$M_{\text{Tot}} = K_{\text{LM}}F_{\text{LM}} + K_{\text{RM}}F_{\text{RM}} + K_{\text{LD}}F_{\text{LD}} + K_{\text{RD}}F_{\text{RD}} + F_{\text{Damp}} + O_x \tag{3.23}$$

$$x(t+\Delta t) = x(t) + v(t)\Delta t + \frac{F_{\text{Tot}}}{2m}\Delta t^2 \tag{3.24}$$

$$v(t+\Delta t) = v(t) + \frac{F_{\text{Tot}}}{m}\Delta t \tag{3.25}$$

where the total force, F_{Tot}, is determined by the sum of the force components in the x direction, with the addition of O_x to account for lateral force offset and subject specific K_i parameters (i = LD, RD, LM, RM) to account for the difference in muscle sizes and strengths. The horizontal displacement $x(t+\Delta t)$ and velocity $v(t+\Delta t)$ is calculated using the previous displacement, $x(t)$, velocity, $v(t)$, and mandible mass, m. The horizontal motion also requires its own damping component that accounts for the passive viscous and elastic damping properties of the masticatory system that affect horizontal movement:

$$F_{\text{Damp}} = -\beta \cdot v \tag{3.26}$$

where β is the damping coefficient and v is the horizontal velocity. The total passive elastic muscle response without an active component has an effect in both degree of freedom and its primary function is to be the restorative force within the model, returning it to its resting position when there are no active inputs. In the lateral direction the resting position is at the midline of the body and in the vertical direction the total passive elastic muscle response has similar properties to the elbow joint, but with more muscular influences.

3.3 Hybrid Model of the Masticatory System

The improved understanding of the EMG signals of the six accessible mandibular muscles will allow the musculoskeletal model to be enhanced to better accommodate the available information and apply them to produce more functional movement prediction. The improved model will be built on underlying principles that have not been previously considered in the past by other research groups, particularly in relation to multiple DOF physiological model-based systems. This part presents the formulation of this model and the incorporation of artificial neural networks to present a hybrid approach to movement prediction. The function of the ANN is to help identify the type of movement from the available EMG channels to then allow the physiological model to predict the appropriate movement.

3.3.1 Physiological Model Reconfiguration

It was found that the two DOFs of movement could be independently actuated from the available muscle groups—provided six channels of EMG data were utilised instead of the previous four employed. To accommodate this, the brunt of the changes occurred in the musculoskeletal model where the geometric structure was updated to include an independent DOF of movement and actuating muscles.

The results of the study implied that lateral movements of the mandible could be identifiable from the bilateral temporalii on their own, as long as the activities of the other muscles were isolated. If the other muscles were to be involved in distinguishing lateral movements there would be no discernible difference in the activity patterns that correlate with horizontal shifts of the mandible. Therefore in order to make use of the findings, a completely independent DOF is required that is only affected by the temporalii muscles. Similarly, the temporalii would still not be required to open and close the mandible because that has already been shown to be effectively managed by the masseter and digastric muscles.

Separating the muscles into independent DOFs does not affect the musculotendon models and these remain unchanged as the determiners of active contraction forces from EMG signal inputs. The musculoskeletal model requires significant changes to accommodate the new DOFs and the reinvented model is shown in Fig. 3.13. It shows the different, independent DOFs of the musculoskeletal model and how the musculotendon units are attached within it.

Because the entire mandible is assumed to translate, the positions of the insertion and origin points of the temporalii have no effect on the resulting movement. The only cases where this would be an important consideration would be if the mandible was able to rotate in the frontal plane or forces at the TMJs were of interest. For the current study and model development, these issues are not relevant. In Fig. 3.13b, the bilateral masseter and digastric muscles have not been included because they do not contribute to the movement or the weight of the mandible.

The two independently controlled and driven DOFs are still linked through one parameter—the mass of the mandible. This affects both the weight of the mandible during vertical moments and linear acceleration during lateral movements. To compensate an additional parameter has been introduced to allow the dynamics of each DOF to still operate independently from each other. This is necessary because

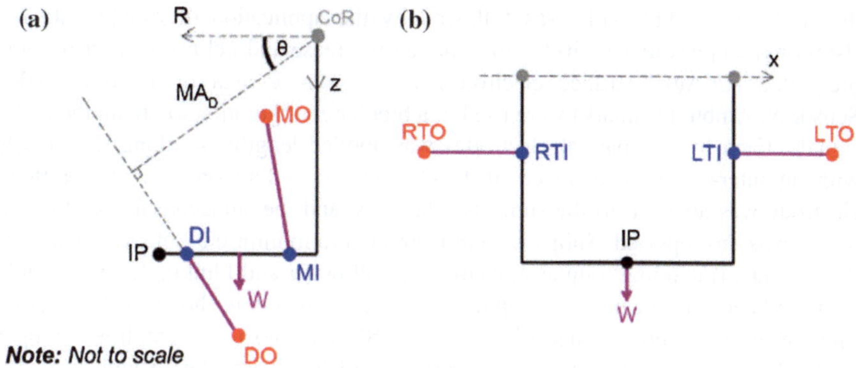

Fig. 3.13 The reconfigured musculoskeletal model of the masticatory system. Note that *left* and *right* masseter and digastric properties are similar and they have no influence on lateral movement. Lateral movement is only affected by the temporalis muscles. **a** Sagittal view. **b** Frontal view (*T* temporalis)

having a single mass value that governs the passive response of vertical motion will not necessarily translate effectively to lateral movements.

The kinematic relationship for vertical movement remains unchanged from the original derivation. The main difference is in the determination of the lateral force from the temporalis muscles and is given by:

$$F_{\mathrm{Tot}} = K_{\mathrm{LT}}F_{\mathrm{LT}} + K_{\mathrm{RT}}F_{\mathrm{RT}} + F_{\mathrm{Damp}} + O_x \tag{3.27}$$

where the total force is now given by the force from the left temporalis, F_{LT} and right temporalis, F_{RT}, with their respective subject-specific coefficients.

3.3.2 Analysis of Mandibular Muscle Based on EMG

The collection of data from subjects involved measurements of EMG signal activity and actual jaw motion. The actual motion of the lower mandible was required to validate any of the physiological models developed to quantify and compare accuracy and performance. Measuring mandibular motion accurately therefore requires more sophisticated and specialised equipment, especially when considering multiple DOFs. One of the most common methods, particularly in speech, masticatory, nutritional or food technology studies, is magnetometry with the use of an Electromagnetic Articulograph (EMA). This system uses an array of magnetic fields to track a sensor attached to a tooth on the mandible. The EMA provides the best access to the mandible for movement recordings but is plagued by significant amounts of noise and copious amounts of data post-processing.

Before applying electrodes, the skin above the muscles of interest was first prepared by rubbing it with an abrasive gel (D.O. Weaver & Co., USA) to remove dirt and excess skin. This was followed by the application of rubbing alcohol (Isopropyl, approximately 70 %) to remove oil, grease and gel residue. Disposable pre-gelled Ag/AgCl surface electrodes with a sensor area of 15 mm^2 (Blue Sensor N, Ambu, Denmark) were used in a bipolar configuration to obtain the EMG signals. Each bipolar pair of electrodes was applied lengthwise along the muscle with an inter-electrode distance of 15–20 mm depending on size. An earthing electrode was attached to the subjects' clavicles, and the subjects sat upright with their heads unsupported. Subjects were instructed to minimise all other movements during trials (including tongue movement, swallowing and blinking). An example of the bilateral arrangement of bipolar electrode channels is shown in Fig. 3.14a. The electrodes were connected to a *g*. USBamp biosignal amplifier (Guger Technologies, Austria), sampled at 1200 Hz and hardware filtered with a 50 Hz notch filter to remove power line interference and 0.1 Hz high pass filter to remove baseline noise while retaining almost all of the information content within the signal.

The EMA system (Carstens, Germany) was originally developed for the study of the mechanics behind the production of human speech and the EMA cube is shown in Fig. 3.14b. Its operation principle is based on induction, where an AC voltage is induced in sensors within a magnetic field. There are six transmitted coils at pre-determined locations around the cube that generate alternating magnetic fields at frequencies ranging between 7.5 and 13.5 kHz and a magnetic flux of between 1.3 and 16.7 T. The sensors within the cube essentially consist of small coils and the alternating magnetic fields induce alternating currents into the sensors in a similar fashion to the transformer effect, and these are registered as analogue signals. The magnitude of the induced current depends on the distance and angle of a

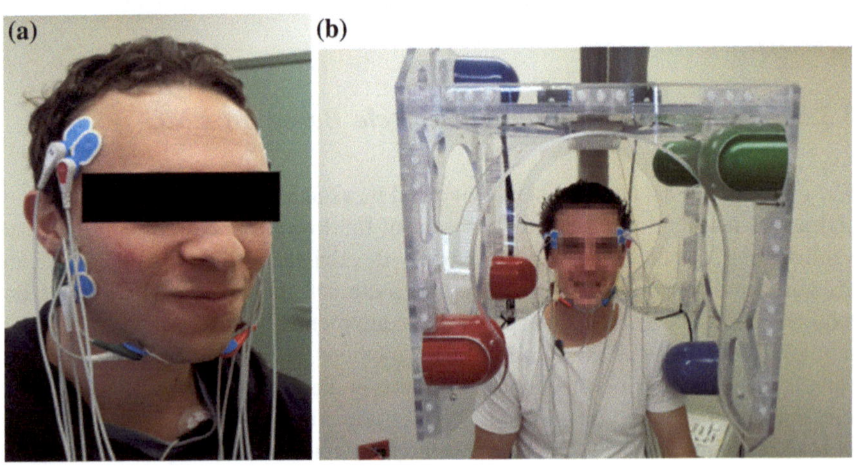

Fig. 3.14 **a** Bipolar electrode channel locations for the masticatory system. Six channels of data are available from (*top* to *bottom*): the bilateral temporalis, masseter and digastric muscles. **b** Subject positioned within the EMA cube. The pairs of coloured nodes are the electromagnetic coils that are used to determine sensor position and orientation

sensor respective to each transmitter coil and because the transmitters are operating at different frequencies, the amplitude of each sensor from all transmitter coils can be obtained simultaneously. The combination of six amplitudes allows the position and orientation of the sensor to be determined (in five DOFs: three translational and two rotational). The optimal measurement location is a 150 mm sphere at the centre of the EMA cube and deviations outside of this region increasingly degrade the accuracy of the measurements.

The EMA system has a synchronisation platform, called Sybox Opto-4, which provides status, trigger and pre-trigger signals from the EMA that can be utilised by up to four other systems for data synchronisation. The signals come in the form of a digital output and these can be used to determine when the EMA is recording data through the sweep and attention signals. The attention signal initially acts as a pre-trigger and becomes active 100 ms before data recording begins. When data is being recorded, the attention signal changes its state every 5 ms to indicate the acquisition of a signal movement sample (at a 200 Hz frequency). The sweep signal only becomes active when a recording is in progress. This signal can be used to synchronise the recording of EMA data with simultaneous EMG signal data acquisition. The complete hardware configuration and setup is shown in Fig. 3.15. Note that data from the EMA is stored on the PC controlling the EMA system while EMG data is stored on the PC connected to the EMG recording system.

The full process that occurs to record both sets of data and then combine them is shown in Fig. 3.16. Each system is initialised manually but it is the recording of EMG data that is automatically governed by the EMG system through the Sybox and triggering mechanism. During trials, the data is recorded on the different PC systems and in post processing they are combined into single data files. This meant that data could not be feasibly verified on-the-y or immediately after being recorded due to time constraints with subjects.

Fifteen healthy young adults (9 men and 6 women), aged 21–34 years (mean 25.4 years, SD 3.1), volunteered for data collection. The study was approved by the

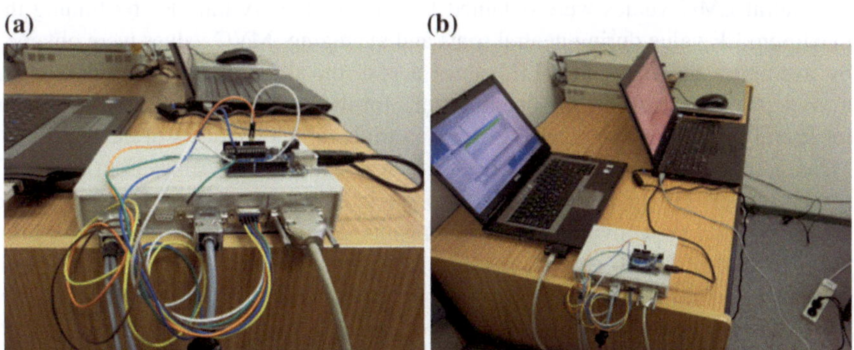

Fig. 3.15 Complete hardware setup with the Sybox to synchronise the two systems recording data independently from each other. **a** Close up of Sybox and Arduino microcontroller on top. **b** Left PC records EMA data while right PC records EMG data, and they are linked through the Sybox

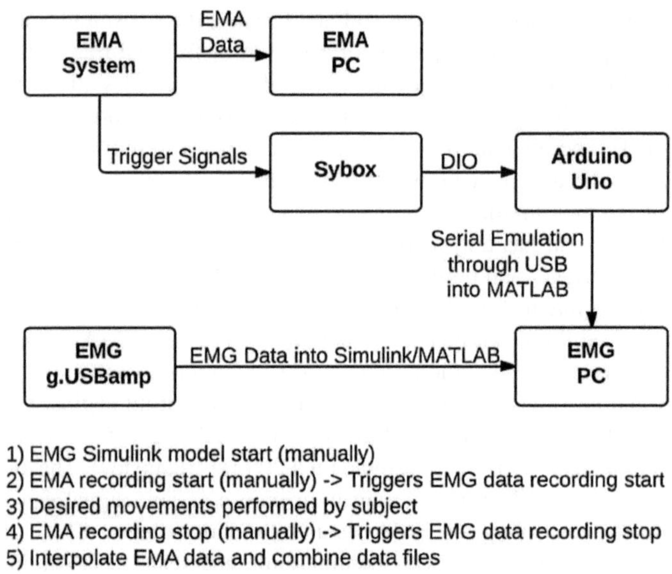

Fig. 3.16 Synchronised data recording process. Schematic of the system and procedure to record and sync data

University of Auckland Human Participants Ethics Committee (Reference #2011/7557) and subjects were briefed in detail on the experimental protocol. Subjects were instructed to perform prescribed movements (without food) to obtain EMG signal and EMA data. Before each movement type, subjects were given clear instructions on how to perform the movement with a demonstration and allowed to practise before actual data acquisition. EMG channels were recorded from the bilateral masseter, anterior temporalis and digastric muscles, while the subjects were seated in the EMA cube.

Neutral EMG values were obtained for each of the six muscles by finding the maximum LE value during neutral trials and averaging. MVC values were obtained by averaging the maximum LE values across the three clenching trials for the masseters and temporalii, and opening trials for the digastrics. Pseudo MVC values for lateral movements were averaged across trials for 1 s windows of mean activity. Mean activity values were used because it was common for subjects to have difficulty in performing a singular, controlled lateral movement and spikes in the signals would have provided misleading results should maximum values have been used. A total of 30–40 cycles for each type of movement were acquired for each subject and muscle contributions were visually identified within a 30 ms window size. The peak contributions of the muscles during opening, closing, lateral left and lateral right movements were identified visually for analysis, examples of which are shown in Fig. 3.17.

For each subject, the mean muscle activations across all 30–40 cycles for each movement type were determined. These were then converted into an activation

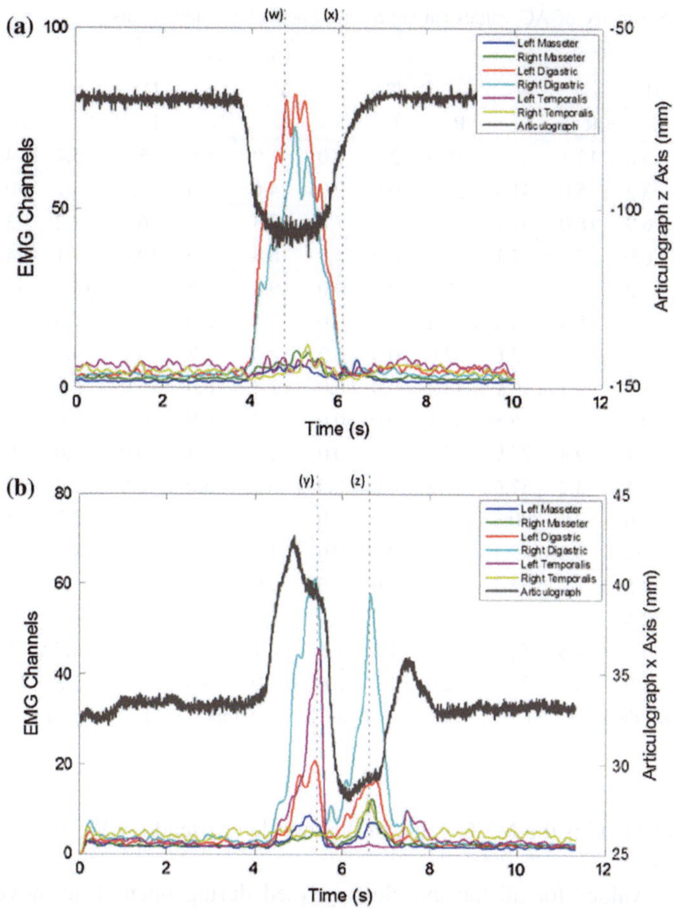

Fig. 3.17 Data selection based on peak contributions. Plots contain processed linear envelopes from six channels of EMG data along with jaw movement as measured from the EMA (unfiltered in the relevant z and x directions). **a** Example of peak activity samples selected for an (w) opening movement and (x) a closing movement. **b** Example of peak activity samples selected for a lateral movement to the (y) *left* and (z) *right*

coefficient (AC, unit %), which is being used as an index of the activation level of the muscle above neutral as a percentage of MVC, and given by the following piecewise function:

$$\mathrm{AC} = \begin{cases} 0 & \text{if } V_\mathrm{M} - V_\mathrm{N} \leq 0 \\ V_\mathrm{M}/\mathrm{MVC} & \text{if } V_\mathrm{M} - V_\mathrm{N} > 0 \end{cases} \tag{3.28}$$

where V_M is the average activity of each muscle across all cycles of a subject during either an opening, closing or lateral movement, V_N is the neutral activity of the

Table 3.1 Summary of AC values (in %) during open–close movements

Open jaw							Close jaw					
	M		D		T		M		D		T	
Subject	L	R	L	R	L	R	L	R	L	R	L	R
A	5.0	12.1	41.7	45.0	2.0	0.0	7.0	8.9	5.8	5.4	4.2	4.7
B	3.2	5.0	41.8	23.0	0.0	0.0	4.6	4.3	7.8	5.1	0.0	0.0
C	6.9	18.0	57.1	57.8	6.5	7.0	7.3	14.3	6.8	7.2	3.4	6.4
D	6.9	7.9	67.1	42.2	0.0	5.9	6.8	3.9	10.6	3.1	4.4	6.0
E	15.2	22.7	80.1	76.5	9.6	0.0	19.8	32.5	12.2	13.2	54.7	27.6
F	8.3	5.8	74.2	70.2	3.6	0.0	4.1	2.0	10.5	7.0	4.8	4.0
G	5.3	5.2	83.6	62.6	0.0	6.2	2.0	2.7	6.7	4.8	0.0	0.0
H	1.9	3.1	46.9	48.2	0.0	0.0	2.3	0.0	5.0	6.0	4.5	0.0
I	0.0	0.0	65.8	68.1	0.0	0.0	0.0	0.0	0.0	0.0	0.0	0.0
J	6.1	9.4	77.9	87.2	0.0	0.0	2.8	4.4	0.0	0.0	0.0	0.0
K	1.1	3.2	37.6	9.7	0.0	0.0	0.8	5.0	8.6	2.4	0.0	2.1
L	0.0	2.9	20.3	26.2	0.0	0.0	0.0	0.0	2.1	2.3	1.9	0.0
M	2.5	3.3	45.4	37.6	0.0	0.0	1.9	3.1	5.8	4.0	7.2	4.1
N	2.5	1.0	34.7	33.7	0.0	0.0	0.0	1.1	5.4	5.6	0.0	3.6
O	2.6	2.7	19.2	18.0	0.0	0.0	2.3	5.8	5.7	4.3	0.0	0.0
Average	4.5	6.8	52.9	47.1	1.5	1.3	4.1	5.9	6.2	4.7	5.7	3.9
SD	3.9	6.4	21.1	22.9	2.9	2.6	5.0	8.3	3.6	3.2	13.8	7.0

SD—standard deviation, M—masseter, D—digastric, T—temporalis, L—left and R—right

muscle and MVC is the MVC value of the muscle or pseudo MVC value for lateral movements.

The AC values for all the muscles analysed during open-close movements is shown in Table 3.1. It is immediately evident that the digastrics are heavily involved in opening movements with an average activation of 52.9 and 47.1 % for the left and right sides respectively, compared to the other muscles which mostly have less than 5 % activation increases. The temporalii have very little involvement during opening movements, with both sides rising above a neutral activation for only one subject (subject C), while other subjects have either one side or none with activations above zero. For closing movements all muscles have between a 4 and 6.5 % activation involvement, which suggests that before occlusion the closing movement is primarily caused by passive elastic muscle activities.

The Lilliefors test on the data provided enough evidence that data for the left masseter, and left and right digastric muscles followed a normal distribution, but the remainder did not for both opening and closing movements. This may have been because of a limiting sample size and the usage of the AC affected the test when replacing below neutral activations with zeroes. However, since the main muscles of interest followed a normal distribution ANOVA tests were still performed.

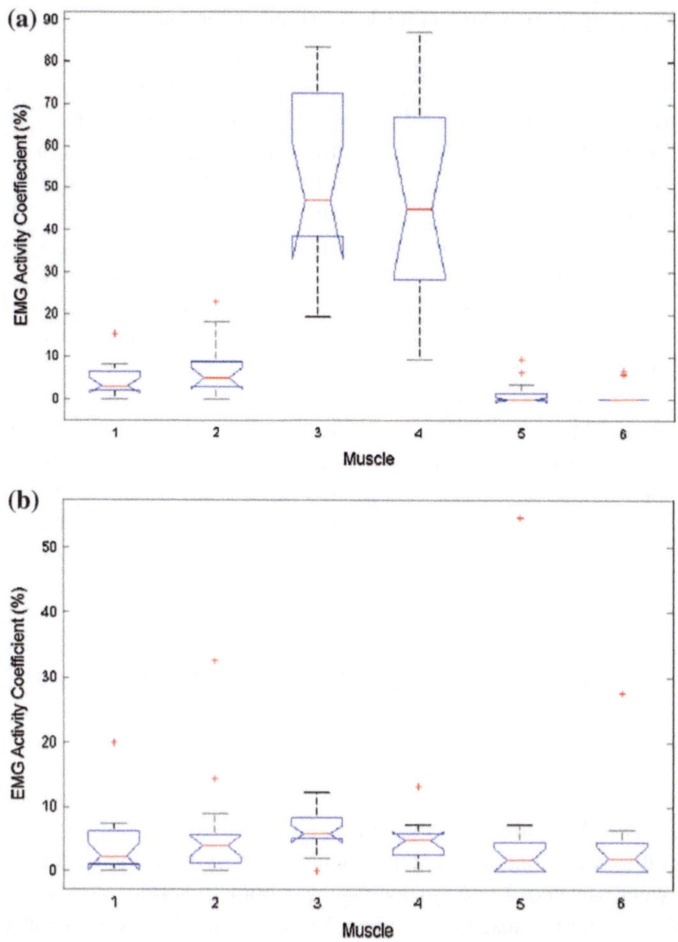

Fig. 3.18 ANOVA plots of activation **coefficients** for opening and closing movements across all the subjects. The numbers correspond to muscles as follows: *1* left masseter, *2* right masseter, *3* left digastric, *4* right digastric, *5* left temporalis and *6* right temporalis. **a** Opening movement, *p*-value of 0. **b** Closing movement, *p*-value of 0.94

The result of one-way ANOVA for the opening and closing movements across all the subjects is shown in Fig. 3.18. The *p*-value of 0 very strongly suggests that the means of digastric activity during opening are significantly different from that of the masseters and temporalii and the *p*-value of 0.94 very strongly suggests that there is no significant difference between the AC values of all the muscles during closing movements (although the limitations of the Lilliefors test results must still be considered).

Table 3.2 Summary of AC values (in %) during lateral movements

Open jaw							Close jaw					
	M		D		T		M		D		T	
Subject	L	R	L	R	L	R	L	R	L	R	L	R
A	87.2	127.8	52.1	43.8	42.4	0.0	0.0	146.8	40.6	42.0	0.0	47.3
B	84.4	53.1	72.6	60.8	0.0	0.0	54.7	59.1	42.7	24.1	0.0	43.8
C	57.1	104.3	74.0	83.6	66.8	0.0	89.0	22.3	54.5	49.4	0.0	112.4
D	9.9	50.4	28.4	40.8	67.7	0.0	64.8	10.5	120.4	82.8	0.0	103.1
E	70.6	85.5	72.6	83.7	88.5	0.0	0.0	52.2	60.4	62.8	0.0	119.3
F	0.0	104.3	84.5	85.9	0.0	0.0	104.1	0.0	45.5	51.0	0.0	107.2
G	70.4	39.3	0.0	0.0	0.0	0.0	0.0	0.0	0.0	0.0	0.0	0.0
H	44.0	56.0	62.1	91.3	0.0	0.0	68.5	34.6	96.7	165.7	0.0	54.7
I	37.4	0.0	47.7	50.0	35.4	0.0	48.9	0.0	161.9	96.5	0.0	63.3
J	83.4	91.0	69.7	87.8	0.0	0.0	81.1	0.0	0.0	0.0	0.0	0.0
K	99.4	69.0	93.3	46.6	101.7	0.0	40.4	89.2	87.7	0.0	0.0	0.0
L	66.3	77.9	58.5	71.7	65.3	0.0	32.6	46.7	73.7	75.2	0.0	36.9
M	91.0	77.4	85.4	88.8	162.8	0.0	66.5	91.4	90.7	90.1	0.0	93.1
N	107.7	97.5	88.7	93.8	0.0	0.0	88.8	118.3	81.2	111.8	0.0	0.0
O	29.4	60.7	34.9	53.5	75.7	0.0	76.0	71.5	58.9	66.7	0.0	153.1
Average	62.5	72.9	61.6	65.5	47.1	0.0	54.4	49.5	67.6	61.2	0.0	62.3
SD	32.4	31.5	25.6	26.4	48.9	0.0	33.9	46.6	42.2	45.9	0.0	50.3

SD—standard deviation, M—masseter, D—digastric, T—temporalis, L—left and R—right

The AC values for left and right motions during lateral movements are shown in Table 3.2. The AC values of the temporalis have a 0 % average for the side contralateral to directional movements, while the activity of the remaining muscles range between 47 and 73 % on average for both directions of movement. The higher values occur because the pseudo MVC values used are significantly less than actual MVC values for the muscles and AC values above 100 % are not unexpected.

Unlike the open-close movement data, the Lilliefors test provided evidence that most of the mandibular muscles followed a normal distribution, except for right digastric and left temporalis muscles, but only during the lateral left movement—again this is believed to be attributed to zero substitutions and a limited sample size. One-way ANOVA for the left and right movements across all the subjects are shown in Fig. 3.19. The p-values of both cases are 0.0001 or less, which strongly suggests that the means of muscle activity are significantly different. However, this is being influenced by the zero values of the right temporalis during left movements and the left temporalis during right movements. If these muscles are removed from the ANOVA, the p-values become 0.34 and 0.82 for the left and right movements respectively. However, lateral data could be determined from temporalii data and there is enough evidence to suggest that there is a difference in temporalii activations that corresponds to the direction of movement.

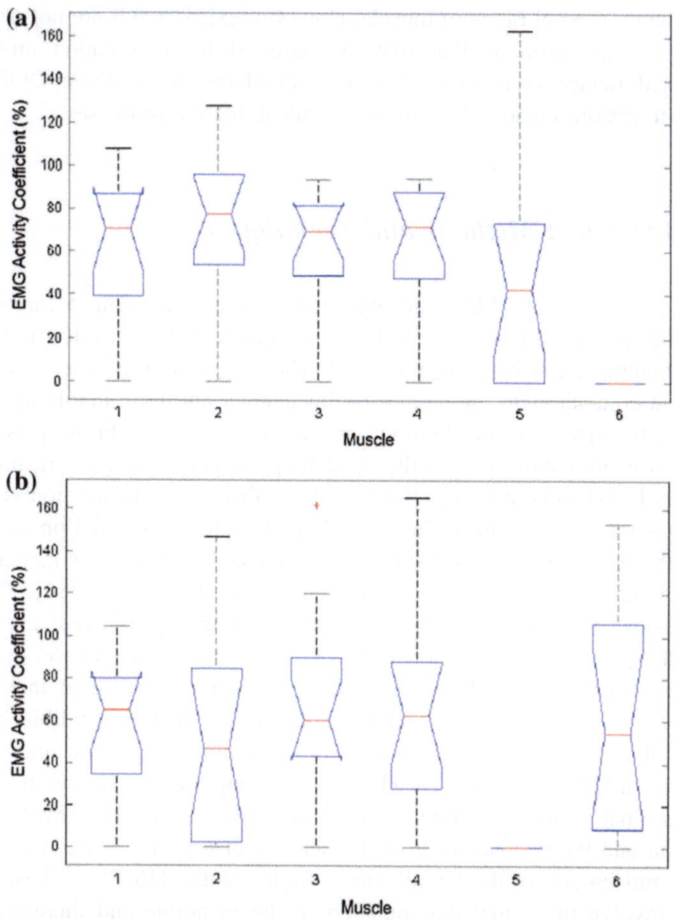

Fig. 3.19 ANOVA plots of activation coefficients for lateral movements across all the subjects. The numbers correspond to muscles as follows: *1* left masseter, *2* right masseter, *3* left digastric, *4* right digastric, *5* left temporalis and *6* right temporalis. **a** Lateral left movement, *p*-value of 0.0001. **b** Lateral right movement, *p*-value of 0.0001

3.4 Jaw Rehabilitation

There is no specific medical condition called 'jaw motion disorder' and for the scope of this chapter, jaw motion disorder will be used to describe a deviation from ideal or normal function of the masticatory system, due to a single factor or combination of pathologies that affect mandibular movement. The causes of this dysfunctional movement can be from temporomandibular joint disorder (TMJD), which is an affliction of the TMJ, or paralysis or weakening of mandibular muscle. The therapy has to be tailored to a particular patient and should suit their specific needs. Passive motion therapy followed by active therapy can help strengthen and increase the movement range of muscle. However, existing aids are not sufficient at emulating all the motions that may be required for mastication and a more sophisticated device is required that accommodates the multiple DOFs of the mandible to restore mandibular function in rehabilitative processes.

3.4.1 Treatment Methods and Techniques

The high prevalence of TMJD and other muscular disorders mean careful assessment of the individual patient's condition is required before any form of rehabilitation or treatment can be prescribed [13]. The jaw motion disorder treatments of interest that coincide with the themes of this chapter are those involving the usage of physical therapy to restore joint and muscle function [14]. From questionnaires and clinical examination, one of the most frequent jaw disabilities resulting from TMJD was found to be chewing (64.5 %) [15]. Physical rehabilitation is largely a manual process and early muscular rehabilitation techniques relied on the therapist showing the patient how to perform actively assisted exercises for increasing performance in areas such as range of motion and lateral movements [16]. Since then, other methods such as electrotherapy, relaxation training and biofeedback have also been used in the management of TMJD [17]. Medlicott and Harris presented a systematic review of the effectiveness of these different physical therapies and found that active exercises and manual mobilizations of the mandible, and combinations of active exercises, manual therapy, postural correction and relaxation techniques could both be effective [17]. This is supported by Nicolakis et al. who determined that exercise therapy seemed valuable for treating myofascial pain dysfunction and the displacement of the anterior disc in the TMJ, and found that restricted movement could be alleviated significantly [18–20]. These exercise therapies involve the actual manipulation of the mandible and therefore involve varying amounts of motion. The efficacy of isometric exercise, which mostly relates to strengthening bite force (in the masseters and temporalii) is less certain. Thompson et al. determined that increases in maximum bite force is easily attainable with training but targeting the strengthening of individual jaw muscles is more difficult to achieve [21]. Furthermore, there is some evidence that suggests jaw exercises do not reduce symptoms and signs of TMJD in patients with chronic whiplash-associated disorders [22]. However, the differences caused by the TMJD being induced from whiplash are not fully explored and the relevance of physical therapy may be questionable. The majority of the literature, with supporting data and evidence, has touted the efficacy of exercise therapy methods in improving masticatory system function.

The manual and labour intensive components of exercise therapy involves muscle stretching, guided opening and closing movements, manual joint distraction and disc/condyle mobilisation [20]. These movements are either performed passively or actively and with or without the assistance of a therapist. They mirror similar properties of the rehabilitation methods, which are used for the rehabilitation of other limbs, such as the upper arm, and during gait. This suggests that the application of exoskeletons could also benefit the jaw rehabilitation process. In this case, however, the physical load on the therapist is less because the masticatory system is of a significantly smaller scale than the upper or lower limb. Instead, the focus is on relieving the physical stress on the patients, who are often given exercises to perform in their homes, without a therapist [16, 18, 21]. In this capacity an exoskeleton is able to provide active assistance in place of the therapist or the patient themselves, and this is particularly advantageous if the patient suffers from muscular pathologies that are not localised to the craniofacial region, such as the wider effects of a stroke. The other advantage such a device would offer is the ability to perform pre-determined trajectories and function on an assist-as-needed basis or with a resistance based control system.

3.4.2 Existing Jaw Exoskeletons and Interfaces

Research involving both the masticatory system and features of robotics has been heavily focussed on the development of chewing robots to assess food texture [23], a jaw robot to emulate mastication [24], a 6-DOF anthropomorphic robotic jaw intended as a prosthesis [25] and a large, bulky rehabilitative robot for lateral movement training [26], examples of which are shown in Fig. 3.20. It is evident from the figure that the current trajectory of research, involving robotics and masticatory studies, is not heading towards an optimal design environment for jaw exoskeletons and rehabilitation. Existing methods use incredibly large, bulky devices that are not designed with the patient's best interests and comfort in mind. The field of masticatory robotics is specifically targeting studies on chewing behaviour and methods to characterise and reproduce that behaviour [27]. Some of these chewing models utilise physiological models, but the primary motivation of the models is to emulate chewing behaviour and the associated active and reactive forces [28–30]. This means that they are not developed around the physical limitations of the masticatory system and instead incorporate them for modelling accuracy, making them unsuitable for control or dynamic applications.

The development of exoskeletons for the jaw is in a non-existent state, with a search of the available literature revealing no significant developments of such a system. The only available example that fits within the criteria of a practical exoskeleton designed for the purposes of jaw rehabilitation is being developed concurrently to the research presented in this chapter for the rehabilitation of temporomandibular disorder by Wang et al. [31]. The exoskeleton has a single active DOF and operates with a four-bar linkage system as its main driving mechanism, and is shown in Fig. 3.21. The device is still in the early stages of development, having undergone several prototypal stages and finite element analysis to ensure it is structurally sound. The movement it is able to produce corresponds closely with actual trajectories of the TMJ at the condylar process and incisor point, without causing stress or damage to the TMJ in simulations. This device does not match the

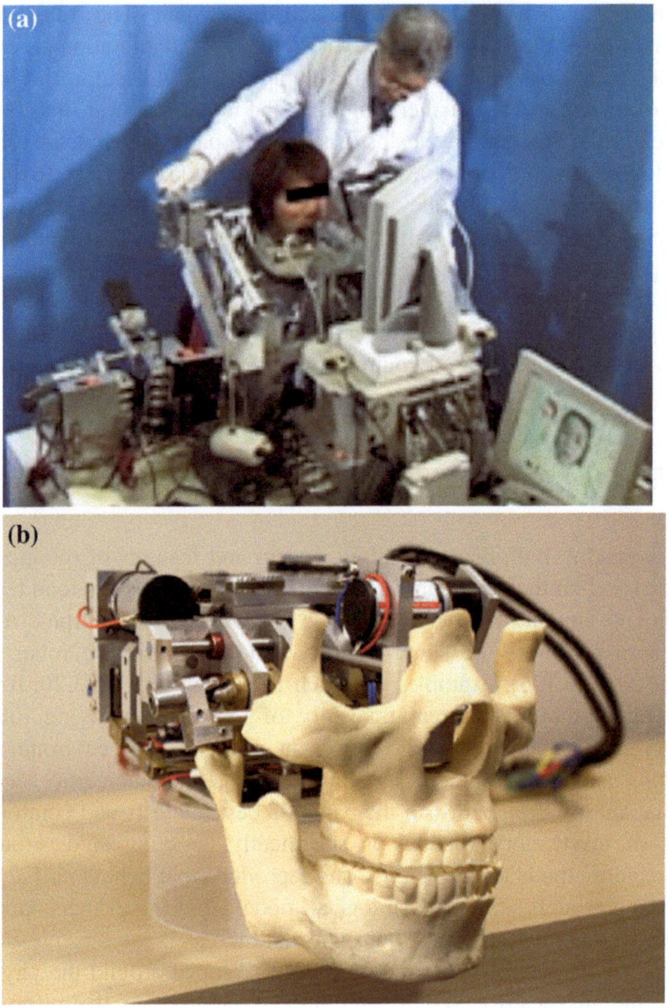

Fig. 3.20 Examples of masticatory robots. These robots were developed with the main purpose of reproducing chewing behaviour. **a** WY masticatory robot [27]. **b** Anthropomorphic robotic jaw [25]

sophistication of the advanced 6-DOF chewing robots because it suffers from additional limitations such as the reduced amount of space for actuators and the considerations for patient comfort and safety when using the device. Further work is being carried out to finalise and improve the performance of the device to ensure that it is light, safe and can accommodate the needs of the patient. The neuromuscular interface for the jaw developed as a result will enable the jaw exoskeleton to be controlled via the patient's mandibular muscle EMG signals, and enable a more intuitive and effective approach for TMJD rehabilitation.

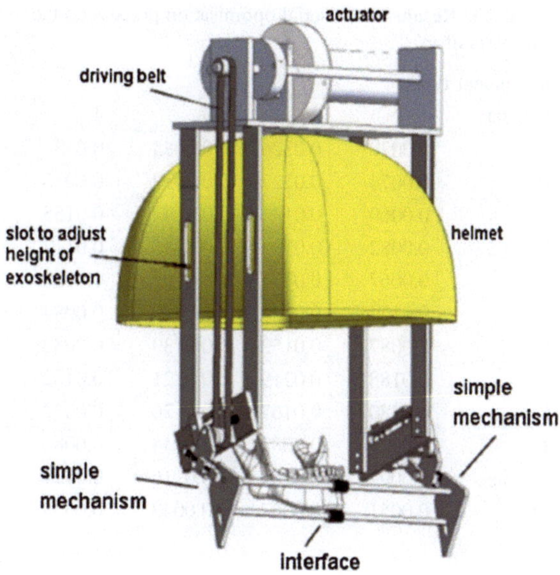

Fig. 3.21 A jaw exoskeleton that is currently under development [7]

In the past, the EMG signals of the mandibular muscles have mostly been used to evaluate robotic therapy treatment of the jaw [32] or study the effects on the mandibular muscles from TMJD [33, 34], but not to drive a robot or facilitate rehabilitation through a neuromuscular interface. Biomechanical models have been developed for the prediction of static bite forces for the purposes of understanding joint loading [28, 35] and the usage of the EMG signal as a predictor has only gone so far as to be included in these models to drive bite force prediction [36]. The EMG signals of the masticatory system have also been modelled and preliminary attempts have been made at movement recognition using the EMG signal with artificial neural networks [37, 38]. However, these methods have focussed on the identification of bruxism or determining forceful closing movements, and only utilised the EMG signals from the bilateral temporalis and masseter muscles. There have been no developments that apply the EMG signal for the purpose of driving a physiological model of the masticatory system with multiple degree of freedom for simulation, study or interfacing applications.

3.4.3 Neuromuscular Interface: Conjecture

Table 3.3 shows a summary of the performance of the hybrid model with the averaged RMSE values across each type of movement for the subjects. The average RMSE value ranges from 9.7 to 18.9 mm across the movements of different complexities. These results demonstrate levels of accuracy that in absolute terms are comparable with other movement prediction methods (the physiological model of

Table 3.3 Results of the serial optimisation process on the hybrid model. Data values are RMSE with units of m

Movement type							
Subject	1	2	3	4	5	6	7
A	0.0070	0.0326	0.0085	0.0134	0.0104	0.0182	0.0641
B	0.0074	0.0127	0.0039	0.0080	0.0107	0.0199	0.0127
C	0.0060	0.0171	0.0147	0.0155	0.0143	0.0137	0.0150
D	0.0082	0.0133	0.0183	0.0117	0.0161	0.0137	0.0092
E	0.0067	0.0135	0.0105	0.0128	0.0157	0.0127	0.0098
F	0.0124	0.0133	0.0070	0.0084	0.0137	0.0122	0.0138
G	0.0087	0.0152	0.0139	0.0082	0.0104	0.0130	0.0180
H	0.0188	0.0219	0.0121	0.0182	0.0402	0.0194	0.0170
I	0.0180	0.0167	0.0126	0.0072	0.0173	0.0144	0.0116
J	0.0039	0.0082	0.0144	0.0080	0.0116	0.0166	0.0102
Average	0.0097	0.0164	0.0116	0.0111	0.0160	0.0154	0.0181
SD	0.0051	0.0067	0.0042	0.0038	0.0088	0.0029	0.0164

the elbow joint yielded results between 6 and 22.4 mm RMSE). However, it should also be considered that the masticatory system has a smaller range of motion and what might be a small error for the elbow joint could be more significant in this case.

The following figures demonstrate the effect of the hybrid model for the various kinds of movements that were presented to it. The predicted movement is the result of having all parameters tuned, including the lateral, vertical, offset and ANN parameters. It appears that a significant effect the ANN has on the output of the model is to introduce a little high frequency noise. This might be a result of the ANN output changing rapidly when it misclassifies a state. The effect might not reduce performance when the hybrid model is implemented in an NI because of physical system damping or the ability to post process the output further with additional smoothing techniques. It may also be mitigated through the improvement of the ANN implementation, which at this initial stage is fairly rudimentary.

However, despite this the hybrid model still performs well with RMSE values below 10 mm for all movement types. The model appears to struggle with chewing movements, which may be because of the high frequency of movement and changes affecting the ANN (in Fig. 3.22). This may also be due to the ANN currently only being capable of producing three states of output, and not considering a movement consisting of a vertical and lateral component. A more sophisticated ANN is required to deal with these deficiencies (Fig. 3.23, 3.24 and 3.25).

In some cases, for example Fig. 3.22 and 3.26, it seems that the model has been tuned to perform optimally at the expense of a single DOF of movement. Note that in these cases the result is not from the inability of the physiological model to identify movement but from the ANN suppressing the other DOF. This is best explained through the latter example, which is for continuous cycles of lateral

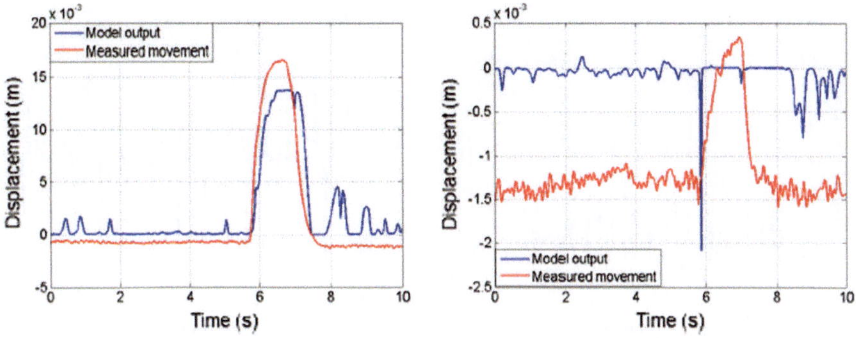

Fig. 3.22 Typical results of serial tuning of the hybrid model for a single open–close movement. Total RMSE = 0.0034 m

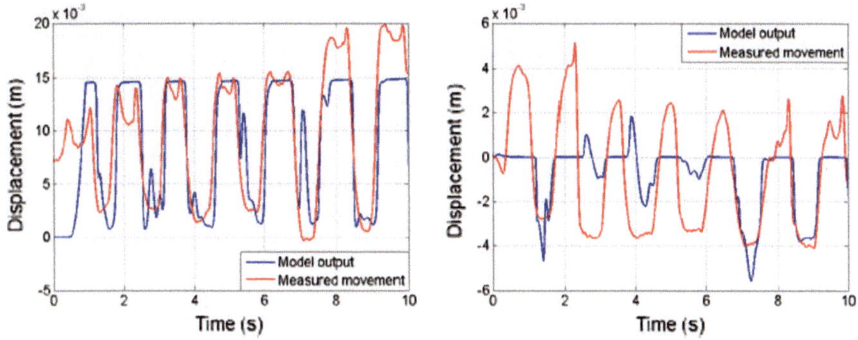

Fig. 3.23 Typical results of serial tuning of the hybrid model for continuous open−close movements. Total RMSE = 0.0064 m

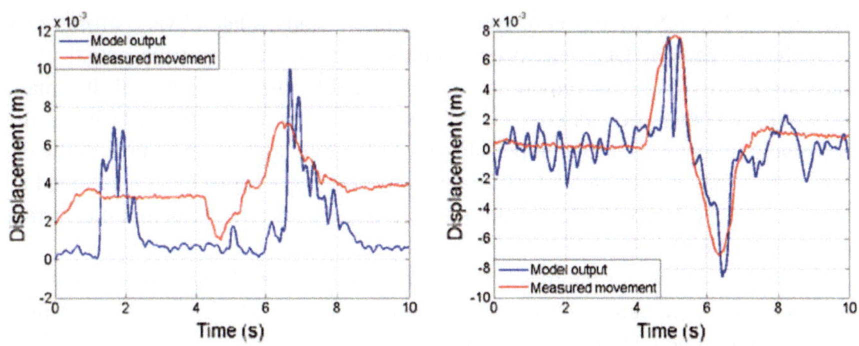

Fig. 3.24 Typical results of serial tuning of the hybrid model for a single lateral movement. Total RMSE = 0.0042 m

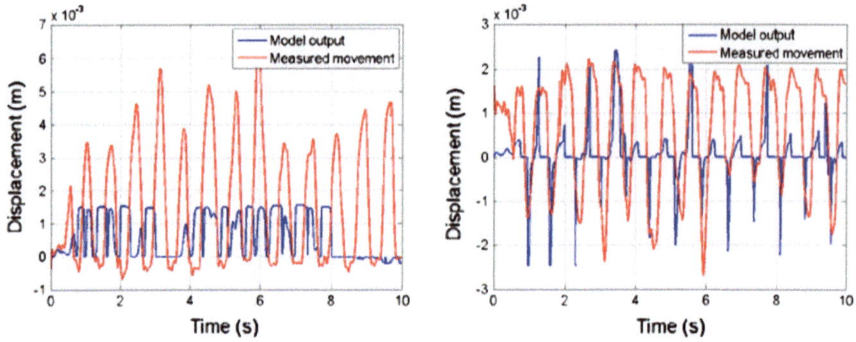

Fig. 3.25 Typical results of serial tuning of the hybrid model for continuous chewing movements. Total RMSE = 0.0034 m

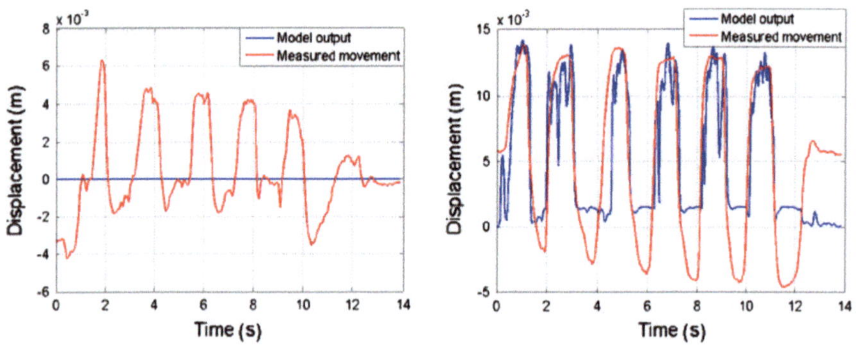

Fig. 3.26 Typical results of serial tuning of the hybrid model for continuous lateral movements. Total RMSE = 0.0065 m

movement. The ANN has identified the movement state as lateral very strongly and as such, the vertical DOF has been suppressed completely and the actual minor fluctuations in vertical movement are not recreated by the hybrid model. It remains to be seen whether such an effect is more desirable for rehabilitation or predicting movement trajectories, as it can possibly provide more control to the user of the end device than they would have of their own body (i.e. if the subject had performed the lateral cycles perfectly, there should not have been any vertical fluctuations in their actual movement).

The hybrid model for the masticatory system has not yet been implemented with the necessary hardware components to form a neuromuscular interface. This is mostly due to time restraints, and the design, fabrication and assembly of an NI and test platform for the masticatory system would be beyond the scope of this chapter. However, some insights and the outlook on the development of the NI will be discussed in this section.

Converting the Simulink/MATLAB model into a form usable by an embedded system will not be overly complicated by the introduction of the ANN because its relatively simple structure can be represented simply in code. Also, the addition of four more channels of EMG signal data will only require additional signal processing circuitry and the previous microcontroller should be able to handle the additional input channels without slowing in performance.

Problems may arise from the additional bulk of the electronic components and leads if there is no wireless signal capability. If wireless communication were to be included care must also be made to ensure that the transmission speed (of all the relevant data) is fast enough. Ideally, the signal acquisition module for the masticatory system would be able to communicate with the same central processing module as the signal acquisition module for the elbow joint. This would lead to a centralised processing unit that is capable of handling all inputs from around the body in one system. It is believed that such an NI for the masticatory system is feasible, especially given the ability of the previously developed prototypal systems for the elbow joint. The development of the final hardware system and improvement to the hybrid model is suggested as ongoing and future work.

3.5 Summary

This chapter introduced the masticatory system and its associated numerous complexities, and a new physiological model with two DOFs was developed for it. This model was able to identify movements but was easily affected by co-activation of muscles and the random nature of muscle activities made it difficult to perform consistently. An in-depth study was therefore performed on the mandibular muscles to properly characterise all accessible mandibular muscle EMG signals from which to base the physiological model. The results of the analysis identified a feasible configuration for the model of the masticatory system but still did not completely provide a solution to deal with muscles that displayed EMG activity during multiple movements of interest. Based on the findings of the EMG signal study, the physiological model of the masticatory system was reconfigured and the concept of a hybrid model consisting of the physiological model and ANN was introduced. The effectiveness of the hybrid model was proven through experimental data from multiple subjects and was analysed offline.

References

1. B.S. Kraus, R.E. Jordan, L. Abrams, *A Study of the Masticatory System: Dental Anatomy and Occlusion* (The Williams and Wilkins Company, Maryland, 1969)
2. K.H. Harib, K.A. Moustafa, A.S. Ullah, S. Zenieh, Parallel, serial and hybrid machine tools and robotics structures: comparative study on optimum kinematic designs, in *Serial and*

Parallel Robot Manipulators—Kinematics, Dynamics, Control and Optimisation (InTech, 2012)
3. J.H. Koolstra, Dynamics of the human masticatory system. Crit. Rev. Oral Biol. Med. **13**, 366–376 (July 2002)
4. W.E. McDevitt, *Functional Anatomy of the Masticatory System* (Butterworth & Co, 1989)
5. P.D.S. Calderon, E.M. Kogawa, J.R.P. Lauris, P.C.R. Conti, The influence of gender and bruxism on the human maximum bite force. J. Appl. Oral Sci. **14**, 448–453 (2006)
6. J.P. Okeson, *Management of Temporomandibular Disorders and Occlusion*, 6th edn. (Elsevier Mosby, Missouri, 2008)
7. X. Wang, W. Xu, K. Etzel, J. Potgieter, O. *Diegel, Mechanism Design and Analysis of a Wearable Device for Rehabilitation of Temporomandibular Disorder*, in 2010 Ieee International Conference on Robotics and Biomimetics, Tianjin, China (Dec 2010), pp 1674–1679
8. W. Xu, J. Bronlund, J. Potgieter, K. Foster, O. Rohrle, A. Pullan, J. Kieser, Review of the human masticatory system and masticatory robotics. Mech. Mach. Theory **43**(11), 1353–1375 (2008)
9. C. Peck, A. Hannam, Human jaw and muscle modelling. Arch. Oral Biol. **52**(4), 300–304 (2007)
10. S. Fels, F. Vogt, K. van der Doel, J. Lloyd, I. Stavness, E. Vatikiotis-Bateson, Artisynth: a biome-chanical simulation platform for the vocal tract and upper airway, Tech. Rep. TR-2006-10, University of British Columbia (2006)
11. I. Stavness, A. Hannam, J. Lloyd, S. Fels, Towards predicting biomechanical consequences of jaw re-construction. Ann. Int. Conf. IEEE Eng. Med. Biol. Soc. (EMBS) **2008**, 4567–4570 (2008)
12. W. Xu, J.E. Bronlund, *Mastication Robots* (Springer, Berlin, 2010)
13. R. Ohrbach, Disability assessment in temporomandibular disorders and masticatory system rehabilita-tion. J. Oral Rehabil. **37**(6), 452–480 (2010)
14. A. Van Der Bilt, Assessment of mastication with implications for oral rehabilitation: a review. J. Oral Rehabil. **38**(10), 754–780 (2011)
15. A. Yap, E. Chua, J. Hoe, Clinical tmd, pain-related disability and psychological status of tmd patients. J. Oral Rehabil. **29**(4), 374–380 (2002)
16. W.H. Bell, W. Gonyea, R.A. Finn, K.A. Storum, C. Johnston, G.S. Throckmorton, Muscular rehabilitation after orthognathic surgery. Oral Surg. Oral Med. Oral Pathol. **56**(3), 229–235 (1983)
17. M.S. Medlicott, S.R. Harris, A systematic review of the effectiveness of exercise, manual therapy, electrotherapy, relaxation training, and biofeedback in the management of temporomandibular disorder. Phys. Ther. **86**(7), 955–973 (2006)
18. P. Nicolakis, B. Erdogmus, A. Kopf, A. Djaber-Ansari, E. Piehslinger, V. Fialka-Moser, Exercise therapy for craniomandibular disorders. Arch. Phys. Med. Rehabil. **81**(9), 1137–1142 (2000)
19. P. Nicolakis, B. Erdogmus, A. Kopf, G. Ebenbichler, J. Kollmitzer, E. Piehslinger, V. Fialka-Moser, Effectiveness of exercise therapy in patients with internal derangement of the temporomandibular joint. J. Oral Rehabil. **28**(12), 1158–64 (2001)
20. P. Nicolakis, B. Erdogmus, A. Kopf, M. Nicolakis, E. Piehslinger, V. Fialka-Moser, Effectiveness of exercise therapy in patients with myofascial pain dysfunction syndrome. J. Oral Rehabil. **29**, 362–368 (2002)
21. D. Thompson, G. Throckmorton, P. Buschang, The effects of isometric exercise on maximum volun-tary bite forces and jaw muscle strength and endurance. J. Oral Rehabil. **28**(10), 909–917 (2001)
22. L. Klobas, S. Axelsson, K. Tegelberg, Effect of therapeutic jaw exercise on temporomandibular disorders in individuals with chronic whiplash-associated disorders. Acta Odontol. Scand. **64**(6), 341–347 (2006)
23. W.L. Xu, J.S. Pap, J. Bronlund, Design of a biologically inspired parallel robot for foods chewing. IEEE Trans. Ind. Electron. **55**(2), 832–841 (2008)

24. A. Takanishi, T. Tanase, M. Kumei, I. Kato, Development of 3 dof jaw robot wj-2 as a human's mastication simulator, in *Fifth International Conference on Advanced Robotics (ICAR)* (June 1991), pp. 277–282
25. E. Flores, S. Fels, and E. Vatikiotis-Bateson, Chew on this: design of a 6dof anthropomorphic robotic jaw, in *The 16th IEEE International Symposium on Robot and Human interactive Communication (RO-MAN)* (Aug 2007), pp. 648–653
26. A. Okino, T. Inoue, H. Takanobu, A. Takanishi, K. Ohtsuki, M. Ohnishi, Y. Nakano, A clinical jaw movement training robot for lateral movement training, in *IEEE International Conference on Robotics and Automation* (*ICRA*), vol. 1 (Sept 2003), pp. 244–249
27. W. Xu, J. Bronlund, J. Potgieter, K. Foster, O. Rohrle, A. Pullan, J. Kieser, Review of the human masticatory system and masticatory robotics. Mech. Mach. Theory **43**(11), 1353–1375 (2008)
28. L. Iwasaki, P. Petsche, W. McCall Jr, D. Marx, J. Nickel, Neuromuscular objectives of the human masticatory apparatus during static biting. Arch. Oral Biol. **48**(11), 767–777 (2003)
29. D. Xie, W. Xu, K. Foster, J. Bronlund, Object-oriented knowledge framework for modelling human mastication of foods. Expert Syst. Appl. **36**(3), 4810–4821 (2009)
30. J. Margielewicz, W. Chladek, T. Lipski, Kinematical analysis of mandibular motion in a sagittal plane. Acta Bioeng. Biomech. **10**(1), 9–19 (2008)
31. X. Wang, W. Xu, K. Etzel, J. Potgieter, O. Diegel, Mechanism design and analysis of a wearable device for rehabilitation of temporomandibular disorder, in *IEEE International Conference on Robotics and Biomimetics (ROBIO), 2010*, Tianjin, China (Dec 2010), pp. 1674–1679
32. W. Xu, F. Fang, J. Bronlund, J. Potgieter, Generation of rhythmic and voluntary patterns of mastication using matsuoka oscillator for a humanoid chewing robot. Mechatronics **19**(2), 205–217 (2009)
33. Z. Liu, K. Yamagata, Y. Kasahara, Electromyographic examination of jaw muscles in relation to symptoms and occlusion of patients with temporomandibular joint disorders. J. Oral Rehabil. **26**(1), 33–47 (1999)
34. L. Dahlstrom, Electromyographic studies of craniomandibular disorders: a review of the literature. J. Oral Rehabil. **16**(1), 1–20 (1989)
35. J. Koolstra, T. van Eijden, W. Weijs, M. Naeije, A three-dimensional mathematical model of the human masticatory system predicting maximum possible bite forces. J. Biomech. **21**(7), 563–576 (1988)
36. V.F. Ferrario, C. Sforza, G. Zanotti, G. Tartaglia, Maximal bite forces in healthy young adults as predicted by surface electromyography. J. Dent. **32**(6), 451–457 (2004)
37. B. Fu, Classification of multi-channel emgs for jaw motion recognition by signal processing and artificial neural networks, Master's thesis, The University of British Columbia, 2004
38. C.L. Long, Pattern recognition using surface electromyography of the anterior temporalis and masseter muscles, Master's thesis, The University of British Columbia, 2004

24. A. Takanobu, T. Yanase, M. Kaneko, L. Kato, Development of a new jaw robot and a human's mastication simulator, in *[illegible] International Conference on Advanced Robotics (ICAR)* ([illegible]), pp. 277–282
25. [illegible] Flores, S. Bell, and B. Watkins-Bateson [illegible] on the [illegible] (RO-MAN) [illegible]
26. [illegible]
27. [illegible]
28. [illegible]
29. [illegible]
30. [illegible]
31. [illegible]
32. [illegible]
33. [illegible]
34. [illegible]
35. [illegible]
36. [illegible]

Chapter 4
Modelling Human Shoulder and Elbow

The human upper limb can be considered a serial manipulator with three segments connected through three joints. The wrist joint connects the hand to the forearm, the elbow joint connects the forearm to the upper arm and the shoulder joint connects the upper arm to the torso. The wrist joint is modelled as three revolute joints intersecting at one point yielding a 3-DOF spherical joint. The elbow joint is modelled as a simple 1-DOF hinge joint. In this chapter, the physiological model of the elbow joint developed in the previous chapter was coupled with linear envelope processing and experimentally validated with data from multiple subjects.

4.1 Anatomy of the Human Upper Limb

4.1.1 The Human Shoulder

The human shoulder joint is one of the most complex joints in the human skeleton and is fundamentally a mechanism consisting of three joints, the glenohumeral, the sternoclavicular and the acromioclavicular joints [1, 2] as shown in Fig. 4.1. These three joints allow the upper arm to move with extraordinary mobility over a large range of motion. It is formed by the articulation between the head of the humerus, which is the "ball" and the glenoid fossa of the scapula, which is the "socket". The connection between these two bones is relatively small due to the shallowness of the glenoid fossa which gives the joint its tremendous mobility.

The movements of the two remaining joints, the sternoclavicular and the acromioclavicular joints, are much smaller compared to the glenohumeral joint. The sternoclavicular joint articulates the medial end of the clavicle onto the manubrium at the top of the sternum. The acromioclavicular joint is formed by the articulation between the acromion of the scapula and the distal end of the clavicle. These two joints cause translations of the glenohumeral head and also increase the rotational range of motion of the shoulder. Motions of the humerus involve the simultaneous motions of the glenohumeral, acromioclavicular and sternoclavicular joints [3]. An example of this simultaneous movement is in the shoulder abduction movement shown in Fig. 4.2.

S.(S.Q.) Xie, *Advanced Robotics for Medical Rehabilitation*,
Springer Tracts in Advanced Robotics 108, DOI 10.1007/978-3-319-19896-5_4

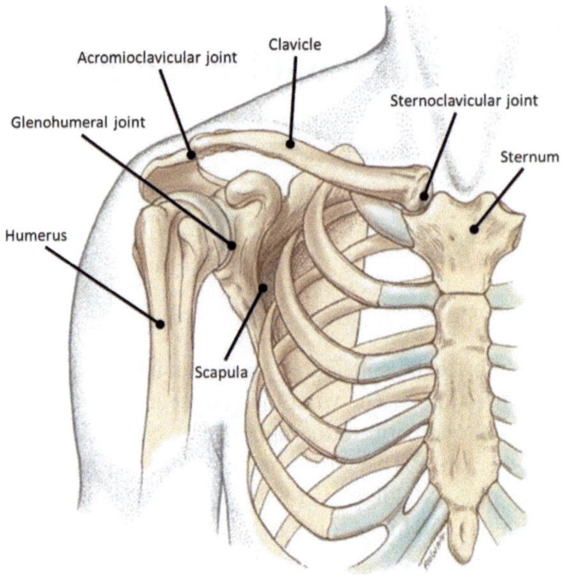

Fig. 4.1 Anatomy of the human shoulder. The three joints responsible for shoulder movements are the glenohumeral, sternoclavicular and acromioclavicular joints

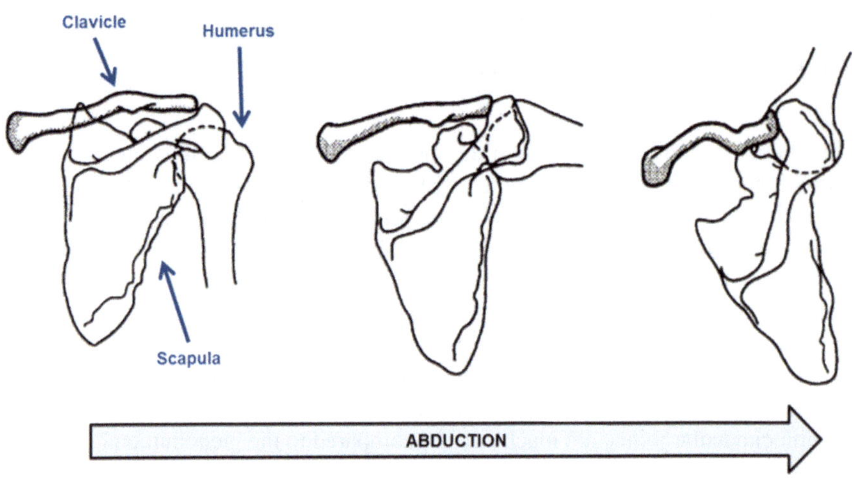

Fig. 4.2 Shoulder abduction requires simultaneous movement of the glenohumeral, sternoclavicular and acromioclavicular joints [3]. It can be seen that the clavicle, scapula and humerus all move during abduction

In the kinematic sense, the movements of all three joints (the glenohumeral, sternoclavicular and acromioclavicular joints) can be combined and simplified into 5-DOF [2]. This includes 3-DOF for the spherical and axial rotation of the upper

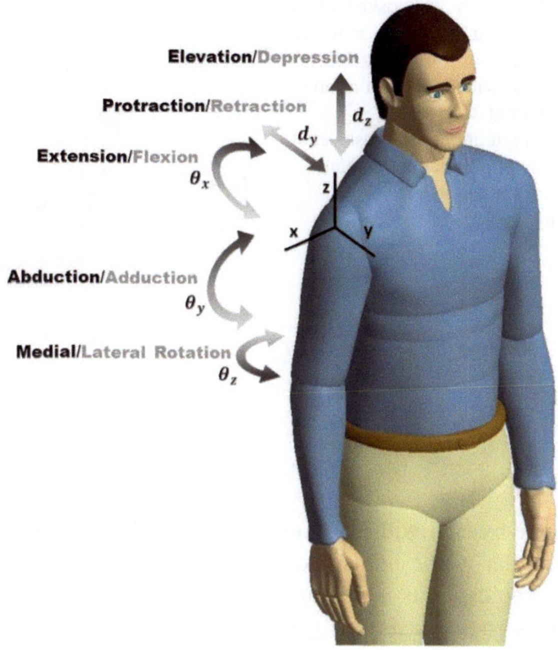

Fig. 4.3 Movements of the 5-DOF shoulder joint

arm about the shoulder ICOR and 2-DOF for the translations of the ICOR along the vertical axis and along the anterior–posterior axis. The 3-DOF of rotational motion is commonly referred to as shoulder abduction and adduction, flexion and extension, and medial and lateral rotation. The 2-DOF of translational motion is referred to as elevation and depression and retraction and protraction. This 5-DOF of the shoulder is illustrated in Fig. 4.3.

Independently moving the 2-translational DOF with an exoskeleton is particularly challenging as the user's torso, shoulder and upper arm must be rigidly attached to the exoskeleton. Furthermore, shifts in the user's body posture can cause relatively large inaccuracies in translation movements of the shoulder. In this research, the 2-translational DOF of the shoulder is not considered in the exoskeleton design. Exclusion of this 2-DOF does not cause significant issues since the range of motion of this DOF is relatively small and full shoulder rotation can still be achieved. Shoulder translations are also less important compared to shoulder rotations in positioning the hand. These small translations can still be performed while using an exoskeleton due to the soft strap and human tissue.

4.1.2 Spherical Wrist Mechanism for Exoskeleton Shoulder

An exoskeleton has a kinematic structure that resembles the human limb, with robot joint axes that align with the limb joint axes. This robot is designed to operate

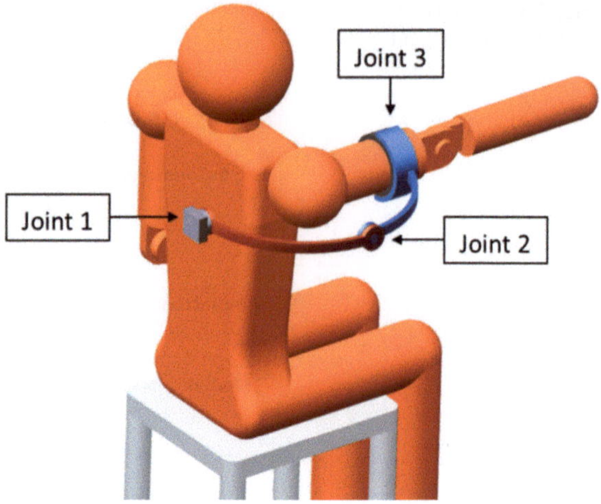

Fig. 4.4 A 3R exoskeleton in a singular configuration where the axis of rotation of Joint 3 aligns with the axis of rotation of Joint 1. In this configuration, the exoskeleton cannot produce horizontal flexion and extension movements of the shoulder

side-by-side with the human upper limb and therefore must produce movements similar to the human counterpart. The human shoulder joint is one of the most complex joints in the human body and designing an exoskeleton for this joint is a challenging task. The shoulder joint has a very large range of motion, capable of rotating the upper arm in 3-DOF in a spherical motion over approximately half of the entire workspace (i.e. the upper arm has a semi-spherical workspace).

Hence, a shoulder exoskeleton is also required to have 3-DOF of spherical motion. However, it is not feasible to implement a true ball-and-socket spherical joint for an active exoskeleton as it cannot be aligned with the user's shoulder joint and is difficult to actuate. Therefore, exoskeletons in the past use a 3R spherical wrist mechanism often with 90° links to replicate the spherical movement [4–8]. Most shoulder exoskeletons have a structure similar to that shown in Fig. 4.4, where a most distal joint (Joint 3) is incorporated into a revolving mechanism around the upper arm. However, the 3R mechanism behaves like a gimbal and consequently possesses problematic singular configurations [8, 9]. These singular configurations occur when the axes of rotation of two rotary joints align with each other, resulting in the loss of 1-DOF. The human shoulder joint behaves like a spherical joint which does not possess any singular configurations and therefore does not experience this problem. The 3R mechanism, however, has two distinct singular configurations which occur when the axis of rotation of the base joint (Joint 1) align with the axis of rotation of the distal joint (Joint 3). One singular configuration occurs when the axis of Joint 3 is in the same direction as the axis of Joint 1. The second singular configuration occurs when the axis of Joint 3 is 180° opposite to that of the first configuration as shown in Fig. 4.4.

When the 3R mechanism approaches a singular configuration, the mechanism has difficulty performing rotations about the axis that is lost. A slow rotation of the shoulder about the affected axis requires high velocities from the 3R joints. The worst case is when two of the 3R joints completely align with one another, i.e. a

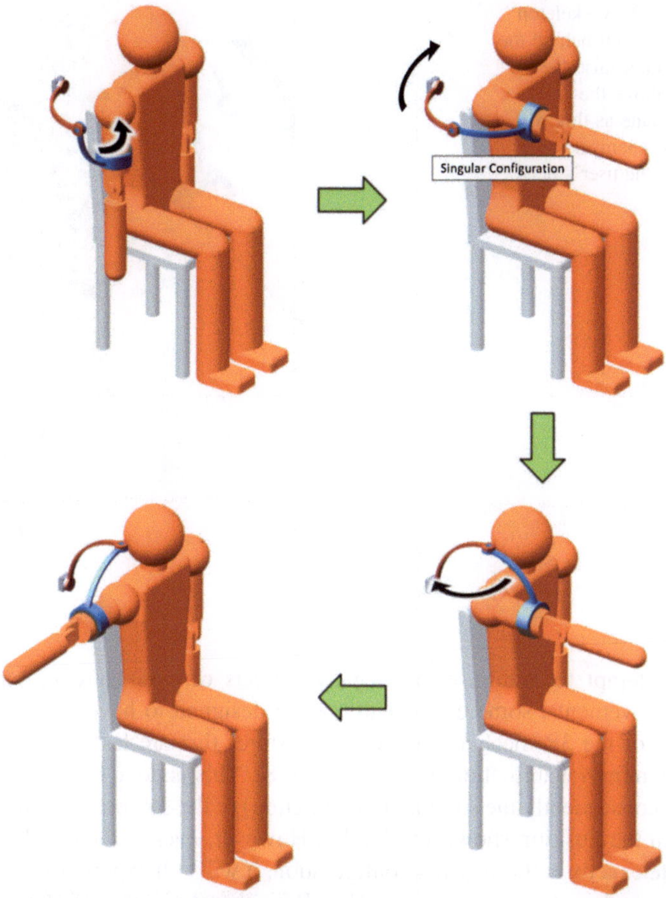

Fig. 4.5 A 3R exoskeleton moves into a singular configuration shown in the *top right* figure, where the axis of rotation of Joint 3 aligns with the axis of rotation of Joint 1. In this configuration, the exoskeleton cannot produce horizontal flexion and extension of the shoulder unless Joint 1 is adjusted into the position shown in the *bottom right* figure

singular configuration occurs. In this situation, the 3R mechanism needs to change its configuration instantaneously in order to produce smooth shoulder rotations about the lost axis (see Fig. 4.5). This is not possible in practice as there will always be a time delay to move the 3R mechanism into the necessary configuration. This causes the exoskeleton to produce jerky movements which can hinder the user's shoulder movement and cause injuries or discomfort. The design shown in Fig. 4.4 is the simplest design of the 3R exoskeleton with the base joint of the 3R mechanism positioned directly behind the shoulder. However, this exoskeleton design has a very limited range of motion due to the limited space available for the movement of the mechanism's links. It is not possible for this exoskeleton to raise the user's upper arm above the horizontal plane as this will cause part of the 3R mechanism to collide with the user's head. This problem is illustrated in Fig. 4.6.

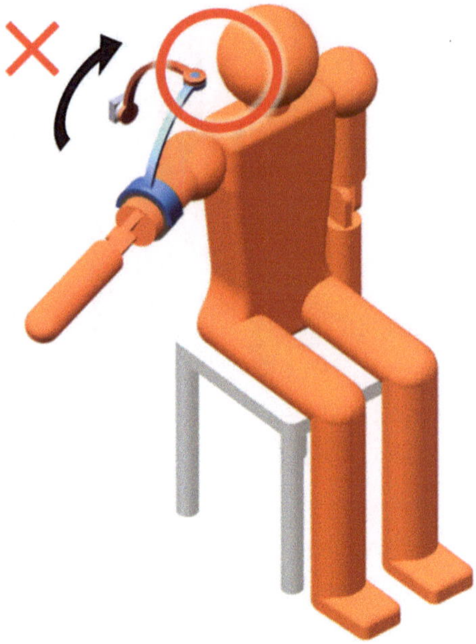

Fig. 4.6 A 3R exoskeleton with the base joint behind the shoulder cannot raise the upper arm above the horizontal plane as this will cause the mechanism to collide with the user's head

In an attempt to minimise the negative effects of singular configurations on shoulder movements, some exoskeletons were designed to have the singular configurations of the 3R mechanism occur at postures that are less likely to interfere with performing rehabilitation exercises [5, 7, 8]. This is done by moving the base joint (and consequently the singular configuration) of the 3R mechanism laterally so that it is in the position shown in Fig. 4.7. However, even if the exoskeleton does not operate exactly at the singular configuration, it will still experience a decrease in performance when it operates nearby. The 3R mechanism with a 45° lateral offset of the base joint can achieve a larger range of motion than the simpler design in Fig. 4.4, as it is possible to raise the user's arm above the horizontal plane. However, the 3R mechanism will still move dangerously close to the user's head when the upper arm is raised above the horizontal plane. In addition, raising the upper arm backwards will make the arm dangerously close to the base joint of the 3R mechanism as shown in Fig. 4.8.

It is possible to avoid the singular configurations and keep the mechanism away from potential collisions if a redundant joint is introduced into the 3R mechanism. The resulting 4R spherical wrist mechanism (Fig. 4.9) has one redundant joint which can be used to keep the system away from singular configurations. This 4R spherical wrist concept has been considered for generic robot manipulators in the past [10–13], but it has not been utilised in the design of an exoskeleton's shoulder mechanism. This mechanism has been used in limited studies, possibly because there are better alternatives to using a replicated spherical joint for a generic robot manipulator. A shoulder exoskeleton, however, has very limited joint design possibilities due to the workspace constraints and the necessity to replicate the

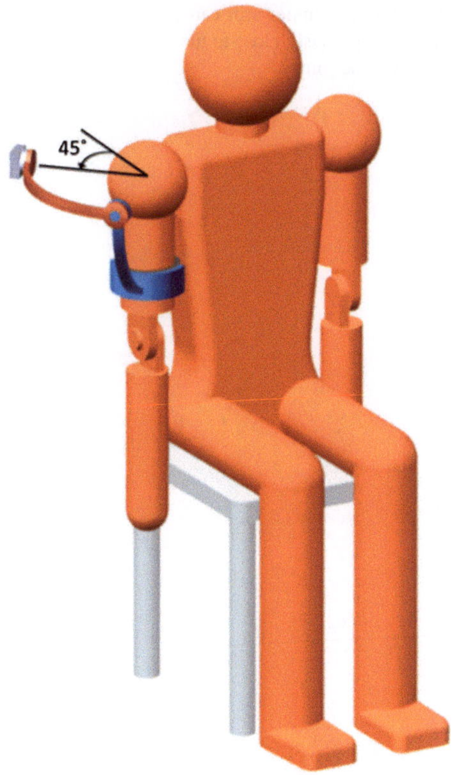

Fig. 4.7 The 3R exoskeleton design with the base joint offset laterally by 45° from behind the shoulder

shoulder's spherical movements. In this case, a 4R mechanism is very suitable. In this research, the 4R mechanism is considered for the design of an upper limb exoskeleton's shoulder complex.

4.2 The 4R Mechanism for the Exoskeleton Shoulder

The 4R mechanism has four revolute joints and is therefore considered a 4-DOF robot. However, the 4R mechanism is only capable of moving the end-effector in 3-DOF of spherical motion about the ICOR. Hence, the 4R mechanism can be described as a 4-DOF redundant robot with 3-DOF of spherical motion. This kinematic redundancy is required to avoid singular configurations of the mechanism and prevent mechanical interference with the user while achieving the entire shoulder workspace.

The fundamental 4R mechanism consists of a stationary base, an end-effector and three links (L_1, L_2, L_3) connected in series through four revolute joints (θ_1, θ_2, θ_3, θ_4) as shown in Fig. 4.10. Each of the four revolute joints has an axis of rotation that intersects with the ICOR. The joints are positioned a suitable distance away

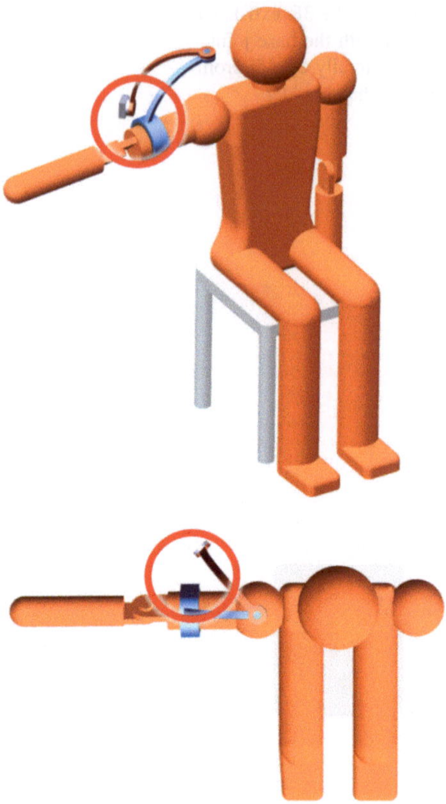

Fig. 4.8 The upper arm can move dangerously close to the shifted base joint

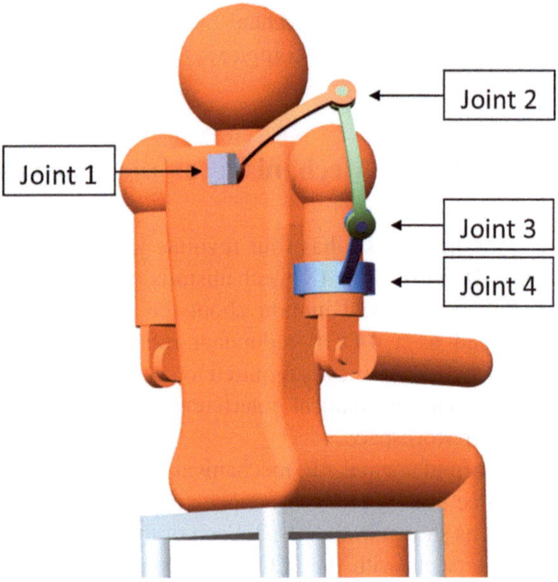

Fig. 4.9 The 4R shoulder mechanism concept

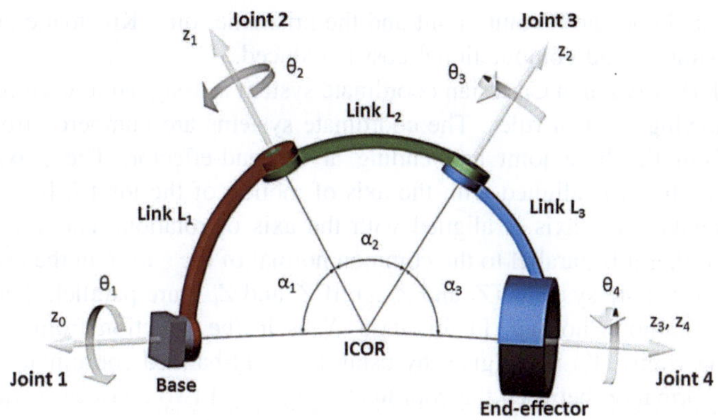

Fig. 4.10 Parameters of the 4R mechanism

from the ICOR so that they do not interfere with the user's shoulder. This allows the 4R mechanism to operate alongside the human upper arm and mimic the spherical movements of the human shoulder joint. Due to the characteristics of the mechanism design, the position and orientation of the end-effector directly reflects the posture of the user's upper arm.

The following terms are used to describe the various aspects of this mechanism:

ICOR	The centre of spherical rotation. All joints of the 4R mechanism intersect at this point. The ICOR of the 4R coincides with the ICOR of the human shoulder joint.
Link angle (α)	The angle between the two joints in the arc-shaped link about the ICOR.
Joint angle/angular position (θ)	The angle of rotational displacement of the revolute joint from the default position.
Joint/end-effector position	The location of the joint/end-effector with respect to the ICOR.
Joint configuration	A combination of joint positions that achieves a certain end-effector position.

4.2.1 Kinematic Modelling of the 4R Mechanism

The kinematics of the multilink 4R mechanism is modelled using the Denavit–Hartenberg (DH) notation [14]. The main advantage of the DH notation is that only four parameters are required for each joint whereas six parameters are normally required for 6-DOF of a rigid body in 3D space. This is made possible by kinematic constraints present in the two types of 1-DOF robotic joints that can be used in a serial manipulator, the revolute joint and the prismatic joint. Kinematic analysis is therefore simpler and computational cost is reduced.

In the DH notation, a Cartesian coordinate system is assigned to each robot joint while following a set of rules. The coordinate systems are numbered from 0 to n starting from the base joint and ending at the end-effector. The z-axis (Z_i) is assigned so that it is aligned with the axis of motion of the joint i. In the case of revolute joints, the z-axis is aligned with the axis of rotation. The x-axis (X_i) is assigned so that it is parallel to the common normal of the z-axes in the current and precious coordinate systems (Z_i and Z_{i-1}). If Z_i and Z_{i-1} are parallel, then there is no unique common normal. In this case, X_i is in the direction from Z_{i-1} to Z_i. Finally, the y-axis (Y_i) is assigned by using the right-handed coordinate system.

A transformation between the coordinate systems of two consecutive joints in a serial robot is described by one transformation associated with the joint $[J]$ and a second transformation associated with the link $[L]$. The coordinate transformation along a serial robot is then a sequence of these transformations. For a robot with n links, the complete kinematics equation of the robot is given by (4.1) where $[T]$ is the transformation from the base joint to the end-effector.

$$[T] = [J_1][L_1][J_2][L_2]\ldots[J_n][L_n] \tag{4.1}$$

By defining the coordinate systems using the DH notation outlined above, the transformations can be defined by (4.2) and (4.3), where θ_i is the angle about Z_{i-1} from X_{i-1} to X_i and is the joint variable if joint i is rotary; d_i is the distance along Z_{i-1} from the origin of the $(i-1)$th coordinate system to the common normal of Z_{i-1} and Z_i and is the joint variable if joint i is prismatic; a_i is the length of the common normal of Z_{i-1} and Z_i from the Z_{i-1} axis to the Z_i axis; and α_i is the angle about the common normal of Z_{i-1} and Z_i from the Z_{i-1} axis to the Z_i axis.

$$[J_i] = \begin{bmatrix} \cos\theta_i & -\sin\theta_i & 0 & 0 \\ \sin\theta_i & \cos\theta_i & 0 & 0 \\ 0 & 0 & 1 & d_i \\ 0 & 0 & 0 & 1 \end{bmatrix} \tag{4.2}$$

$$[L_i] = \begin{bmatrix} 1 & 0 & 0 & a_i \\ 0 & \cos\alpha_i & -\sin\alpha_i & 0 \\ 0 & \sin\alpha_i & \cos\alpha_i & 0 \\ 0 & 0 & 0 & 1 \end{bmatrix} \tag{4.3}$$

These transformations are a sequence of translations and rotations where

$$[J_i] = \mathrm{Trans}_{J_i}(d_i)\mathrm{Rot}_{J_i}(\theta_i) \tag{4.4}$$

$$[L_i] = \mathrm{Trans}_{L_i}(a_i)\mathrm{Rot}_{L_i}(\alpha_i) \tag{4.5}$$

$$\mathrm{Rot}_{J_i}(\theta_i) = \begin{bmatrix} \cos\theta_i & -\sin\theta_i & 0 & 0 \\ \sin\theta_i & \cos\theta_i & 0 & 0 \\ 0 & 0 & 1 & 0 \\ 0 & 0 & 0 & 1 \end{bmatrix} \tag{4.6}$$

$$\mathrm{Rot}_{L_i}(\alpha_i) = \begin{bmatrix} 1 & 0 & 0 & 0 \\ 0 & \cos\alpha_i & -\sin\alpha_i & 0 \\ 0 & \sin\alpha_i & \cos\alpha_i & 0 \\ 0 & 0 & 0 & 1 \end{bmatrix} \tag{4.7}$$

The coordinate systems of two consecutive joints are related as

$$T_i^{i-1} = [J_i][L_i] \tag{4.8}$$

This gives the DH transformation matrix as

$$T_i^{i-1} = \begin{bmatrix} \cos\theta_i & -\cos\alpha_i \sin\theta_i & \sin\alpha_i \sin\theta_i & a_i \cos\theta_i \\ \sin\theta_i & \cos\alpha_i \cos\theta_i & -\sin\alpha_i \cos\theta_i & a_i \sin\theta_i \\ 0 & \sin\alpha_i & \cos\alpha_i & d_i \\ 0 & 0 & 0 & 1 \end{bmatrix} \tag{4.9}$$

To interpret the transformation, the matrix can be represented as (4.10), where R is the 3×3 rotation matrix (4.11) which represents the relative orientation between the two coordinate systems (i.e. relates the X_i, Y_i, Z_i axes with the $X_{i-1}, Y_{i-1}, Z_{i-1}$ axes) and r is the 3×1 translation vector (4.12) which represents the relative position between the two coordinate systems.

$$T = \begin{bmatrix} R & r \\ 0^{\mathrm{T}} & 1 \end{bmatrix} \tag{4.10}$$

$$R = \begin{bmatrix} \cos\theta_i & -\cos\alpha_i \sin\theta_i & \sin\alpha_i \sin\theta_i \\ \sin\theta_i & \cos\alpha_i \cos\theta_i & -\sin\alpha_i \cos\theta_i \\ 0 & \sin\alpha_i & \cos\alpha_i \end{bmatrix} \tag{4.11}$$

$$r = \begin{bmatrix} r_x \\ r_y \\ r_z \end{bmatrix} = \begin{bmatrix} a_i \cos\theta_i \\ a_i \sin\theta_i \\ d_i \end{bmatrix} \tag{4.12}$$

Transformation into subsequent coordinate systems is achieved by combining the transformation matrices between each successive coordinate system using (4.13). This allows the determination of the relative position and orientation of any subsequent coordinate system with respect to a previous reference coordinate system and vice versa.

$$T_i^0 = T_1^0 T_2^1 \ldots T_i^{i-1} \tag{4.13}$$

The global coordinate system is located at the ICOR of the right shoulder with the x-axis pointing to the right, y-axis pointing forward and z-axis pointing upward with respect to the user. A coordinate system is defined for each subsequent joint using the DH notation. For simplicity, the coordinate system of each joint is defined with an origin at the ICOR of the 4R mechanism, i.e. the length parameters a_i and d_i for all i are zero. This is acceptable because the axis of rotation of all the joints in the 4R mechanism always intersect at the ICOR. As a result, the occurrence of singular configurations is dependent on only the orientation of the joints and independent of the distance between the joints and the ICOR. The DH parameters for the 4R mechanism are shown in Table 4.1. Note that the first line of parameters is used to define the orientation of the base joint with respect to the global coordinate system. Therefore, the numbering of the parameters in Table 4.1 is delayed by one.

The DH parameters of the 4R mechanism are used to obtain the transformation matrices that represent the geometric relationship between each pair of adjacent coordinate systems

$$T_1^0 = \begin{bmatrix} \cos\varphi_z & -\cos\varphi_x \sin\varphi_z & \sin\varphi_x \sin\varphi_z & 0 \\ \sin\varphi_z & \cos\varphi_x \cos\varphi_z & -\sin\varphi_x \cos\varphi_z & 0 \\ 0 & \sin\varphi_x & \cos\varphi_x & 0 \\ 0 & 0 & 0 & 1 \end{bmatrix} \tag{4.14}$$

$$T_2^1 = \begin{bmatrix} \cos\theta_1 & -\cos\alpha_1 \sin\theta_1 & -\sin\alpha_1 \sin\theta_1 & 0 \\ \sin\theta_1 & \cos\alpha_1 \cos\theta_1 & \sin\alpha_1 \cos\theta_1 & 0 \\ 0 & -\sin\alpha_1 & \cos\alpha_1 & 0 \\ 0 & 0 & 0 & 1 \end{bmatrix} \tag{4.15}$$

$$T_3^2 = \begin{bmatrix} \cos\theta_2 & -\cos\alpha_2 \sin\theta_2 & \sin\alpha_2 \sin\theta_2 & 0 \\ \sin\theta_2 & \cos\alpha_2 \cos\theta_2 & -\sin\alpha_2 \cos\theta_2 & 0 \\ 0 & \sin\alpha_2 & \cos\alpha_2 & 0 \\ 0 & 0 & 0 & 1 \end{bmatrix} \tag{4.16}$$

Table 4.1 DH parameters of the 4R robot

Link i	a_i	α_i	d_i	θ_i
1	0	φ_x	0	φ_z
2	0	$-\alpha_1$	0	θ_1
3	0	α_2	0	θ_2
4	0	α_3	0	θ_3
5	0	0	0	θ_4

$$T_4^3 = \begin{bmatrix} \cos\theta_3 & -\cos\alpha_3\sin\theta_3 & \sin\alpha_3\sin\theta_3 & 0 \\ \sin\theta_3 & \cos\alpha_3\cos\theta_3 & -\sin\alpha_3\cos\theta_3 & 0 \\ 0 & \sin\alpha_3 & \cos\alpha_3 & 0 \\ 0 & 0 & 0 & 1 \end{bmatrix} \quad (4.17)$$

$$T_5^4 = \begin{bmatrix} \cos\theta_4 & -\sin\theta_4 & 0 & 0 \\ \sin\theta_4 & \cos\theta_4 & 0 & 0 \\ 0 & 0 & 1 & 0 \\ 0 & 0 & 0 & 1 \end{bmatrix} \quad (4.18)$$

These transformation matrices are used to transform coordinates between the various coordinate systems in the 4R mechanism.

4.2.2 *Forward Kinematics*

Forward kinematics involves the use of known kinematic parameters of a robot's joints and structure to compute the position and orientation of its end-effector. In the case of a shoulder exoskeleton based on a spherical wrist mechanism, forward kinematics utilises the angles of each exoskeleton joint to determine the position and orientation of the end-effector which is effectively the user's upper arm. However, only the orientation is considered during analysis since position does not affect singularity of the mechanism. Also, the position of the upper arm with respect to the shoulder is directly related to its orientation. Therefore, positional information can be omitted to simplify the problem during the analysis of the spherical wrist.

Forward kinematics of the 4R mechanism is achieved by the multiplication of the DH transformation matrices

$$T_5^0 = T_1^0 T_2^1 T_3^2 T_4^3 T_5^4 \quad (4.19)$$

The resulting matrix represents the orientation of the coordinate system coupled to the upper arm with respect to the global coordinate system.

4.2.3 *Inverse Kinematics*

Inverse kinematics is the process of determining a set of required robot joint angles to reach a specified end-effector position. Solving the inverse kinematics problem is more challenging than the forward kinematics problem, particularly for a kinematically redundant system like the 4R mechanism.

There are infinite solutions to the inverse kinematics problem for any given end-effector position due to the kinematic redundancy of the 4R mechanism. However, if the desired end-effector position and the joint angle of one of the three proximal joints are known, the angles of the remaining joints can be derived using inverse kinematics. In this work, the angle of Joint 1 (θ_1) is generated by an algorithm. Therefore, the inverse kinematics problem now involves finding the configuration of a non-redundant 3R mechanism (i.e. the angular positions θ_2, θ_3 and θ_4) which has a finite number of solutions. However, θ_4 only affects the axial rotation of the end-effector and not the position since the end-effector is located in the same position as Joint 4. This means that the end-effector position (i.e. shoulder flexion and extension and abduction and adduction) is dependent on θ_1, θ_2 and θ_3 while the end-effector axial orientation (i.e. shoulder medial and lateral rotation) is dependent on θ_4. The resulting inverse kinematics problem is then to find θ_2 and θ_3 to achieve a desired end-effector position with a given value of θ_1.

The inverse kinematics problem for the 4R robot is solved using a heuristic iterative method based on the Forward and Backward Reaching Inverse Kinematics (FABRIK) algorithm [15]. The FABRIK algorithm has the advantage of converging to a solution with few iterations and has low computational cost.

An iteration of the FABRIK method is a two stage process that begins at the last joint in the chain and works inwards, adjusting the position of each joint along the way. This process is then repeated outwards in the second stage to complete a full iteration. Each iteration moves the end-effector closer to the target position. Hence, the iterations are repeated until the end-effector is sufficiently close to the specified target position. A graphical representation of a full iteration of the FABRIK algorithm applied to a planar manipulator is presented in Fig. 4.11.

For manipulators that move in 3D space, the orientations of each revolute joint's axis must also be considered when applying the FABRIK algorithm described above to ensure the constraints imposed by the links' structures are enforced. This becomes a tedious task since both position and orientation must be considered. However, the characteristics of the 4R mechanism allow a simplified method to be used. For the 4R mechanism, which has all its joints rotate about an ICOR, inverse kinematics is effectively used to find the orientation of each joint axis with respect to the ICOR. Therefore, the FABRIK algorithm has been modified for this research to utilise angular positions rather than linear positions.

First, the conditions which cause a target end-effector position to be unreachable by the 4R mechanism are identified since there will not be an inverse kinematics solution. In the case of the 4R, the distance of the end-effector from the ICOR is always constant. Therefore, the unreachable angular directions of the end-effector are determined using the link angles. The end-effector of the 4R cannot reach a target position if any one of the following geometric conditions is true. These are when the angle at the ICOR between Joint 2 and the target end-effector position φ_t is greater than the sum of the link angles α_2 and α_3 (4.20) or smaller than the difference between the link angles α_2 and α_3 (4.21). Examples of these two conditions are shown in Figs. 4.12 and 4.13.

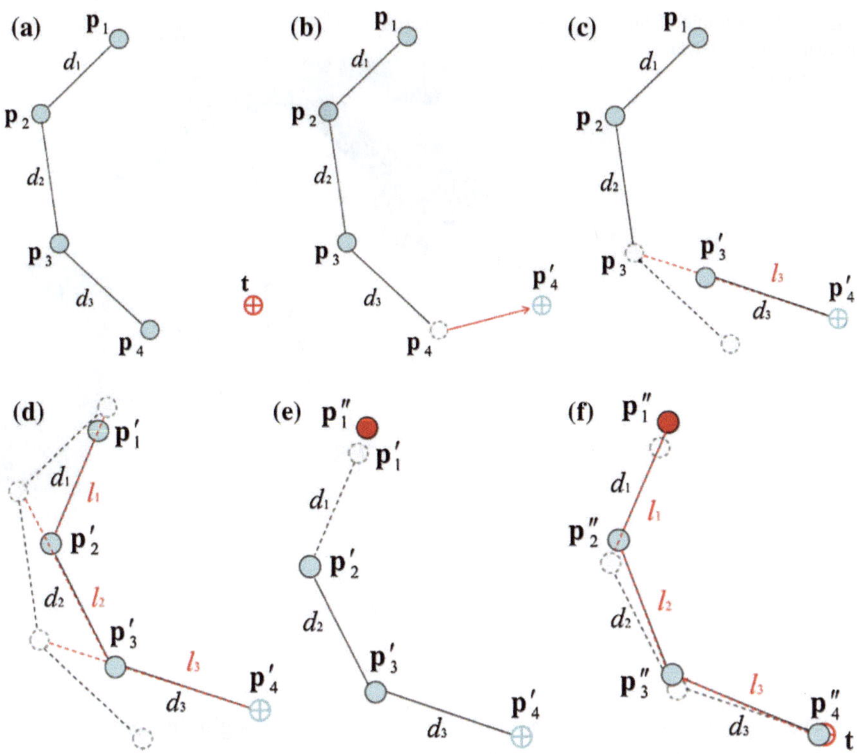

Fig. 4.11 An example of a full iteration of the FABRIK algorithm for a three-jointed planar manipulator [15]. **a** The initial position of the manipulator and the target, **b** move the end-effector $\mathbf{p}_4$ to the target **t**, **c** find the joint $\mathbf{p}_3'$ which lies on the line l_3 that passes through the points $\mathbf{p}_4'$ and $\mathbf{p}_3$, and has distance $\boldsymbol{d}_3$ from the joint $\mathbf{p}_4'$, **d** continue the algorithm for the rest of the joints, **e** the second stage of the algorithm begins by moving the base joint $\mathbf{p}_1'$ to its initial position, **f** repeat the same procedure, but this time start from the base and move outwards to the end-effector. The algorithm is repeated until the position of the end-effector gets sufficiently close to the target at the end of the second stage

Fig. 4.12 Example of an unreachable target that satisfies (3.23)

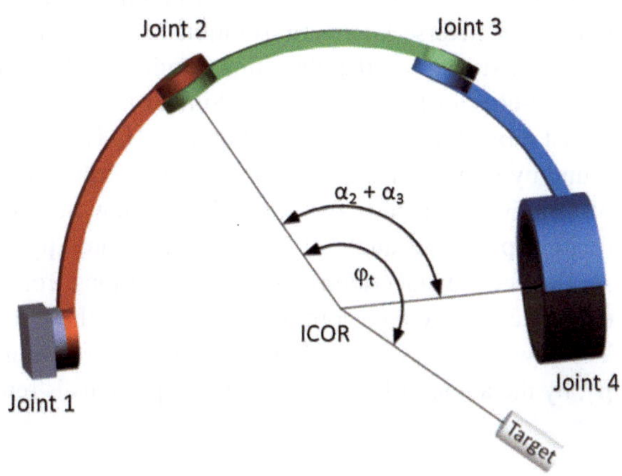

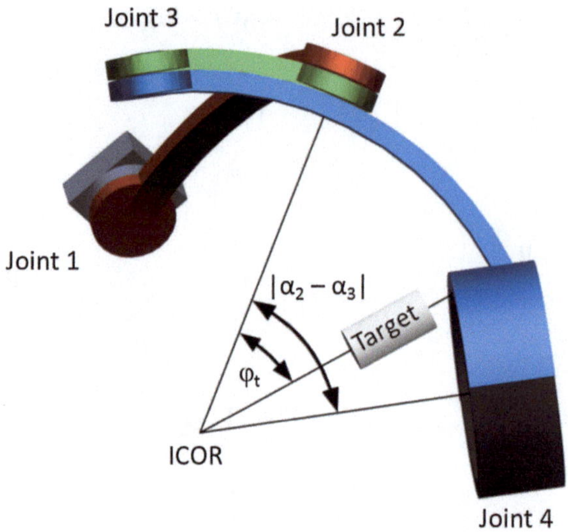

Fig. 4.13 Example of an unreachable target that satisfies (3.24)

$$\varphi_t > \alpha_2 + \alpha_3 \tag{4.20}$$

$$\varphi_t < |\alpha_2 - \alpha_3| \tag{4.21}$$

These conditions apply to the problem specified at the beginning of this section, in which the positions of Joints 1 and 2 and target position of Joint 4 are known and the position of Joint 3 required to achieve the specified position of Joint 4 needs to be determined. In addition, distal joints are not permitted to be positioned under a proximal link. This is to ensure that the links will not interfere with actuators attached on top of the joints.

The parameters in the modified FABRIK algorithm are defined similar to the definition used in the original FABRIK algorithm. $\mathbf{p}_1, \ldots, \mathbf{p}_4$ are the joint positions where $\mathbf{p}_1$ is Joint 1 and $\mathbf{p}_4$ is the end-effector (Joint 4), while $\mathbf{t}$ is the target position for the end-effector and $\mathbf{b}$ is the initial base position. Note that Joint 2 is the base joint in this problem since the angle of Joint 1 is predefined to ensure that a finite number of inverse kinematic solutions can be obtained.

The first stage of the algorithm requires each joint position to be adjusted from the end-effector to the base joint. Similar to the original algorithm, the end-effector is first moved to the target position, $\mathbf{p}'_4 = \mathbf{t}$. The new position of Joint 3, $\mathbf{p}'_3$, is then found by rotating the position of the end-effector, $\mathbf{p}'_4$, about the ICOR by the angle of Link 3, α_3, towards $\mathbf{p}_3$. Similarly, the new position of Joint 2, $\mathbf{p}'_2$, is located by rotating $\mathbf{p}'_3$ by the angle of Link 2, α_2, towards $\mathbf{p}_2$.

The second stage adjusts the joint positions from the base joint (Joint 2) to the end-effector. The base joint is first moved to the initial base joint position, $\mathbf{p}''_2 = \mathbf{b}$. The new position of $\mathbf{p}'_3$, $\mathbf{p}''_3$, is then found by rotating the position of the base joint, $\mathbf{p}''_2$, by the angle of Link 2, α_2, towards $\mathbf{p}'_3$. This is repeated for Link 3 to find a new position for the end-effector. This completes a single iteration of the modified FABRIK algorithm. The iterations are repeated until the end-effector position is sufficiently close to the target position, **t**.

The modified FABRIK algorithm requires the rotation of joint positions about the origin. This is done using Quaternion rotations. Quaternions are a convenient mathematical notation for representing orientations and rotations of objects in 3D space. Euler's rotation theorem states that any rotation or sequence of rotations about a fixed point is equivalent to a single rotation by a given angle about a fixed axis that runs through the fixed point called the Euler axis. The Euler axis is represented by a vector in the Cartesian coordinate system and the angle of rotation is represented by a scalar. A Quaternion is defined by four parameters (4.22), where the three parameters x, y and z describe the axis of rotation and the fourth parameter w indicates the angle of rotation about this axis [16].

$$q(w, x, y, z) \tag{4.22}$$

Rotation quaternions can be used to rotate a point in 3D space about a specified axis by a specified angle. Since only a single rotation is performed, this method does not have the singularity problem that occurs when using a sequence of Euler rotations. For a unit Quaternion, this can be simplified to

$$Q = \begin{bmatrix} 1 - 2y^2 - 2z^2 & 2xy - 2wz & 2xz + 2wy \\ 2xy + 2wz & 1 - 2x^2 - 2z^2 & 2yz - 2wx \\ 2xz - 2wy & 2yz + 2wx & 1 - 2x^2 - 2y^2 \end{bmatrix} \tag{4.23}$$

This transformation matrix is applied to the Cartesian joint position to rotate it about the axis defined by x, y and z with an angle of w to find the position of the adjacent joint

$$p_{n-1} = Qp_n \tag{4.24}$$

Using the first step of the modified FABRIK algorithm as an example: the axis of rotation defined by x, y and z is orthogonal to the plane formed between $\mathbf{p}'_4$, $\mathbf{p}_3$ and the ICOR. The angle of rotation w is the angle size of Link 3, α_3. Applying the Quaternion rotation transforms the new position of the end-effector, $\mathbf{p}'_4$, into the coordinates of the new position of Joint 3, $\mathbf{p}'_3$.

The modified FABRIK algorithm always requires a starting configuration to converge from. However, there are configurations that can cause the algorithm to fail in converging to a solution. This occurs when the second stage of the algorithm returns the joint configuration to the state prior to the first stage. The starting configurations that cause this have all three joints positioned in the same plane, i.e. Links 2 and 3 are parallel with each other. Therefore, to avoid this problem, a starting configuration is generated which has Link 3 positioned orthogonal to Link 2. Algorithm first checks if the angle between the target end-effector position and the base joint (Joint 2) position about the ICOR is equal to either the sum or the difference of the two link angles. If this is the case, then the inverse kinematics solution is simply a configuration with the two links pointing towards the target end-effector position and the modified FABRIK algorithm does not need to be applied. In this research, the modified FABRIK algorithm is terminated once a configuration is obtained with an end-effector position error of less than one.

4.2.4 Range of Motion of Joint 4 and Shoulder Axial Rotation

Joint 4 in the 4R mechanism is implemented using a curved rail mechanism around the upper arm. It is important to keep the range of motion of Joint 4 small to minimise the size of the rail used for this joint. A smaller rail makes the device easier for the user to don and reduces the invasiveness of the mechanism. Joint 4 can independently control shoulder axial rotation. Therefore, range of motion of this joint need to match the shoulder axial rotation.

It has been realised that there are two possible inverse kinematic solutions in most cases, even when the position of Joint 2 is given. An example of this is shown in Fig. 4.14. The two possible solutions are symmetrical to each other with the plane of symmetry intersecting the axis of Joint 2 and the end-effector position. The only case in which there is only one inverse kinematic solution is when Joint 3 also lies in this plane of symmetry.

However, the range of motion of both Joint 4 and the human shoulder axial rotation drifts depending on the end-effector (or upper arm) position in the workspace [17]. In the case of Joint 4, this drift depends on the kinematic design of the

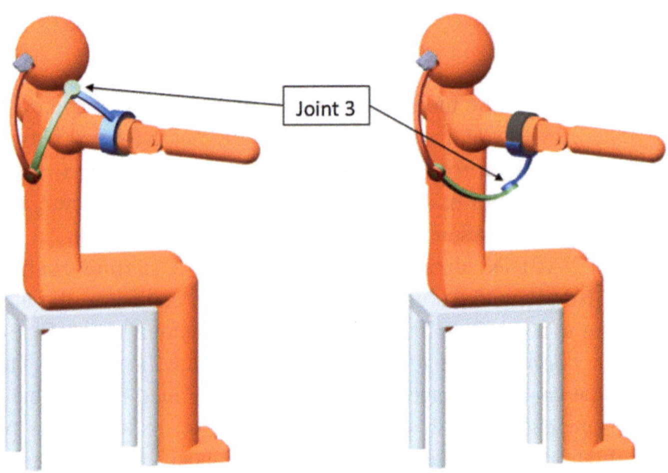

Fig. 4.14 Example of two inverse kinematic solutions in which the 4R mechanism has the same Joint 1, 2 and 4 (end-effector) positions but different Joint 3 position

4R spherical wrist mechanism. Therefore, it is necessary to compare the angular position drift of the exoskeleton's Joint 4 with the corresponding drift of the shoulder's axial rotation. A deviation between the two drifting angular positions will require Joint 4 to have a larger range of motion to ensure that the exoskeleton can reach the extreme limits of shoulder axial rotation. The maximum deviation between the two drifting angular positions in both the positive and negative rotational direction determine the additional range of motion required in Joint 4.

4.3 Physiological Model of the Elbow Joint

4.3.1 Elbow Model Development

This section presents the conceptualisation and development of the model as one of the core components of the NI for the elbow joint [18, 19]. The physiological model consists of three main parts or sub-models: the musculotendon model, the musculoskeletal model and the kinematic model. The interactions between the sub-models are shown in Fig. 4.15. The musculotendon model takes the normalised muscle activation level obtained from a signal filtering process to estimate the resulting muscle force by using a Hill-type muscle model. This model resulted from the developments of Hill, who characterised the dynamic behaviour of muscles by investigating the heat produced during dynamic contractions [20]. The musculotendon model is a mechanical analogy to a biological system that has been validated with experimental data, and there is a musculotendon model for each actuating muscle group.

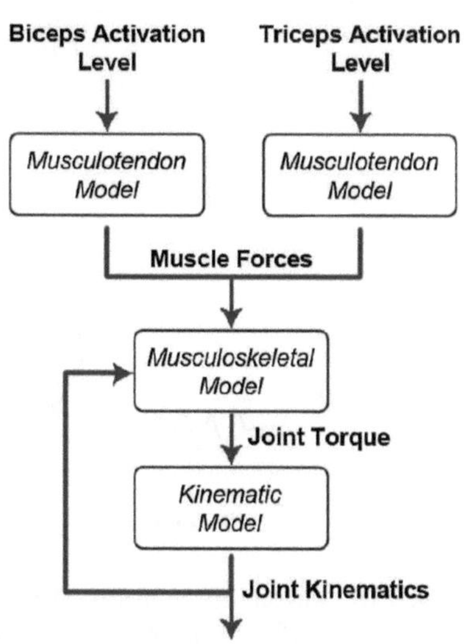

Fig. 4.15 Sub-models and relationships within the physiological model of the elbow. Activation level inputs are the processed EMG signals

4.3.1.1 Musculotendon Models

The purpose of the musculotendon model is to determine the forces being produced by the underlying muscles from the surface EMG signal activation levels. It consists of the main muscle belly, which provides the main contraction force, and tendons at opposite ends, which attach the muscle to the insertion and origin points on the skeletal structure (see Fig. 4.16 for the main sections). This requires a model of the contraction dynamics of the muscle and a Hill-type muscle model was employed.

Hill-type muscle models are built on experimental data and as a result have many different incarnations with variable responses, and are not always relevant to a broad spectrum of movement types. However, because the fundamental approach and methodology are similar, the musculotendon model can be developed from Hill-type muscle models that demonstrate desirable behaviours that are relevant to this specific application. The elbow joint only has two main muscle activation groups for flexion and extension, and the accuracy of the dynamic modelling of the musculotendon system will have a smaller effect on the overall system.

Each musculotendon unit was biomechanically modelled as a muscular unit containing three parallel components: an active contractile element, a non-linear passive elastic component and a passive damping component (to emulate the fluid-filled connective tissues), and two tendon units in series [21]. This mechanical system analogy presents a representation of muscle that reflects its dynamic behaviour. The pennation angle of the muscle (ϕ) was assumed to be 0° so that tendon force was equivalent to muscle force. It was also assumed that tendon stiffness was high enough that changes in length of the tendon were negligible, and a stiff-tendon muscular model would not be significantly detrimental to model performance [22]. The total muscle force (for a single musculotendon unit) is therefore given by the summation of active, passive and viscous forces and found as follows:

$$F_{\mathrm{Tot}} = F_{\mathrm{CE}} + F_{\mathrm{PE}} + F_{\mathrm{VE}} \tag{4.25}$$

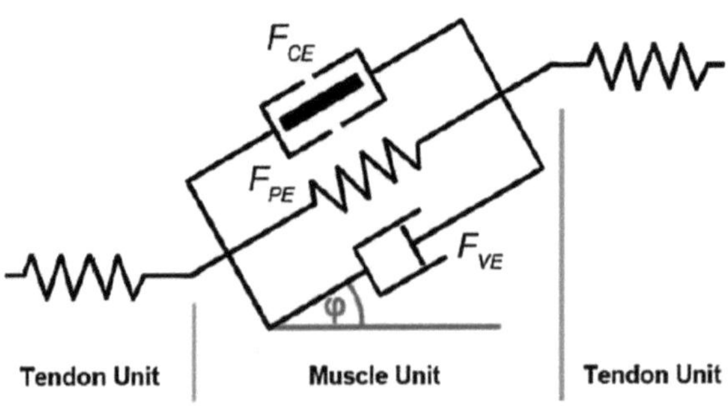

Fig. 4.16 Musculotendon model. The muscle unit consists of a contractile force element (F_{CE}), passive elastic force (F_{PE}) and viscous force (F_{VE})

The force from the contractile element of the muscle can be found as

$$F_{\text{CE}} = R \cdot f(l) \cdot f(v) \cdot A \cdot F_{\text{Max}} \tag{4.26}$$

where R is a subject-specific parameter that accounts for differences in muscle size and strength, A is the normalised activation level of the muscle that is the output from signal processing, F_{Max} is the maximum force that can be produced by the muscle (averaged from the literature) and f(l) and f(v) are the muscle force-length and force-velocity relationships, respectively.

The passive elastic component of the musculotendon model represents the lumped elastic properties of the muscle and tendon. This is based on the relationship determined by [23]

$$F_{\text{PE}} = F_{\text{Max}} \cdot \exp\left(10 \cdot C_{\text{pass}}(l_n - 1)\right)/\exp(5) \tag{4.27}$$

where C_{pass} is a term that allows adjustment to suit subject-specific passive elastic properties and this also contributes to the behaviour of the model after active inputs are removed. Figure 4.17 shows the response of the passive elastic force component and the effect of increasing C_{pass}. Lower values of C_{pass} cause a more gradual increase of passivity and are suggested for muscles that have a wide range of movement. Higher values of C_{pass} cause a more rapid increase in passive elastic force, and this seems applicable to shorter muscles in response to extraneous movements.

The inclusion of a passive damping component has been a point of discussion with some groups determining its inclusion as unnecessary and as a result, excluded it [23, 24], while others have concluded that muscle viscosity is important for the contractile process and passive damping is necessary for muscle stability [25–27]. The muscular viscous element is based on work by [21] and is given as

$$F_{\text{VE}} = F_{\text{Max}} \cdot B \cdot v_n \tag{4.28}$$

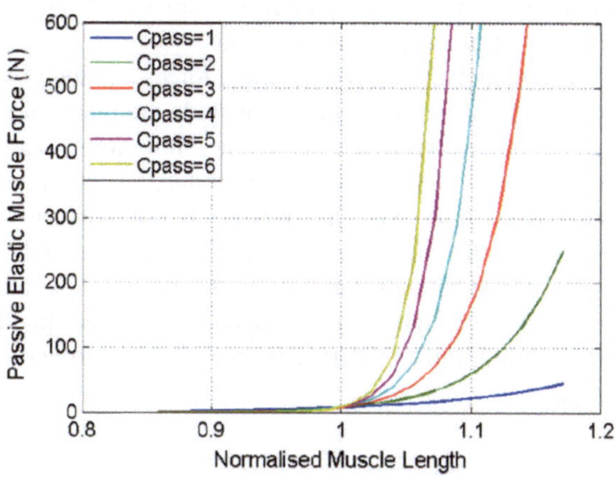

Fig. 4.17 Passive elastic force component response to changes in C_{pass}. In this example, the maximum force of the muscle has been set to 1212 N with an optimal muscle length of 0.26 m

where B is the damping coefficient for the viscosity. Although the damping coefficient is also a function of muscle shortening velocity [27], in this case it will be assumed to be constant.

4.3.1.2 Musculoskeletal Model

The musculoskeletal model consists of an amalgamation of muscle architecture and bone structure of the elbow joint, upper arm and forearm. The elbow joint can be approximated as a single hinge joint with a fixed centre of rotation with respect to joint angle and a constant resting angle [28]. The resting angle of the elbow joint should not be confused with the carrying angle, which is defined as the angle of natural misalignment between the humerus and forearm when the elbow is extended with the palm facing upwards [29]. The resting angle refers to the natural bend at the elbow joint when all muscle activation levels are relaxed and near zero. This is caused by the passive forces in the elbow joint, and more specifically in the biceps group, which when relaxed applies a small amount of tension that causes the forearm to lift slightly, despite its weight.

Figure 4.18 shows a schematic of the musculoskeletal model, which was developed for forearm movements in the sagittal plane and elbow flexion corresponds to a positive displacement (angle d). The bones of the upper and lower arm: humerus (of length Hum and assumed to remain in the vertical position during all movements) and combined ulna and radius (of length L_{Arm} from centre of rotation to end point), are represented by solid black line segments and the active muscle groups that contract as a result of EMG signal activity are in solid blue. These are the biceps (Bi) and triceps (Tr) groups, which attach to the same shoulder "point" at the top of the humerus and on either side of the centre of rotation of the elbow at distances U_{Bi} and U_{Tr}, respectively. It is assumed that bones and lines of muscle action are linear and that the attachments of muscle to bone occur at a single point. Attachment sites and muscle lengths are difficult to measure in vivo and even less when they are presented with underlying physical simplifications. Therefore, many of the musculoskeletal parameters are based on anthropometry data or approximated with reasonable assumptions.

The model also shows the main forces and their directions (in red) that affect the movement of the forearm, and include the biceps force, F_{Bi} and triceps force, F_{Tr}. Unlike other considerations of the elbow joint, which restrict joint motion to the transverse (horizontal) plane by abducting the shoulder to 90° when performing movements [30, 31] this model focuses on movement in the sagittal plane. Therefore, the combined weight of the forearm and hand F_{Arm} acts on the forearm and needs to be considered when determining the total joint torque. It is difficult to measure the weight of the lumped forearm and hand in vivo, so it was estimated from anthropometric data and approximated to act at the midpoint of the forearm ($L_{\mathrm{Arm}} = 2$).

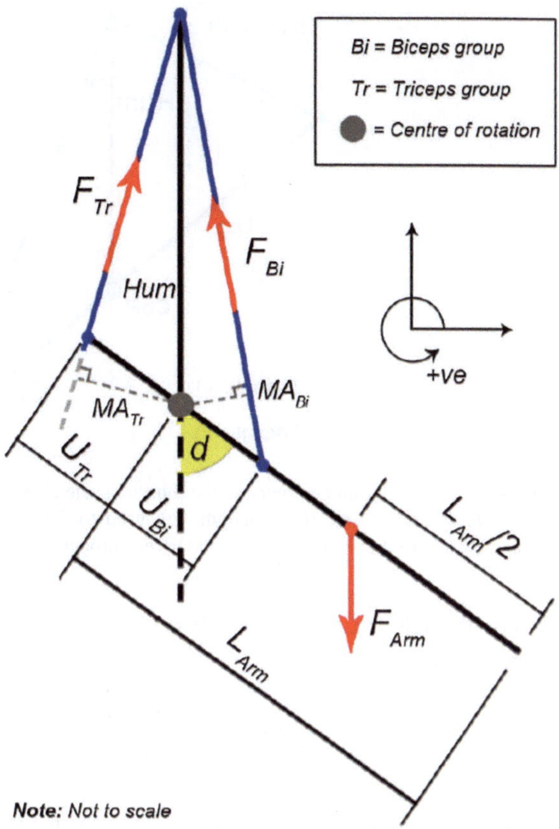

Fig. 4.18 Musculoskeletal model of the elbow joint. The arm is in the sagittal plane, where Hum is the humerus length, U_{Tr} and U_{Bi} are the distances between the centre of rotation and triceps and biceps groups attachment points, respectively, L_{Arm} is the length of the forearm and d is the angle between the forearm and vertical axis

Elbow flexion is considered a positive moment and the moment arms for torque calculations are labelled as $\mathrm{MA_{Bi}}$ and $\mathrm{MA_{Tr}}$. The estimated geometry, such as U_{Bi}, U_{Tr}, Hum and L_{Arm}, can be used to determine the other important geometric properties, including the moment arms and current muscle lengths (distance between their origin and insertion attachment points). Figure 4.19 shows a more detailed portion of the geometry around the centre of rotation, and the corresponding angles that can be used to determine the lengths of the moment arms and the lengths of the approximated muscle groups as follows:

$$\alpha = \pi - d \tag{4.29}$$

For Triangle (a), the cosine rule is applied to determine the current length of the biceps group, applying the cosine rule again to find angle Br

$$\mathrm{Br} = \cos^{-1}\left(\frac{\mathrm{biLength}^2 + U_{\mathrm{Bi}}^2 - \mathrm{Hum}^2}{2 \cdot \mathrm{biLength} \cdot U_{\mathrm{Bi}}}\right) \tag{4.30}$$

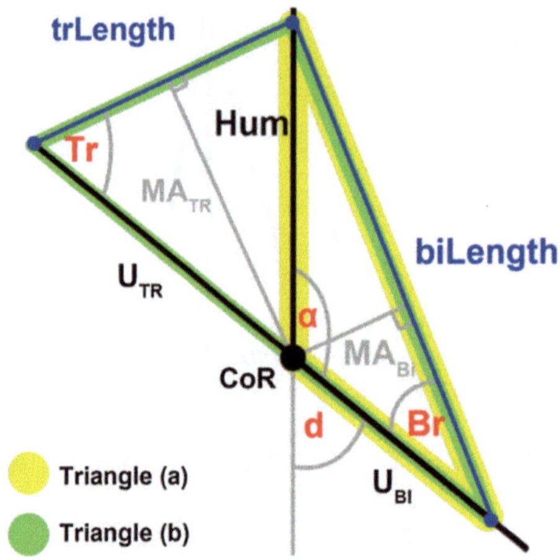

Fig. 4.19 Detailed joint geometry of the musculoskeletal model. The geometric angles (*red*), and bone (*black*) and muscle (*blue*) lengths are used to determine moment arms (*grey*). Triangles (*a*) and (*b*) are used to identify biceps and triceps properties, respectively (see following equations)

For Triangle (b), the cosine rule is applied to determine the current length of the biceps group,

$$\mathrm{Tr} = \cos^{-1}\left(\frac{\mathrm{trLength}^2 + (U_{\mathrm{Bi}} + U_{\mathrm{Tr}})^2 - \mathrm{biLength}^2}{2 \cdot \mathrm{trLength} \cdot (U_{\mathrm{Bi}} + U_{\mathrm{Tr}})}\right) \tag{4.31}$$

Once the entire geometry of the musculoskeletal structure of the joint is known, the length of the moment arms at that instance of time can be determined as

$$\mathrm{MA}_{\mathrm{Bi}} = U_{\mathrm{Bi}} \cdot \sin(\mathrm{Br}) \tag{4.32}$$

$$\mathrm{MA}_{\mathrm{Tr}} = U_{\mathrm{Tr}} \cdot \sin(\mathrm{Tr}) \tag{4.33}$$

4.3.1.3 Kinematic Model

To determine the acceleration, velocity and displacement of the elbow joint the musculoskeletal and musculotendon models need to be combined to determine the overall joint torque. So far, the models have only considered the passive elastic and viscous forces within the muscle, and not the overall joint passivity. It is important to distinguish between muscle force viscosity and an effective viscosity which characterises global mechanical behaviour [32]. These passive forces include elastic and viscous effects from tendons, ligaments and joint components such as the synovial fluid and articular surfaces. A relationship for the total passive joint moment was determined by Stroeve and is provided as follows [31]:

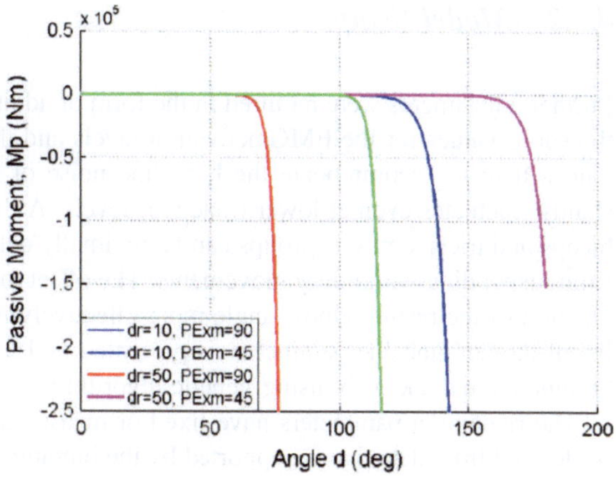

Fig. 4.20 Stroeve's passive joint moment relationship. Shown are the effects of altering the resting angle of the elbow, dr, and range of motion, PE_{xm}

$$M_P = -\beta\omega - \text{sgn}(d - d_r) \cdot M_{Max}/(\exp(PE_{ah} - 1)) \times \exp(PE_{sh}/PE_{xm}|d - d_r|) - 1 \quad (4.34)$$

where β is the elbow joint damping coefficient, sgn is the signum function, d is the current forearm angle, d_r is the resting angle of the forearm, M_{Max} is the maximum elbow moment, PE_{sh} is the passive element shape and PE_{xm} is the range of motion. This relationship is shown in Fig. 4.20 with additional configurations around the nominal values of $d_r = 10$ and $PE_{xm} = 90$.

When the measured and derived musculoskeletal geometry is combined with the musculotendon models discussed in the previous sections and other forces, the total torque about the joint can be determined as

$$M_{Tot} = K_{Bi} \cdot MA_{Bi} \cdot F_{Bi} - K_{Tr} \cdot MA_{Tr} \cdot F_{Tr} - M_W + M_P + O \quad (4.35)$$

where the subscripts Bi and Tr represent the biceps and triceps groups, respectively, M_W is the moment caused by gravity acting on the forearm and hand, K_{Bi} and K_{Tr} are constants which account for inaccuracies in the musculoskeletal model and O is an offset which specifies the resting angle of the forearm due solely to passive elastic forces (M_P accounts for the overall viscous damping forces of the joint). The specification of the resting angle is important because it defines the neutral position that the arm should return to every time the muscle activation level returns to zero or rest. The determination of O depends on the passive torque outputs from the model assuming no muscle activation input and zero movement velocity.

4.3.2 Model Setup

Further adjustments were required in the form of additional parameters. These were threshold values for the EMG activation levels and the offset value. The threshold values help to accommodate the base line noise of the EMG signal, which constantly fluctuates even at lower (inactive) levels. A threshold value for each of the biceps and triceps muscle groups can be optimally determined to prevent the model from responding with jittery movements. The offset torque was applied to adjust the position of the resting elbow angle more effectively in the absence of dr. The final list of the ten tuneable parameters is presented in Table 4.2. These parameters will be tuned simultaneously using genetic algorithms.

The remaining parameters have fixed or measured values and therefore need to be derived from data that is supported by the literature. The muscle attachment sites around the centre of rotation were based on the estimated lengths of muscles attached beyond the elbow joint (from tendons). The biceps group was estimated to attach 0.05 m along the radius/ulna, and the triceps less than this at 0.04 m because of the exaggerated protrusion from the ulna for muscle insertion. Passive elastic and damping coefficients for the musculotendon models (C_{pass} and C_{damp}) were based on desired resting position behaviour and determined through an iterative process of estimation and fine tuning. The lumped forearm and hand mass was determined from data reported by Lemay and Crago [33].

The determination of maximum muscle forces (F_{Max}) and optimal muscle lengths (l_{Opt}) is dependent on the structure of the physiological model. The optimal muscle length can be assumed to occur when the elbow is flexed to a 90° angle [30], which is when the weight of the forearm and hand is producing the greatest amount of torque. Other groups have reported maximum muscle forces and optimum muscle lengths ranging from 850 to 1550 N and 0.062–0.7 m, respectively, which demonstrates the dependence that these values have on the specific model being used [30, 31]. Therefore, to obtain the best representations of maximum muscle forces specific to the model presented in this chapter, the values will be

Table 4.2 Final list of elbow model parameters for tuning

Parameters for tuning	Description
β	Overall damping coefficient
F_{ArmCOM}	Centre of mass of the forearm and hand
L_{Farm}	Length of the forearm
K_{Bi}	User-specific for skeletal error in biceps
K_{Tr}	User-specific for skeletal error in triceps
R_{Bi}	User-specific for biceps muscle size
R_{Tr}	User-specific for triceps muscle size
Thre_{Bi}	Threshold for biceps activation level
Thre_{Tr}	Threshold for triceps activation level
O	Offset value for the passive resting angle of the forearm

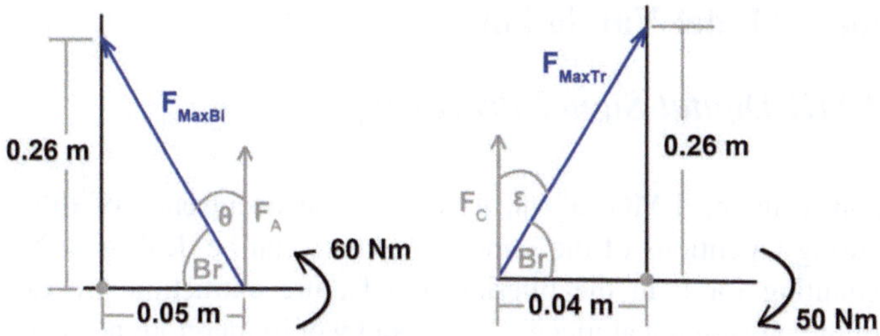

Fig. 4.21 Optimal muscle length geometries. This occurs when the forearm is perpendicular to the upper arm and $d = 90°$

derived from the available musculoskeletal model and measures of maximal elbow torque provided by Winters and Stark: 60 Nm for elbow flexion and 50 Nm for elbow extension [34]. The optimal muscle lengths produce the maximum torques when $d = 90°$, which results in the forearm being positioned perpendicular to the upper arm as shown in Fig. 4.21.

Finally, the corresponding muscle lengths can be determined from the simple application of Pythagoras' theorem

$$l_{\mathrm{OptBi}} = 0.265\,\mathrm{m}, \quad l_{\mathrm{OptTr}} = 0.263\,\mathrm{m}, \tag{4.36}$$

The final list of the fixed parameter values used is provided in Table 4.3. These parameters remain the same for all subjects and any adjustments are made through changes in the tuneable parameters.

Table 4.3 Parameters to be used for model validation

Parameter	Description	Value	Unit
U_{Bi}	Attachment distance to CoR from biceps	0.05	m
U_{Tr}	Attachment distance to CoR from triceps	0.04	m
F_{MaxBi}	Maximum biceps force	1220	N
F_{MaxTr}	Maximum triceps force	1260	N
l_{OptBi}	Optimal biceps muscle length	0.265	m
l_{OptTr}	Optimal triceps muscle length	0.263	m
C_{passBi}	User-specific for biceps elasticity	1	–
C_{passTr}	User-specific for triceps elasticity	3	–
β_{Bi}	User-specific for biceps viscosity	0.1	Ns/m
β_{Tr}	User-specific for triceps viscosity	0.1	Ns/m

These parameters were estimated with support from the literature where possible, and were neither measured or adjusted for subject specificity or involved in the tuning process

4.4 Elbow Model Validation

4.4.1 EMG Digital Signal Processing

The variability in the EMG signal, especially the occurrence of different signal patterns during repetitions of the same movement, can be dealt with by the NI by either accounting for it in the filtering and feature extraction process or in the exibility of the physiological model. The model would therefore need an element of tolerance and be able to identify similar movements from relatively diverse EMG signal inputs, and it is believed that this level of uncertainty can be accommodated within model development. Therefore, the design of an advanced signal processing algorithm is unnecessary within this research and a proven approach was selected from the literature that would be suitable for interfacing applications and muscle activation level estimation. This method is known as linear envelope processing (LEP) and is a cascaded filtering process that can be performed analogously (in hardware) or digitally (in software). Digital implementations of the filtering process were designed in MATLAB using the Filter Design and Analysis Tool (fdatool) as part of the Signal Processing Toolbox.

Linear Envelope Processing (LEP) is commonly found in the literature, providing an average and estimate of muscle activation level in both exoskeletal and prosthetic applications [23, 35–38]. The advantage of LEP is that it is relatively simple to implement, both digitally and in hardware because it consists of several stages of common filter configurations. Assuming that power line interference has previously been removed from the raw EMG signal, via a notch filter with 50/60 Hz cut-off frequency, obtaining a linear envelope is done through three standard and two optional stages, and these are described and demonstrated with examples below (the original raw EMG signal is shown in Fig. 4.22a

1. High-pass filtering: Motion artefacts in the EMG signal are caused by the movement of electrode leads and fluctuations at the skin-electrode interface, and as a result have lower frequencies. The usage of a high-pass filter (HPF) helps to reduce the effects of movement artefacts and Fig. 4.22b shows this effect.
2. Full wave rectification: The negative components of the signal are then inverted so that the signal activity is entirely reflected in the positive domain, as shown in Fig. 4.22c.
3. Low-pass filtering: The application of a low-pass filter (LPF) removes the high-frequency noise from the signal to produce a smooth LE, shown in Fig. 4.22d. This smoothing effect is similar to the effects of a moving average and the cut-off and order of the filter affect the degree of smoothing.
4. Normalisation: The first optional stage of LEP is to scale the smoothed signal to a normalised activation value as shown in Fig. 4.22e (there is no change to the shape of the envelope). This is commonly done against maximum voluntary contraction (MVC), which is the highest amplitude EMG signal attainable without pain or discomfort when the muscle is contracted isometrically.

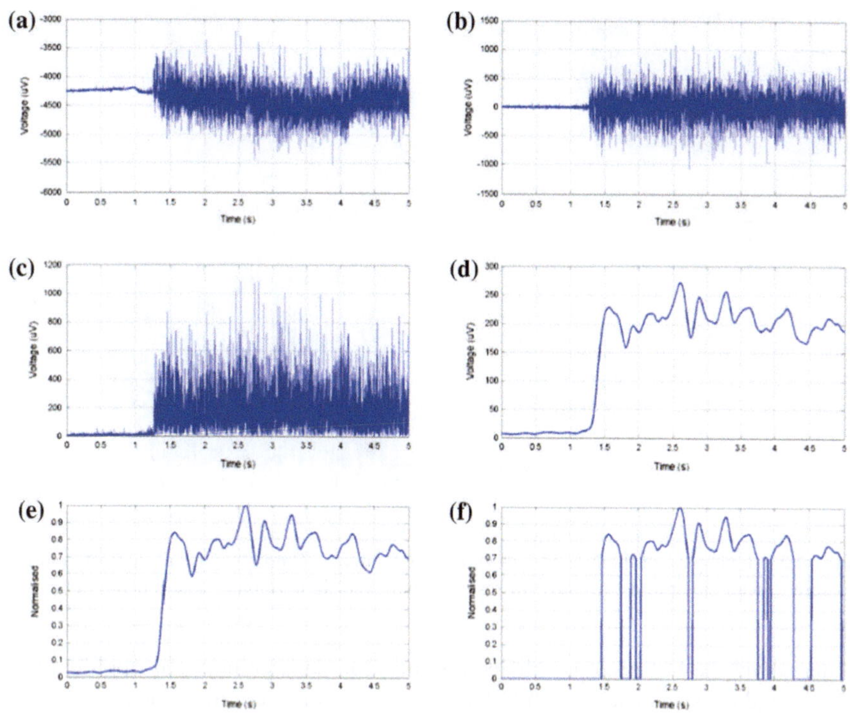

Fig. 4.22 Example of the linear envelope processing technique. The sub-figures show each stage of the process in order. **a** Raw signal, **b** high-pass filtered, **c** full wave rectified, **d** low-pass filtered, **e** normalised, **f** thresholded (in his example at 0.7)

5. Thresholding: The final (and optional) stage of LEP is to provide a threshold below which the LE is floored to zero, shown in Fig. 4.22f, with a threshold value arbitrarily set at 0.7 (or 70 % activation against MVC). This is to account for neutral or ambient activity that is always present in the EMG signal, even when there are no active contractions present.

The selection of filter parameters for the HPF is a straightforward process because the variability in frequencies of movement is relatively limited. De Luca et al. performed a comprehensive study on the effectiveness of HPFs and the influence of their order and cut-off frequency on removing movement artefacts. They were able to narrow down potential filter configurations and recommended a second order Butterworth filter with 20 Hz cut-off for general HPF applications [39].

The main difficulty with LEP is similar to that of moving averages. To improve the smoothing effect of the low-pass filter, the effective length of the sampling window is increased, resulting in a slower response or rise time. This means that very smooth activation profiles can only be achieved at the expense of delayed responses, an unwanted trade-off given the real-time requirements of the NI.

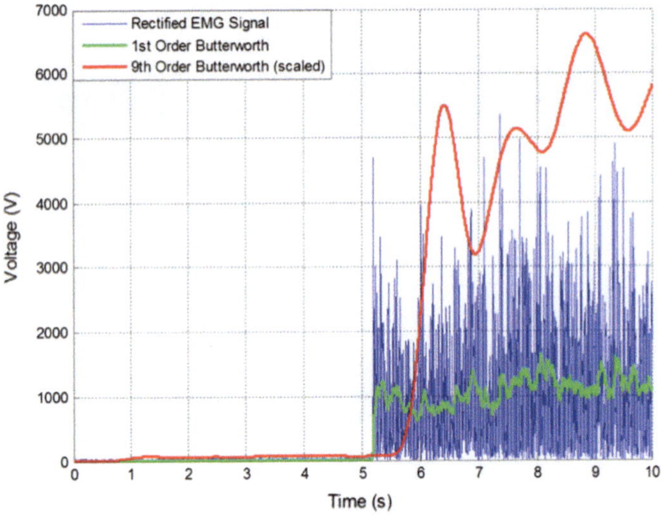

Fig. 4.23 Examples of high- and low-order filter effects. These two results are at opposite extremes, with either a fast response or response with very little rippling, and mutually exclusive

Alternatively, a fast response elicits a profile that has a pronounced rippling effect that would cause an end system to have oscillatory or jittery movement, and fail to closely represent the activation dynamics of the muscle. Examples of these two extremes are shown in Fig. 4.23 and a compromise is therefore required in order to achieve a response time that is fast enough but still has a manageable amount of rippling in the signal. Different groups have suggested their own filter specifications, based on their own experiments and the work of others, and frequency cut-offs can range from 2 to 8 Hz [23, 35].

The selection of appropriate low-pass filter parameters for LEP, therefore depends on a compromise between the rate of response and the amount of rippling in the filtered EMG signal. The determination of an optimal combination of filter order and cut-off frequency that satisfies an objective function was performed through enumeration. The objective was to minimise the weighted combination of rise time and spread in response to a step input. This brief optimization study determined that suitable parameters were of lower order and a cut-off frequency of no more than 5 Hz. The most common configuration in the literature is a fourth order Butterworth filter with 4 Hz cut-off frequency [40, 41] and the results of the brief optimisation study were in agreement with these settings, so this was used for the remainder of the EMG signal processing.

4.4.2 Physiological Model Validation

The physiological model of the elbow joint requires experimental validation with multiple subject data to quantify and characterise the performance of the model. This section describes the process, including the collection of EMG signal and motion data from multiple subjects, the experimental paradigm and the results of the movement predictions from the model when compared to the actual movement [19]. Note that at this stage, the data is processed and analysed offline.

The acquisition of EMG signals is achieved using a g.USBamp biosignal amplifier (Guger Technologies, Austria) and disposable Red Dot Paediatric electrodes (3 M, USA) placed approximately 2 cm apart over the belly of each muscle in a bipolar configuration. The bipolar configuration (alternative to a monopolar configuration) provides a differential signal, and its main advantage is that it has a higher propensity to reject common noise interferences picked up by both electrodes to improve the information quality of the signal. Before the application of electrodes, the skin surface is prepared by rubbing it with an abrasive gel (D.O. Weaver & Co., USA) to remove dirt, followed by rubbing alcohol (Isopropyl, approximately 70 %) to remove oil and grease. The bipolar EMG channels were sampled at 1200 Hz and hardware filtered with a 50 Hz notch filter to remove power line interference. EMG signals were recorded from two muscles for each subject—the biceps and triceps, and electrode locations were based on recommendations by [42] and confirmed by palpation, as shown in Fig. 4.24.

To validate the output of the physiological model for the elbow joint, a comparison is required between the actual elbow angle and the estimated angle. The Polaris Spectra (Northern Digital Incorporated, USA) is a motion tracking system that can track passive markers with a high degree of accuracy (up to 0.3 mm RMS) at up to 60 Hz.

Data was collected from six healthy subjects (four male and two female) between the ages of 23 and 28. The experimental procedures used in this study were approved by the University of Auckland Human Participants Ethics Committee (Reference #7557) and each subject gave informed consent to participate in the experiments. Each subject was instructed to perform five different sets of movements. These movements occurred in the sagittal plane with the upper arm being held vertically and as still as possible, and while the subjects were in the standing position. All movements occurred with the forearm and hand being relaxed and the palm facing medially to prevent the interference of wrist and finger movements. Before each trial session, the maximum voluntary contraction (MVC) for each muscle group was recorded three times and averaged. This was achieved during isometric contractions where the subject either pulled up or pushed down against a table top for measurement of biceps and triceps MVC, respectively.

Each of the movement trials lasted for about 15–20 s and five trials were performed for each type of movement set. To prevent fatigue, trials were separated by at least a 60 s rest period and subjects were given the freedom to have extended

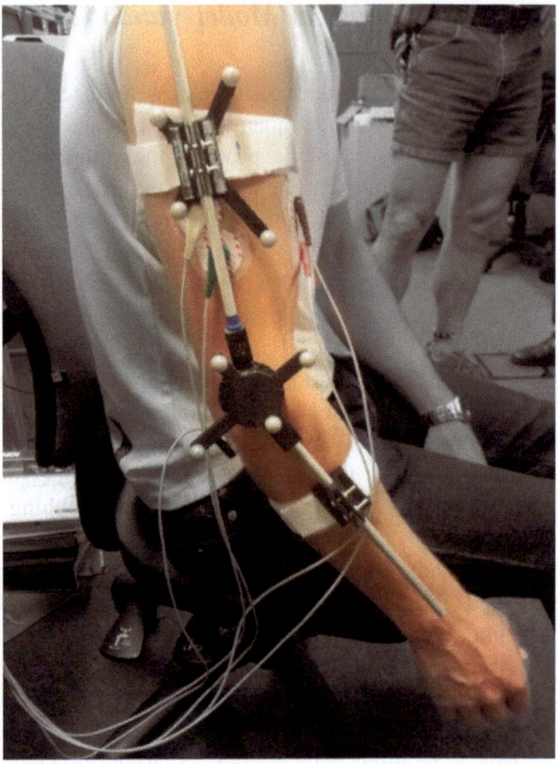

Fig. 4.24 EMG electrode and marker brace attachments to the arm

rests so should they begin to feel the onset of fatigue. The recorded movements were as follows:

1. Single cycle of full flexion and full extension from a neutral, relaxed position at a moderate speed. This is the most basic movement that requires proper limb function.
2. Continuous cycles of full flexion and full extension. The multiple cycles of movement will be used to ensure the repeatability of the model output.
3. Continuous cycles at half the range of capable motion (about 90° elbow angle). This was to not limit the outputs of the model to only the full range of movement.
4. Continuous cycles starting with small amplitude that gradually increases over the course of the trial. This was to determine whether the model can identify different amplitudes.
5. Random movement performed at the discretion of the user with different amplitudes and at varying speeds. This gave the control of movements completely to the user and will provide the most definitive factor in testing the performance of the elbow model.

The early implementation of the elbow model required an offline tuning method that would provide an optimised solution over a relatively large search space and with the tendency to avoid selecting local minima. The genetic algorithm (GA) is based on Darwin's evolution theory and provides an effective way of determining a reasonable solution to a complex problem [43]. The operation of the GA can be described in the following stages [44] and processes are demonstrated with binary genes:

1. [Start] Generate a random population of n chromosomes, where a chromosome is the evolutionary equivalent of a single possible solution.
2. [Fitness] A chromosome contains a fixed random combination of parameter values and when applied to the model for a given data input, these parameters will produce a particular predicted movement. The RMSE between this predicted movement and the actual movement yields the associated cost, which ideally will be zero. The cost is the fitness $f(x)$ of a chromosome and it is evaluated for each chromosome in the population.
3. [New population generation] A new population is created through the repetition of the following evolutionary processes until a completely new population exists: (a) [Selection] Select two parent chromosomes from a population according to their fitness. Chromosomes with higher fitness have a bigger chance of being selected. (b) [Crossover] Probability determines the size and likelihood of the event where parameter values are exchanged between parents to form new offspring (children), see Fig. 4.25a. If no crossover is performed, the offspring are an exact copy of its parents. (c) [Mutation] Probability that a mutation causes new offspring at each locus or position in the chromosome, as demonstrated in Fig. 4.25b. (d) [Acceptance] Place new offspring in a new population.
4. [Replace] Use the newly generated population from this point onwards and prepare it for another iteration of the algorithm.
5. [Test] If the end condition is satisfied, i.e. fitness criteria have been met, stop and return the optimal solution in the current population.
6. [Loop] Otherwise, go back to step 3.

The GA options in the global optimisation toolbox were tested to determine whether there were any significant improvements on the rate of convergence or quality of the optimised solution. It was found from comparing a small sample of data across multiple subjects that the options in Table 4.4 for the GA algorithm and parameter search space (ranges) yielded the most acceptable responses.

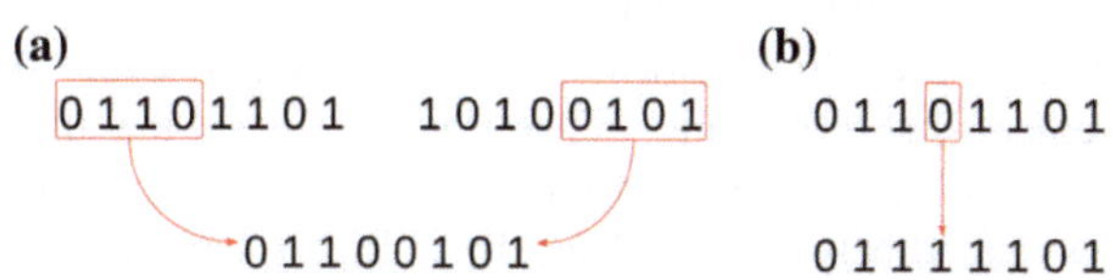

Fig. 4.25 Evolutionary processes examples. **a** Crossover. **b** Mutation

Table 4.4 Genetic algorithm options and parameter ranges

GA_{option}	Value	
Population size	75	
Crossover fraction	0.5	
Elite count	1	
Tolerance function	1.0e−11	
Generations	175	
Parameter	Lower bound	Upper bound
β	0	4
F_{ArmCOM}	0	1
L_{Farm}	0	2
K_{Bi}	0	20
K_{Tr}	0	20
R_{Bi}	0	20
R_{Tr}	0	20
ThreBi	0	1
$Thre_{Tr}$	0	1
O	0	5

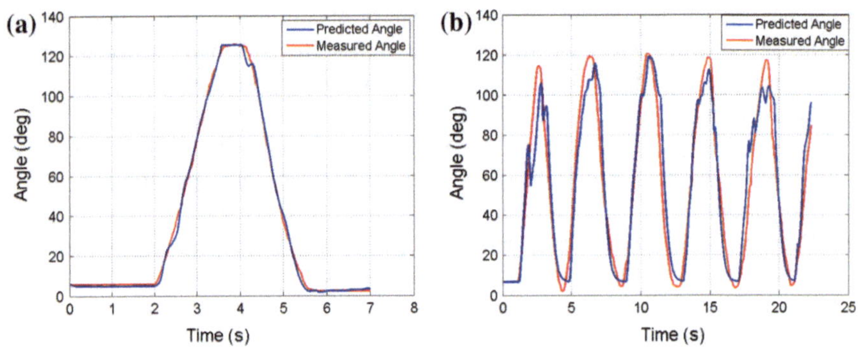

Fig. 4.26 **a** Result of a typical single cycle trial with RMSE of 1.9°. **b** Result of a typical continuous full cycle trial with RMSE of 11.0°

The resulted data after tuning with GAs for all subjects are presented and analysed by movement type below. Note that because each data trial underwent four repetitions through the GA to reduce the chances of identifying local optimum solutions, only the best returned solution was considered because this serves as the most likely global optimum parameter set.

A response from the physiological model to a single cycle of flexion and extension movement is shown in Fig. 4.26a. It was expected that these trials would have the best results after tuning and the values in Table 4.4 confirm this. The subject averages ranged between 4.18° and 10.1° RMSE and this indicates that the model is capable of predicting simple movement trajectories. However, the conditions under which tuning occurs is only optimised for one cycle of motion and it is therefore anticipated that the accuracy of prediction demonstrated in the figure will not be maintained throughout the rest of the movement types and be significantly higher than the 6.53° average over all the subjects.

Figure 4.26b shows the immediate degradation in accuracy when the cycles of movement become continuous. The subject averages range between 15.98° to 36.06° RMSE, which is a large increase from the single cycle of movement. To some degree, the model is still able to identify the sequential movements from EMG data and the figure demonstrates the case of the model performing quite accurately with an 11° RMSE. This is the level of performance required to be consistently obtained if the model was to truly be effective, and the total average of 22.4° RMSE needs to be reduced.

The performance of the model at identifying increasing amplitude movements is slightly worse than the half amplitude cycles, but still better than full amplitude movements with subject averages starting as low as 11.9° and going up to 31.7° RMSE with a 19.5° RMSE total average. The variability in the amplitude can be handled by the model and can be seen in Fig. 4.27a. While the predicted output does not match the actual movement exactly with some overshoot and undershoot, the general trend of increasing amplitude is observable.

Allowing subjects to perform random movements at various amplitudes and speeds is the ultimate performance test for the model, because this is the type of input that would be expected in a real world practical application. Table 4.4 shows that, as would be expected, the model does not perform as well for this type of movement with subject averages ranging from 17.1° to 28.9° RMSE and total average of 22.4° RMSE. However, the standard deviation across all subjects is the lowest except for single cycles of movements at 5.0°. This result superficially may seem to be the worst but results such as the one demonstrated in Fig. 4.27b show that the model is capable of following randomly generated movement.

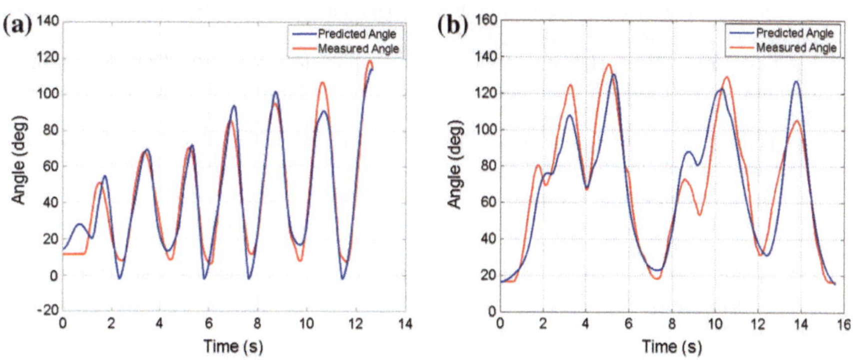

Fig. 4.27 **a** Result of a typical increasing amplitude trial with RMSE of 7.9°. **b** Result of a typical random movement trial with RMSE of 13.0°

4.5 Summary

This chapter proposes a kinematically redundant 4R spherical wrist to overcome the limitations of the 3R. The kinematics of the 4R mechanism is modelled using the DH notation and methods to solve the forward and inverse kinematic problems are developed. To obtain an inverse kinematic solution, it is proposed that a value is set for the angular position of Joint 1 in the 4R mechanism so that the remaining joints form a non-redundant 3R mechanism. A modified FABRIK algorithm is proposed and developed to solve the inverse kinematic problem of the 4R mechanism. This chapter has also presented an EMG-driven physiological model of the elbow joint that was developed in the sagittal plane, and consists of Hill-type musculotendon models and a uniquely defined musculoskeletal system to predict joint motion. In this chapter, the physiological model of the elbow joint developed in the previous chapter was coupled with linear envelope processing and experimentally validated with data from multiple subjects.

References

1. B. Tondu, Estimating shoulder-complex mobility. Appl. Bion. Biomech. **4**, 19–29 (2007)
2. J. Yang, K. Abdel-Malek, K. Nebel, Reach envelope of a 9-degree-of-freedom model of the upper extremity. Int. J. Robot. Autom. **20**, 240–259 (2005)
3. F.C.T. Van Der Helm, Analysis of the kinematic and dynamic behavior of the shoulder mechanism. J. Biomech. **27**, 527–550 (1994)
4. T. Nef, M. Guidali, R. Riener, ARMin III—arm therapy exoskeleton with an ergonomic shoulder actuation. Appl. Bion. Biomech. **6**, 127–142 (2009)
5. C. Carignan, J. Tang, S. Roderick, Development of an exoskeleton haptic interface for virtual task training, in *IEEE/RSJ International Conference on Intelligent Robots and Systems*, 2009, pp. 3697–3702
6. Y. Ren, H.S. Park, L.Q. Zhang, Developing a whole-arm exoskeleton robot with hand opening and closing mechanism for upper limb stroke rehabilitation, in *IEEE International Conference on Rehabilitation Robotics*, 2009, pp. 761–765
7. S.J. Ball, I.E. Brown, S.H. Scott, MEDARM: a rehabilitation robot with 5DOF at the shoulder complex, in *IEEE/ASME International Conference on Advanced Intelligent Mechatronics*, 2007
8. J.C. Perry, J. Rosen, S. Burns, Upper-limb powered exoskeleton design. IEEE/ASME Trans. Mechatron. **12**, 408–417 (2007)
9. D. Naidu, R. Stopforth, G. Bright, S. Davrajh, A 7 DOF exoskeleton arm: shoulder, elbow, wrist and hand mechanism for assistance to upper limb disabled individuals, in *IEEE AFRICON Conference*, 2011
10. G.L. Long, R.P. Paul, W.D. Fisher, Hamilton wrist: a four-revolute-joint spherical wrist without singularities, in *IEEE International Conference on Robotics and Automation*, 1989, pp. 902–907
11. C.R. Carignan, R.D. Howard, A skew-axis design for a 4-joint revolute wrist, in *IEEE International Conference on Robotics and Automation*, 2002, pp. 3636–3642
12. D. Chablat, J. Angeles, The computation of all 4R serial spherical wrists with an isotropic architecture. Trans. ASME J. Mech. Des. **125**, 275–280 (2003)

13. K. Farhang, Y.S. Zargar, Design of spherical 4R mechanisms: function generation for the entire motion cycle. Trans. ASME J. Mech. Des. **121**, 521–528 (1999)
14. J. Denavit, R.S. Hartenberg, A kinematic notation for lower pair mechanisms based on matrices. ASME J. Appl. Mech. **23**, 215–221 (1955)
15. A. Aristidou, J. Lasenby, FABRIK: a fast, iterative solver for the Inverse Kinematics problem. Graph. Models **73**, 243–260 (2011)
16. J.B. Kuipers, *Quaternions and rotation sequences: a primer with applications to orbits, aerospace and virtual reality* (Princeton University Press, Princeton, 2002)
17. X. Wang, M. Maurin, F. Mazet, N.D.C. Maia, K. Voinot, J.P. Verriest, M. Fayet, Three-dimensional modelling of the motion range of axial rotation of the upper arm. J. Biomech. **31**, 899–908 (1998)
18. J. Pau, H. Saini, S. Xie, A. Pullan, G. Mallinson, An emg-driven neuromuscular interface for human elbow joint, in *3rd IEEE RAS and EMBS International Conference on Biomedical Robotics and Biomechatronics* (BioRob), Tokyo, Sept 2010, pp. 156–161
19. J.W.L. Pau, S.S.Q. Xie, A.J. Pullan, Neuromuscular interfacing: establishing an emg-driven model for the human elbow joint. IEEE Trans. Biomed. Eng. **59**(9), 2586–2593 (2012)
20. A.V. Hill, The heat of shortening and the dynamic constants of muscle. Proc. R. Soc. Lond. Series B Biol. Sci. **126**(843), 136–195 (1938)
21. Q. Shao, D.N. Bassett, K. Manal, T.S. Buchanan, An emg-driven model to estimate muscle forces and joint moments in stroke patients. Comput. Biol. Med. **39**(12), 1083–1088 (2009)
22. M. Sartori, D. Lloyd, M. Reggiani, and E. Pagello, A stiff tendon neuromusculoskeletal model of the knee, in *IEEE Workshop on Advanced Robotics and its Social Impacts* (ARSO), Tokyo, Nov. 2009, pp. 132–138
23. T. Buchanan, D. Lloyd, K. Manal, T. Besier, Neuromusculoskeletal modeling: estimation of muscle forces and joint moments and movements from measurements of neural command. J. Appl. Biomech. **20**(4), 367–395 (2004)
24. M. Vilimek, Musculotendon forces derived by different muscle models. Acta Bioeng. Biomech. **9**(2), 41–47 (2007)
25. G.F. Elliott, C.R. Worthington, Muscle contraction: viscous-like frictional forces and the impulsive model. Int. J. Biol. Macromol. **27**(5), 327–332 (2000)
26. L. Schutte, M. Rodgers, F. Zajac, R. Glaser, Improving the efficacy of electrical stimulation-induced leg cycle ergometry: an analysis based on a dynamic musculoskeletal model. IEEE Trans. Rehabil. Eng. **1**(2), 109–125 (1993)
27. A. Martin, L. Martin, B. Morlon, Theoretical and experimental behaviour of the muscle viscosity coefficient during maximal concentric actions. Eur. J. Appl. Physiol. **69**(6), 539–544 (1994)
28. T.K. Koo, A.F. Mak, Feasibility of using emg driven neuromusculoskeletal model for prediction of dynamic movement of the elbow. J. Electromyogr. Kinesiol. **15**(1), 12–26 (2005)
29. K. An, B.F. Morrey, E. Chao, Carrying angle of the human elbow joint. J. Orthop. Res. **1**(4), 369–378 (1983)
30. D. Kistemaker, A. Van Soest, M. Bobbert, A model of open-loop control of equilibrium position and stiffness of the human elbow joint. Biol. Cybern. **96**(3), 341–350 (2007)
31. S. Stroeve, Impedance characteristics of a neuromusculoskeletal model of the human arm i. posture control. Biol. Cybern. **81**(5), 475–494 (1999)
32. A. Desplantez, C. Cornu, F. Goubel, Viscous properties of human muscle during contraction. J. Biomech. **32**(6), 555–562 (1999)
33. M.A. Lemay, P.E. Crago, A dynamic model for simulating movements of the elbow, forearm, and wrist. J. Biomech. **29**(10), 1319–1330 (1996)
34. J.M. Winters, L. Stark, Analysis of fundamental human movement patterns through the use of in-depth antagonistic muscle models. IEEE Trans. Biomed. Eng. **32**(10), 826–839 (1985)
35. A. Au, R. Kirsch, Emg-based prediction of shoulder and elbow kinematics in able-bodied and spinal cord injured individuals. IEEE Trans. Rehabil. Eng. **8**(4), 471–480 (2000)
36. R. Merletti, P. di Torino, Standards for reporting EMG data. Int. Soc. Electrophysiol. Kinesiol. (1999)

37. T. Farrell, R. Weir, The optimal controller delay for myoelectric prostheses. IEEE Trans. Neural Syst. Rehabil. Eng. **15**(1), 111–118 (2007)
38. T. Lenzi, S.M.M. De Rossi, N. Vitiello, M.C. Carrozza, Proportional emg control for upper-limb powered exoskeletons, in *Annual International Conference of the IEEE Engineering in Medicine and Biology Society* (EMBC), Boston, Sept. 2011, pp. 628–631
39. C. De Luca, L. Donald Gilmore, M. Kuznetsov, S. Roy, Filtering the surface emg signal: Movement artifact and baseline noise contamination, J. Biomech. **43**(8), 1573–1579 (2010)
40. K. Manal, T. Buchanan, Use of an emg-driven biomechanical model to study virtual injuries. Med. Sci. Sports Exerc. **37**(11), 1917–1923 (2005)
41. E. Cavallaro, J. Rosen, J. Perry, S. Burns, B. Hannaford, Hill-based model as a myoprocessor for a neural controlled powered exoskeleton arm—parameters optimization, in *Proceedings of the 2005 IEEE International Conference on Robotics and Automation* (ICRA), Apr 2005, pp. 4514–4519
42. J.R. Cram, G.S. Kasman, J. Holtz, *Introduction to Surface Electromyography* (Aspen Publishers Inc., Gaithersburg, Maryland, 1998)
43. C.R. Reeves, *Handbook of Metaheuristics*, vol. 146, Chap. 5 Genetic Algorithms (Springer Link, 2010), pp. 109–139
44. P. Bajpai, M. Kumar, Genetic algorithm—an approach to solve global optimisation problems. Indian J. Comput. Sci. Eng. **1**(3), 199–206 (2010)

Chapter 5
Upper Limb Exoskeleton Development

This chapter discusses the optimisation of the 4R mechanism specifically for a shoulder exoskeleton. The goal of the optimisation was to find an optimal kinematic design of the 4R mechanism and identify the optimal joint configurations for this redundant 4R mechanism to operate. Algorithms are developed to evaluate the performance of a given 4R design in terms of joint velocities during transitions of the end-effector and proximity to singular configurations. The workspace of the human shoulder is considered and factors that can limit the workspace of the 4R are analysed. The concepts behind multi-objective optimisation and the NSGA II algorithm are presented. The optimisation problem is outlined, discussed and a set of optimisation variables and objectives are defined for the algorithm.

5.1 Design Optimisation of a 4R Shoulder Mechanism

Angular displacements of the four joints in the mechanism are examined to ensure they have feasible movements with minimal velocities throughout the workspace. Singularity analysis is done using the Jacobian matrix of the 4R and its condition number. The optimal 4R design obtained from the optimisation process is analysed and its performance discussed compared to other designs.

5.1.1 *Optimisation Algorithms*

A popular multi-objective evolutionary algorithm used by researchers is the Non-dominated Sorting Genetic Algorithm II (NSGA II) [1]. NSGA II has been shown to perform better than other well-known multi-objective evolutionary algorithms including the Pareto-archived Evolution Strategy (PAES) [2] and Strength Pareto Evolutionary Algorithm (SPEA) [3] in terms of finding a diverse set of solutions and in converging near the true Pareto optimal set. Therefore, NSGA II is chosen as the multi-objective evolutionary algorithm for optimising the design of the 4R mechanism in this research.

S.(S.Q.) Xie, *Advanced Robotics for Medical Rehabilitation*,
Springer Tracts in Advanced Robotics 108, DOI 10.1007/978-3-319-19896-5_5

NSGA II is based on genetic algorithm, a popular evolutionary algorithm which uses techniques inspired by the process of natural evolution. An initial population of solutions (or chromosomes) is randomly generated and three natural operators, namely selection, crossover and mutation, are applied to generate a new population of better solutions. This process is repeated iteratively to obtain better and better solutions until a termination condition is reached. A common termination condition is setting a maximum number of iterations to be performed. The selection operator uses a fitness function to determine the quality of the solutions. The evolution mechanism in NSGA II enables exploration of various trade-off solutions which allows an approximation of the Pareto set to be found and preserves the diversity of solutions. These are two key features of multi-objective evolutionary algorithms.

The NSGA II algorithm is illustrated in Fig. 5.1 and has the following steps:

1. **[Start]** Select a termination criterion based on number of iterations.
2. **[Initialize]** Initialize a random population of Q chromosomes (suitable solutions).
3. **[Fitness]** Evaluate the values of various objectives for each chromosome in the population.
4. **[Rank]** Classify population into fronts using non-dominating sorting algorithm and assign non-domination ranks to each solution.
5. **[Offspring]** For the first iteration, create a duplicate copy of the parent population by randomly arranging its solutions and call this offspring population.

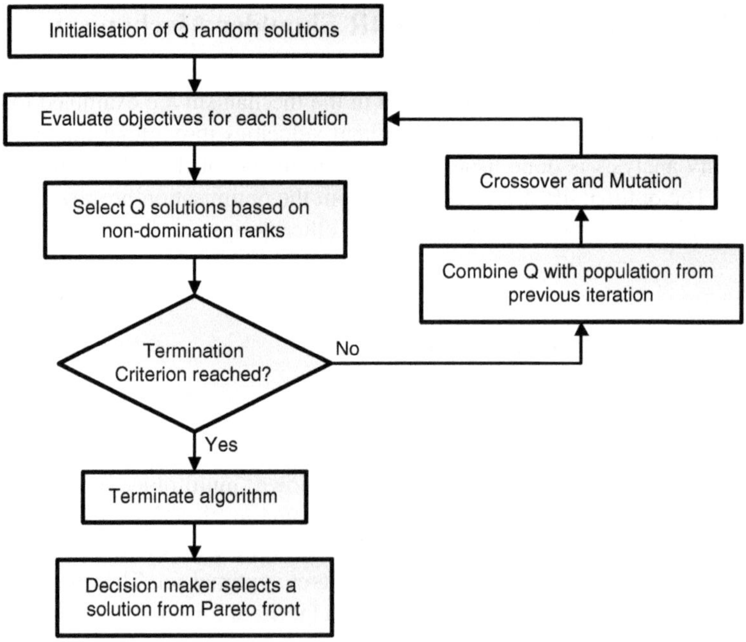

Fig. 5.1 Process diagram of the NSGA II algorithm

6. **[Selection]** Combine offspring with the parent population and select Q solutions based on non-domination rank. Call the resulting population as parents.
7. **[Crossover]** Crossover the parents with a crossover probability to form new offspring.
8. **[Mutation]** Mutate the new offspring with a chosen mutation probability.
9. **[Rank]** Evaluate solutions for their objective values to perform non-dominated sorting and once again classify the population into fronts based on their non-domination ranks.
10. **[Check]** Check for the termination criteria and stop if this is achieved else go to Step 6.
11. **[End]** Stop and return the final population when the termination criterion is reached.

A kinematically redundant 4R mechanism can avoid the undesirable singular configurations that can occur with a 3R mechanism and achieve good performance in the entire shoulder workspace. The goal was to optimise the 4R mechanism to ensure the additional DOF provided by the redundant joint is efficiently utilised to achieve a high performance in a shoulder. This involves finding an optimal 4R design and also a set of optimal joint configurations for the mechanism [4].

The redundant joint in the 4R mechanism allows flexibility in the 4R linkage design. Whereas a 3R mechanism requires all link angles to be 90° in order to achieve the full spherical workspace, the link angles of the redundant 4R mechanism can have a variety of sizes and still achieve the full spherical workspace. Hence, there are a range of possible 4R mechanism designs that can be used in a shoulder exoskeleton. The 4R design can have variations in the sizes of the three link angles and the location of the base joint as shown in Fig. 5.2.

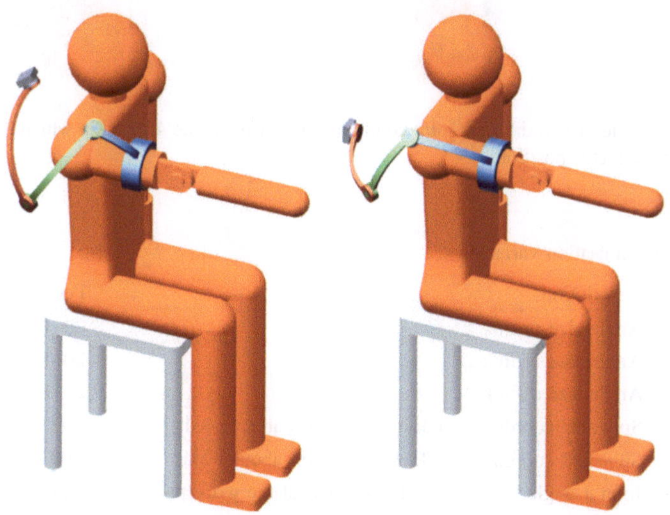

Fig. 5.2 Example of two different 4R designs with different link angle sizes and base joint position

In addition, an issue arising from the redundancy is that it is possible to achieve the same end-effector position with a range of different 4R configurations as shown in Fig. 5.3, i.e. there are infinite inverse kinematics solutions. Therefore, it is also necessary to identify the optimal joint configuration for reaching any given end-effector position in the shoulder workspace. The NSGA II algorithm is used to solve this complex nonlinear optimisation problem.

Six variables are used in this optimisation problem. Descriptions for these variables and their permitted values are shown in Table 5.1. The first five variables describe the design of the 4R mechanism, where α_1, α_2 and α_3 describe the three link angles and φ_z and φ_x describe the position of the base joint relative to the user's shoulder in spherical coordinates. Here, φ_z precedes φ_x in the sequence of Euler rotations and the default position is directly above the user's right shoulder.

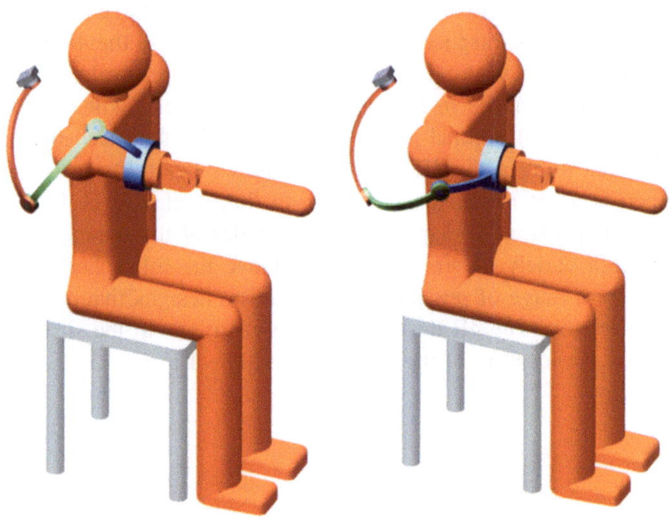

Fig. 5.3 Example of two different joint configurations of the same 4R design which both achieve the same end-effector position

Table 5.1 Optimisation variables

Variable	Description	Permitted value (°)
α_1	Angle size of link 1	20–160
α_2	Angle size of link 2	20–160
α_3	Angle size of link 3	20–160
φ_z	Spherical coordinate of Joint 1 location about *z*-axis	−45 to 45
φ_x	Spherical coordinate of Joint 1 location about *x*-axis	−90 to 90
θ_1^0	Joint 1 angle when the end-effector is at the workspace centre	−180 to 180

The sixth variable θ_1^0 is used to determine the optimal joint configurations of the 4R mechanism. This variable is the angle of Joint 1 (θ_1) when the end-effector is at the centre of the shoulder workspace. These three latter variables are illustrated in Fig. 5.4. A given value of θ_1 is necessary because there are infinite possible joint configurations for achieving a given end-effector position due to the kinematic redundancy. If θ_1 is known, the angular positions of the remaining joints required to achieve the given end-effector position can be determined from inverse kinematics. However, this only gives the configuration for reaching one position in the workspace. Therefore, an expanding algorithm is developed to compute the joint configurations for reaching the remaining workspace.

The NSGA II algorithm produces a population of solutions, each with a value for the six variables within their permitted ranges. Each iteration of the algorithm improves these solutions until a set of Pareto optimal solutions are obtained.

In this optimisation problem, achieving the entire human shoulder workspace without mechanical interference is considered to be a compulsory objective. The other performance objectives are average joint motion, global condition number and maximum condition number. The NSGA II algorithm uses these three performance objectives to evaluate each solution that can reach the entire shoulder workspace and the best performing solutions are selected for producing the next generation of solutions. These objectives are discussed in the subsequent sections.

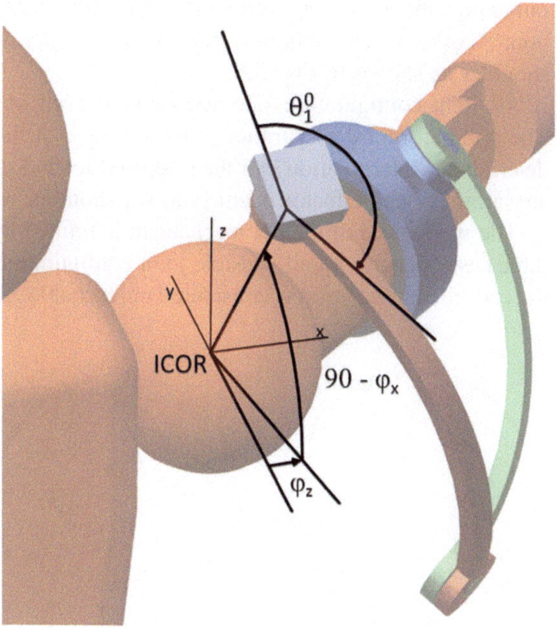

Fig. 5.4 Illustration of the optimisation variables φ_z, φ_x and θ_1^0

5.1.2 Workspace of the 4R Mechanism

The 4R mechanism is intended for a shoulder exoskeleton; therefore, the workspace of the human shoulder needs to be considered during optimisation. The workspace for the human shoulder is approximately half of the spherical workspace (i.e. a semi-sphere) while the 4R exoskeleton can be designed to operate the end-effector in the entire spherical workspace.

The semi-spherical shoulder workspace is discretised into points, each indicating an end-effector position to be analysed. A common method for allocating points on the surface of a sphere is by using the longitude and latitude parameters. However, this method results in a non-uniform distribution of points with a higher density of points at the two poles of the sphere. This causes the performance near the poles to have a larger influence on the overall performance score. Ideally, the points should be uniformly distributed to ensure the workspace is analysed evenly. A set of 89 uniformly distributed points over the semi-spherical workspace is generated using an algorithm proposed by Teanby [5]. This algorithm performs repeated subdivisions of a spherical icosahedron to obtain an increasingly dense grid of evenly distributed points on the surface of a sphere. Figure 5.5 shows the spheres from two consecutive subdivisions.

A sphere of 162 points is selected for representing the end-effector positions as this has a sufficient point density to provide a good representation of the 4R performance over the workspace. Since only the shoulder workspace is required rather than the entire spherical workspace, only 89 of the 162 points are used. These points cover a semi-spherical region in the lateral-anterior region of the user's shoulder as shown in Fig. 5.6.

4R joint configurations are assessed for each of the 89 end-effector positions. The optimal joint configurations to reach each of the 89 end-effector positions are determined. Interpolation can then be used to find the joint configuration to reach any arbitrary end-effector position in the shoulder workspace.

The workspace of the 4R mechanism is limited by three factors. If any of these three cases occur with all possible joint configurations for an end-effector position, the end-effector position is considered unreachable. The first case occurs when there

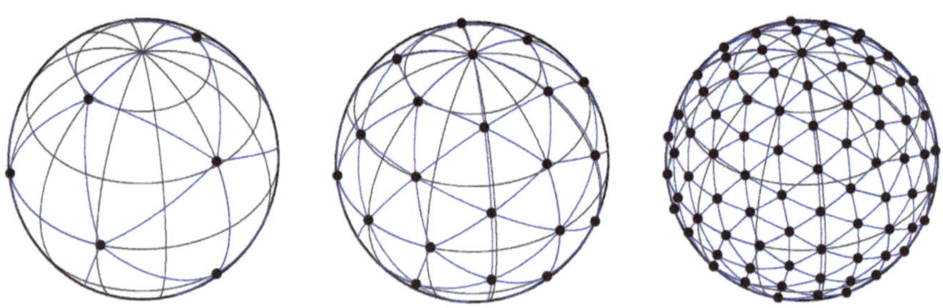

Fig. 5.5 Illustration of two consecutive subdivisions of a spherical icosahedron [5]. The *black dots* represent evenly distributed points on the surface of a sphere

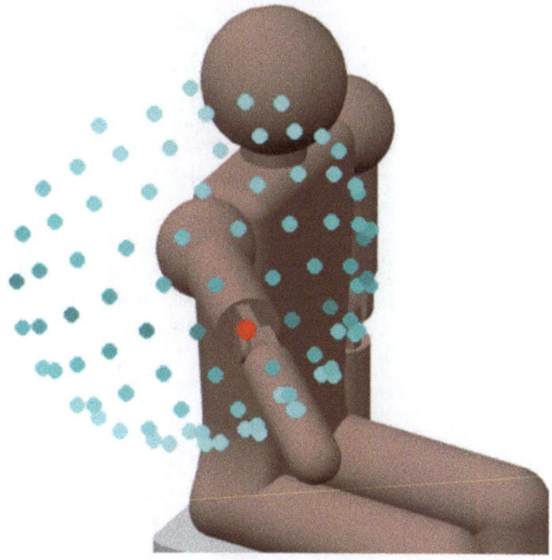

Fig. 5.6 The semi-spherical shoulder workspace is discretised into 89 uniformly distributed points for analysis. The model user shown has a shoulder posture at the *centre* of the workspace, represented by a *red point*

is no inverse kinematics solution for the given end-effector position and Joint 1 angle. This occurs when the end-effector cannot reach the position with the given link dimensions. The second case occurs when the joint configuration is at or very close to a singular configuration. Since there are significant limitations in operating at a singular configuration, the end-effector position that causes the singular configuration cannot be included into the robot workspace. The final case occurs when a part of the 4R structure is required to enter a forbidden region to reach an end-effector position. These include regions that can harm or cause discomfort for the user or cause mechanical interference between different parts of the exoskeleton system.

Therefore, the links must also not enter the user's anterior region. End-effector positions that require the links to enter the user's medial or anterior regions are considered unreachable. The boundary for this region is specified by a vertical plane intersecting the ICOR with a normal axis in the anterior-medial direction, 45° from the anterior axis. In addition, the region near the head and torso is also forbidden, i.e. the region above and below the ICOR. This region is represented by a vertical cylindrical volume with an axis intersecting the ICOR. Figure 5.7 shows the boundary of the region which the 4R mechanism must not enter.

To identify whether the 4R mechanism enters the forbidden region, the locations of Joints 1, 2 and 3 are checked. Joint 4 is at the end-effector which is always located within the upper arm workspace due to the design; therefore, this joint will not cause any forbidden intrusions. To ensure the 4R mechanism does not enter the medial-anterior region of the user, the condition in (5.1) must be met, where x_j and y_j are, respectively, the x and y Cartesian coordinates of the location of joint j in the global coordinate system.

$$x_j > y_j \quad \text{for } j = 1, 2, 3 \tag{5.1}$$

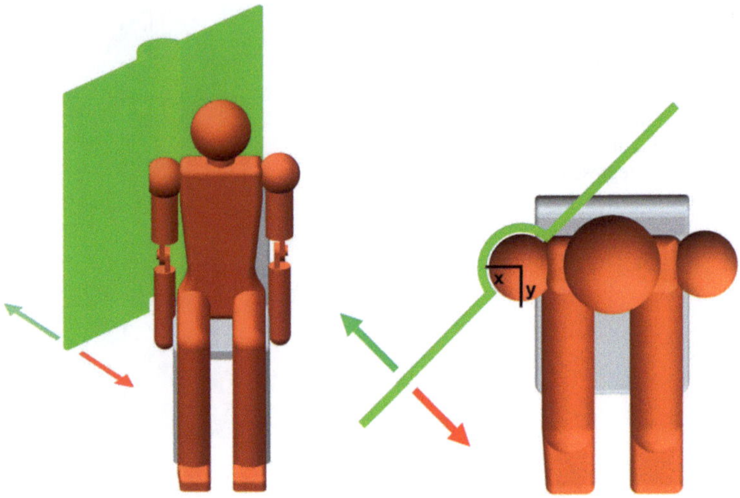

Fig. 5.7 Boundary of forbidden region for the 4R mechanism structure. The *red arrow* indicates the region that is forbidden and the *green arrow* indicates the permitted operating region

Furthermore, the intrusion into the region above and below the shoulder ICOR is also forbidden and (5.2) must also be satisfied, where d is the minimum allowable distance between a 4R joint and the vertical axis intersecting the shoulder ICOR.

$$\sqrt{x_j^2 + y_j^2} > d \quad \text{for } j = 1, 2, 3 \tag{5.2}$$

The coordinates of Joint 1, 2 and 3 with respect to the global coordinate system are derived using the DH transformation matrices of the 4R mechanism. Given that the coordinate systems are defined according to the DH notation and that the axes of rotation of all the joints intersect with the origin of the global coordinate system, the z-axis of the local coordinate system at each joint indicates the direction the joint is located with respect to the global coordinate system. The normalised coordinates of the jth joint's local z-axis with respect to the global coordinate system can be obtained from (5.3), where a_x, a_y and a_z are obtained from the DH matrix (5.4). Equations (5.1) and (5.2) are then used to check whether any joint lies in the forbidden region.

$$(x, y, z)_j = (a_x, a_y, a_z)_j^0 \tag{5.3}$$

$$T_j^0 = \begin{bmatrix} n_x & o_x & a_x & r_x \\ n_y & o_y & a_y & r_y \\ n_z & o_z & a_z & r_z \\ 0 & 0 & 0 & 1 \end{bmatrix} \tag{5.4}$$

In addition, Joint 1 must not be positioned within the shoulder workspace. This is because the position of Joint 1 is fixed and positioning this joint inside the shoulder workspace will prevent the upper arm from entering this region of the workspace. Therefore, the location of Joint 1 is restricted to a region behind the shoulder joint. This is reflected in the ranges of φ_z and φ_x.

An expanding algorithm has been developed to obtain the optimal joint configurations for all 89 end-effector positions in the shoulder workspace while ensuring feasible joint transitions. This makes use of the value θ_1^0 which is generated by the NSGA II algorithm as the sixth variable. This variable is the θ_1 value for reaching the end-effector position at the centre of the shoulder workspace. The expanding algorithm firstly finds the optimal joint configuration for this centre position using the six variable values of the solution provided by the NSGA II algorithm. The algorithm then computes the optimal joint configurations for all the end-effector positions adjacent to this starting position. This is done while ensuring the transition between adjacent end-effector positions are realistic, requires minimal joint displacements, does not cause interference and avoids approaching a singular configuration. This is achieved by generating a range of θ_1 values for the adjacent child position which are within 20° of the parent positions' θ_1 value and analysing the performance of their respective joint configurations. The θ_1 value that gives the best performing joint configuration is then selected as the optimal for the child end-effector position. This is done for each end-effector position that is adjacent to the parent position and has not already been analysed. The process is then applied to the next layer of adjacent end-effector positions and is repeated until all 89 positions in the shoulder workspace have been investigated. Figure 5.8 shows the first two iterations of the expanding algorithm.

By starting from the centre end-effector position in the workspace, the expanding algorithm is completed with the minimum number of iterations. The overall ease of transition between every combination of adjacent end-effector positions is used as part of the average joint motion objective in the optimisation algorithm. This is calculated as the average change in joint angles between the joint configurations of every pair of adjacent end-effector positions $\Delta\theta_{\text{ave}}$. The objective is to minimise (5.5), where $\Delta\theta(i,j,k)$ is the change in joint angle of joint i in moving the end-effector from workspace position j to an adjacent position k, m is the number of end-effector positions adjacent to position j, and n is the total number of workspace positions.

$$\Delta\theta_{\text{ave}} = \frac{\sum_{i=1}^{3}\sum_{j=1}^{n}\sum_{k=1}^{m}|\Delta\theta(i,j,k)|}{3\text{ nm}} \tag{5.5}$$

The resulting set of 89 θ_1 values which achieves optimal joint configurations for reaching the 89 end-effector positions will be used to control the kinematically redundant robot. Interpolation of the 89 θ_1 values can be done to find the optimal joint configuration for any arbitrary end-effector position in the shoulder workspace. This is achieved by interpolating the set of θ_1 data to find the optimal θ_1 value followed by inverse kinematics to compute the corresponding θ_2 and θ_3 values. The

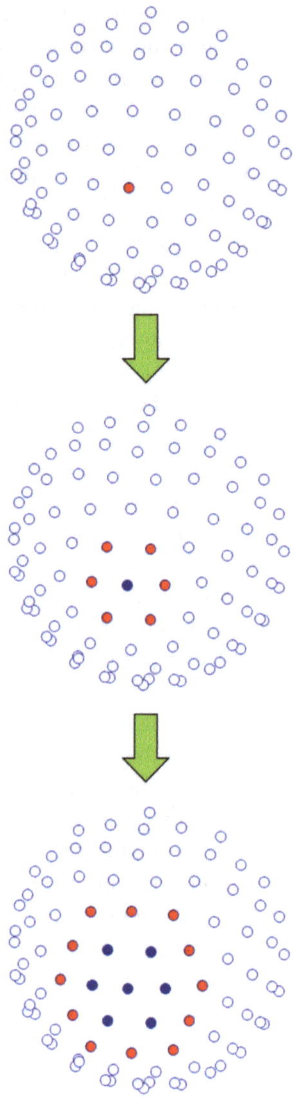

Fig. 5.8 The first two iterations in the expanding algorithm. Each iteration finds the joint configurations for a new layer of end-effector positions. The *red points* represent the positions to be analysed in the current iteration and the *blue points* represent the positions that have already been analysed in a previous iteration

joint angles obtained represent the optimal joint configuration for reaching the specified end-effector position.

In this research work, the range of motion of shoulder axial rotation is assumed to drift linearly up to 45° between the limits of horizontal flexion and extension. It is desirable to minimise the largest clockwise and counter-clockwise angular offset between the angular position of Joint 4 and the angular position of shoulder axial rotation that occurs in the workspace. A small maximum offset will mean that only a small additional range of motion is required for Joint 4 on top of the range of motion of shoulder axial rotation. The objective is to minimise (5.6), where $\Delta\theta^4_{\max}$ is the additional range of motion required for Joint 4, $\theta_0^4(j)$ is the default angular position of Joint 4 at end-effector position j relative to the global coordinate system, and $\theta_0^a(j)$ is the default angular position of shoulder axial rotation at upper arm position j relative to the global coordinate system.

$$\Delta\theta_{\max}^4 = \max\left(\theta_0^4(j) - \theta_0^a(j)\right) - \min\left(\theta_0^4(j) - \theta_0^a(j)\right) \tag{5.6}$$

5.1.3 Singularity Analysis

Singularity analysis is done using Jacobian matrices and its condition number which has often been used as measures of robot manipulability [6–8]. The Jacobian matrix of the robot maps the robot's joint velocities to the angular velocity of the end-effector according to (5.7), where ω is the angular velocity of the end-effector, J is the Jacobian matrix and $\dot{\theta}$ is the joint velocity vector.

$$\omega = J\dot{\theta} \tag{5.7}$$

The Jacobian matrix for the 4R mechanism J is a 3×4 non-square matrix due to the redundant joint. Each column of J represents the relationship between the end-effector and one of the four revolute joints. (5.7) can be written as (5.8), where $J = [\, J_1 \quad J_2 \quad J_3 \quad J_4 \,]$ and is a 3×4 matrix with J_1, J_2, J_3, and J_4 representing the relationships between the angular velocity of the 4R end-effector ω and the angular rates $\dot{\theta}_1, \dot{\theta}_2, \dot{\theta}_3$ and $\dot{\theta}_4$ of Joints 1, 2, 3 and 4, respectively.

$$\omega = [\, J_1 \quad J_2 \quad J_3 \quad J_4 \,] \begin{bmatrix} \dot{\theta}_1 \\ \dot{\theta}_2 \\ \dot{\theta}_3 \\ \dot{\theta}_4 \end{bmatrix} \tag{5.8}$$

Due to the spherical nature of the 4R mechanism and the assignment of the DH coordinate systems at the ICOR, the Jacobian for each joint i can be obtained with (5.9), where n_z, o_z and a_z are obtained from the DH transformation matrix (5.10).

$$J_i = {}^{i}\begin{bmatrix} n_z \\ o_z \\ a_z \end{bmatrix}_5 \tag{5.9}$$

$$T_5^i = \begin{bmatrix} n_x & o_x & a_x & r_x \\ n_y & o_y & a_y & r_y \\ n_z & o_z & a_z & r_z \\ 0 & 0 & 0 & 1 \end{bmatrix} \tag{5.10}$$

By definition, the condition number is given by (5.11), where $\|\cdot\|$ is the norm of the matrix [8].

$$k(J) = \|J\|\|J^{-1}\| \tag{5.11}$$

Given that the vector norms are Euclidean norms, the condition number becomes a measure of the ratio of the largest to the smallest singular value of the Jacobian matrix. These singular values are determined by factorizing J using the singular value decomposition rule in (5.12), where X and Y are the orthogonal matrices and Σ is a diagonal matrix of three singular values related as $\sigma_1 \geq \sigma_2 \geq \sigma_3 \geq 0$ [9].

$$[J]_{4\times3} = \left[X^T\right]_{4\times4}[\Sigma]_{4\times3}[Y]_{3\times3} \tag{5.12}$$

The condition number of the Jacobian matrix $k(J)$ is then defined by (5.13), where the range of the condition number is given by (5.14).

$$k(J) = \frac{\sigma_1}{\sigma_3} \tag{5.13}$$

$$1 \leq k(J) \leq \infty \tag{5.14}$$

The condition number indicates how far away the specified configuration is from the nearest singular configuration. The closer the condition number is to unity, the further away the configuration is to a singular configuration. Therefore, the objective is to optimise the 4R mechanism to operate in configurations with a condition number value close to unity. This is a minimisation problem.

To simplify the calculation, the GCN can be discretely defined as (5.15), where $k(j)$ is the condition number for the jth workspace position and n is the total number of workspace positions.

$$\mathrm{GCN} = \frac{\sum_{j=1}^{n} k(j)}{n} \tag{5.15}$$

The GCN has the same range of possible values as the condition number:

$$1 \leq \mathrm{GCN} \leq \infty \tag{5.16}$$

As with the condition number, a value of GCN near unity is desirable. This indicates the mechanism operates through most of the shoulder workspace without approaching a singular configuration. However, the GCN can overlook the occurrence of undesirable peak condition number values. To ensure these peak values are not overlooked, the maximum condition number value out of the 89 calculated for the workspace $\mathrm{CN}_{\max}$ is also considered in the optimisation process:

$$\mathrm{CN_{max}} = \max(k(1), \ldots, k(n)) \tag{5.17}$$

The singularity objectives are therefore the minimisation of the GCN and $\mathrm{CN_{max}}$.

Design optimisation of the 4R mechanism was carried out using the variables and objectives discussed throughout this chapter. The optimisation problem is formulated as (5.18), where x is a solution in the population of solutions X.

$$\text{minimise } F(x) = (f_{ws}(x), \Delta\theta(x), \mathrm{GCN}(x), \mathrm{CN_{max}}(x)) \tag{5.18}$$

$$\Delta\theta(x) = \Delta\theta_{ave}(x) + \Delta\theta^4_{max}(x) \tag{5.19}$$

Table 5.2 lists 10 Pareto optimal solutions of the NSGA II optimisation for a right shoulder 4R exoskeleton. For a left shoulder exoskeleton, the values for φ_z and θ_1^0 are multiplied by negative one. Note that each solution is considered to perform equally well by the NSGA II algorithm. In this research, the 10th solution is selected for the design of the upper limb exoskeleton. This solution is selected because the sizes of the three links are smaller compared to the other solutions; therefore, an exoskeleton designed with these parameter values will have a lower weight. It is also possible to select a solution based on clinical input.

The optimal variable values of the selected solution are shown in Table 5.3. A 4R exoskeleton designed with these variable values can theoretically achieve 100 % of the shoulder workspace without interfering with the user. Figure 5.9 shows a 4R exoskeleton with these parameter values.

The optimised 4R design has both a GCN and a $\mathrm{CN_{max}}$ value that is closer to unity compared to the other designs. The lower GCN value of 1.7 for the optimised 4R compared to 1.9 for the unoptimised 4R and 2.4 for the 3R indicates that on average this 4R exoskeleton is able to operate further from singular configurations than the other designs when operating in the shoulder workspace. The small $\mathrm{CN_{max}}$

Table 5.2 Ten Pareto optimal solutions

Variables						Objectives		
α_1	α_2	α_3	φ_z	φ_x	θ_1^0	GCN	$\mathrm{CN_{max}}$	Average joint motion
92.1	79.7	64.1	3.9	32.7	−146.5	1.70	2.50	0.162
88.6	81.2	64.0	5.6	35.3	−147.9	1.71	2.42	0.162
77.3	89.6	90.9	41.2	57.3	179.9	1.65	2.83	0.166
94.0	80.2	64.4	−0.4	35.0	−151.6	1.71	2.39	0.162
104.3	79.9	69.1	−13.7	26.1	−132.9	1.70	3.81	0.159
80.5	94.7	74.3	40.4	59.9	−180.0	1.65	2.99	0.167
83.5	90.7	68.1	29.6	73.5	−175.1	1.69	2.57	0.160
77.1	89.6	91.4	41.7	57.0	180.0	1.65	2.88	0.167
95.0	79.7	64.7	6.9	−56.3	−147.2	1.69	2.56	0.163
88.9	79.9	62.9	9.0	35.2	−149.0	1.71	2.41	0.162

Table 5.3 4R variable values of the selected Pareto optimal solution

Design variable	Optimal value (°)
α_1	88.9
α_2	79.9
α_3	62.9
φ_z	9.0
φ_x	35.2
θ_1^0	−149.0

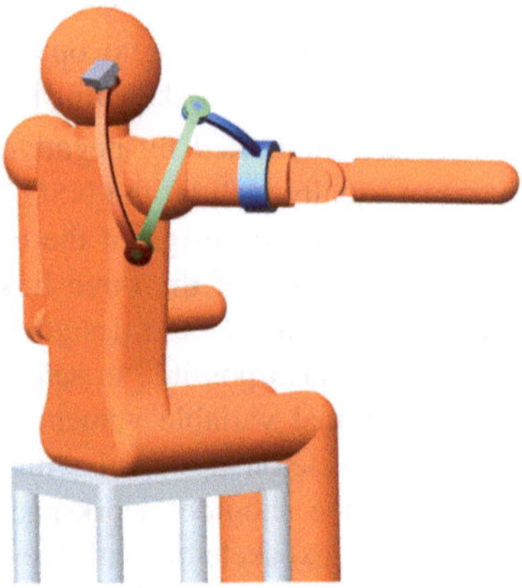

Fig. 5.9 The 4R mechanism design obtained from the NSGA II optimisation

value of 2.4 for the optimised 4R indicates that this design can achieve the entire shoulder workspace with configurations that are all relatively far from a singular configuration. The unoptimised 4R has a higher CN_{max} value of 5.0 and therefore will operate in a configuration that is closer to a singular configuration than any of the optimised 4R configurations. The large CN_{max} value for the 3R exoskeleton confirms that there is a region in the defined shoulder workspace that requires the 3R exoskeleton to operate very close to a singular configuration. This agrees with the analysis that this 3R design cannot avoid operating near a singular configuration in the shoulder workspace. Figure 5.10 shows the condition number values of the 89 positions for each design.

From Fig. 5.10a, it can be seen that the optimised 4R mechanism operates the closest to singular configurations when at the edge of the shoulder workspace. To demonstrate the optimised 4R mechanism's poorest performance, an example of the trajectories of Joints 1, 2, and 3 in performing a circular movement of the upper arm along the edge of the shoulder workspace is presented in Figs. 5.11 and 5.12. This circumduction movement involves approximately 360° rotation of the shoulder and is done with a near-constant velocity of 51.4°/s over 7 s. The peak 4R joint velocity during this movement occurs in Joint 2 at 76°/s which is 48 % higher than the shoulder velocity. Joints 1 and 3 have slightly lower peak velocities at 65 and 63°/s, respectively.

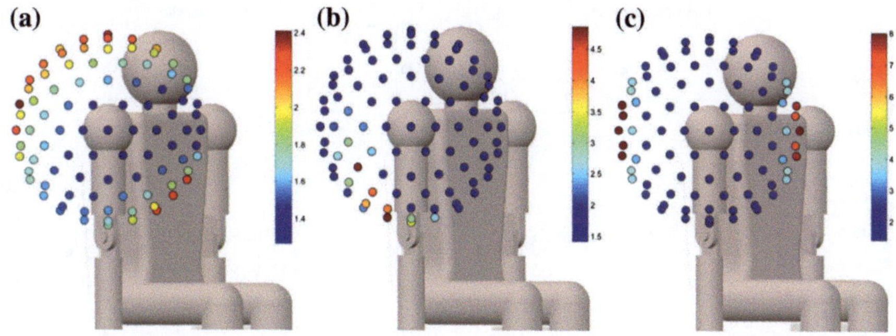

Fig. 5.10 Condition number results for the 89 workspace points of three different designs: **a** optimised 4R, **b** 4R with 90° links and base joint behind the shoulder, and **c** 3R with the base joint rotated 45° laterally from behind the shoulder

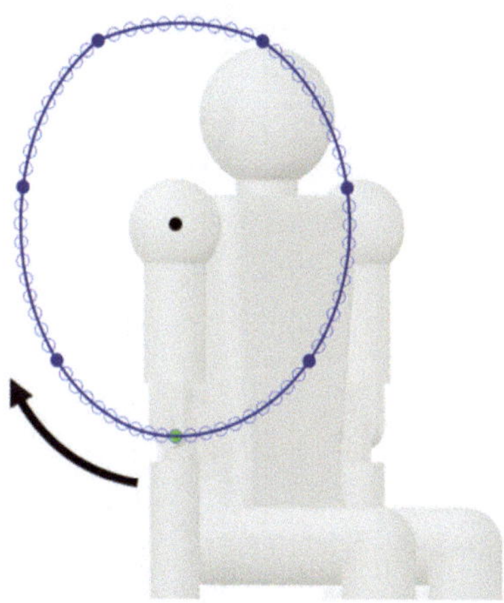

Fig. 5.11 Trajectory path for the optimised 4R mechanism where it operates closest to singular configurations. This movement is a constant velocity shoulder circumduction over 7 s. Each point indicates a position of the upper arm and 4R end-effector. The *green point* indicates the starting and ending position, the solid *blue points* indicate the positions at every time step of 1 s and the *hollow points* indicate the positions at every time step of 0.1 s

In terms of joint movement, the optimised 4R design has a significantly lower average joint motion of 0.162 compared to 0.242 for the unoptimised 4R and 0.250 for the 3R design. This implies that on average the joints of the optimised 4R move at a lower velocity when moving the end-effector through the shoulder workspace compared to the other designs.

Figure 5.13 shows the optimal joint angles of Joints 1, 2 and 3 to reach each of the 89 end-effector positions in the shoulder workspace. These joint angles combine to give the optimal joint configurations selected by the optimisation algorithm for the kinematically redundant 4R mechanism. 3D models of these 89 configurations

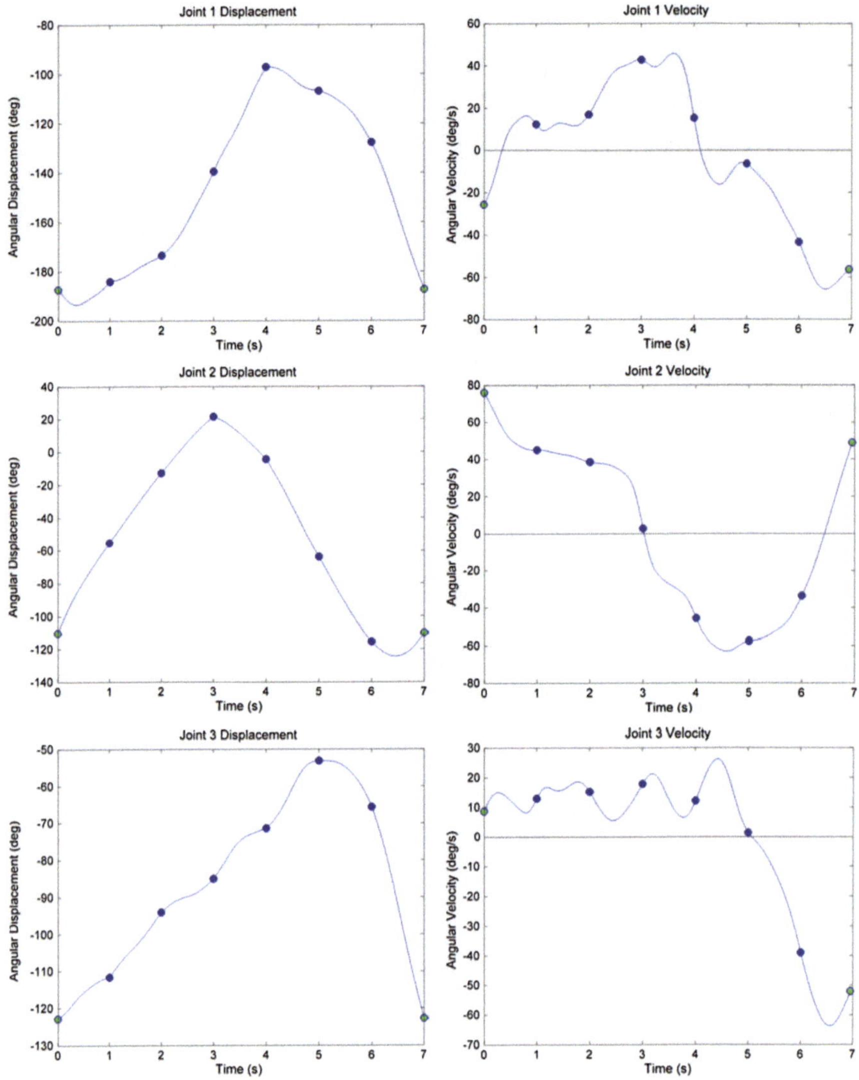

Fig. 5.12 Position and velocity trajectories of Joints 1, 2 and 3 in the optimised 4R mechanism during the 7 s shoulder circumduction illustrated in Fig. 5.11

can be found in Appendix A. From Fig. 5.13, it can be seen that each joint can smoothly transition between adjacent end-effector positions in all directions without requiring sudden changes in joint angle.

Figure 5.13d shows that the offset between the angular positions of Joint 4 and that of shoulder axial rotation is minimal for the majority of the workspace. The larger offset occurs at the workspace boundary in the horizontally extended positions and at the vertical flexed position. These boundary positions are very difficult

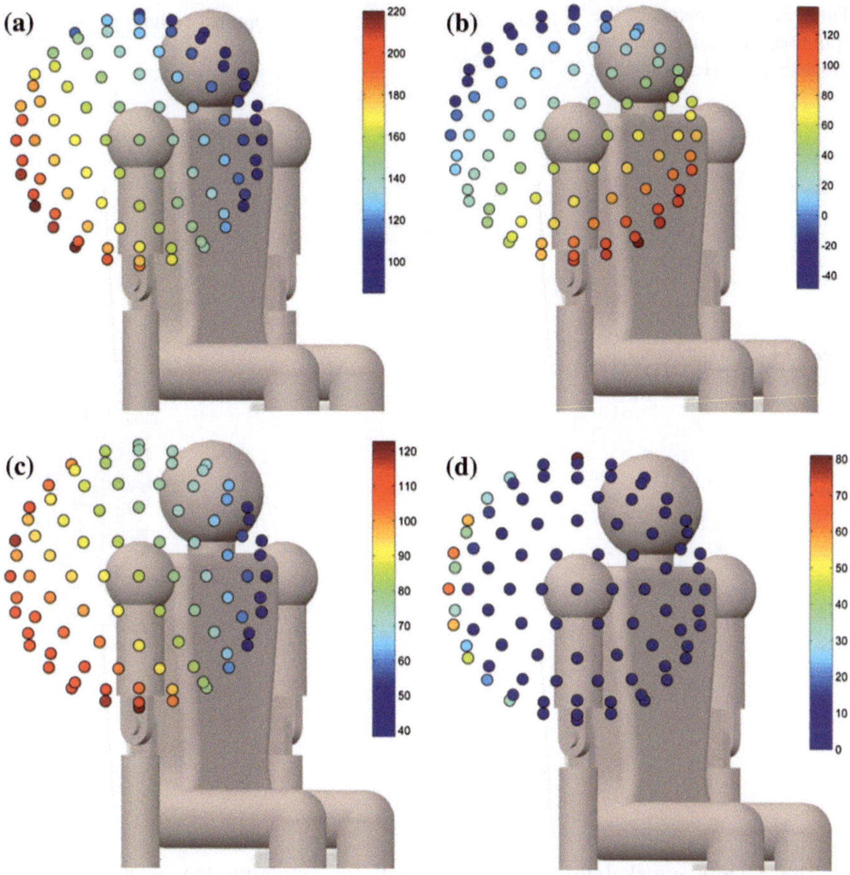

Fig. 5.13 Displacement angles of Joints 1, 2 and 3 to optimally reach each of the 89 end-effector positions. **a** Joint 1 displacements. **b** Joint 2 displacements. **c** Joint 3 displacements. **d** Offset between the *angular position* of Joint 4 and the angular position of shoulder axial rotation

to reach for a typical shoulder and should not be an issue. A small offset means that Joint 4 can be implemented using a small arc-shaped rail with an arc size similar to the range of motion of shoulder axial rotation. A small rail makes the exoskeleton easier for the user to don and does not have the problem that a circular rail has where the rail interferes with the user's torso when the upper arm is lowered.

5.2 Exoskeleton Kinematic Design

The optimised 4R mechanism parameters are used in the design of a 5-DOF active exoskeleton for the left upper limb. The previous parameters were defined for the right shoulder and are converted for the left shoulder in Table 5.4. The 4R mechanism for the left shoulder is shown in Fig. 5.14.

Table 5.4 Parameters of the optimised 4R design for a left shoulder exoskeleton

Design variable	Optimal value (°)
α_1	88.9
α_2	79.9
α_3	62.9
φ_z	−9.0
φ_x	35.2
θ_1^0	149.0

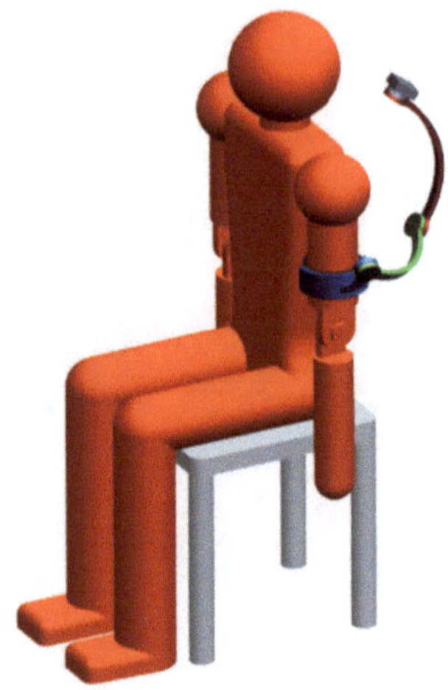

Fig. 5.14 The optimised 4R mechanism concept for the *left shoulder*

The 5-DOF exoskeleton includes 4-DOF for actuating the 3-DOF spherical motion of the shoulder joint and 1-DOF for actuating elbow movements. In other words, the exoskeleton can perform shoulder flexion and extension, abduction and adduction, medial and lateral rotation and elbow flexion and extension movements. These 4-DOF produce the largest movements in the upper limb and recovery of these movements is considered highly important in improving upper limb function. The 3-DOF spherical movements of the wrist and 2-DOF translational movements of the shoulder contribute less to upper limb movements and are not implemented in the present exoskeleton prototype. Figure 5.15 shows a CAD model of the exoskeleton and Fig. 5.16 shows a photograph of the exoskeleton used by a healthy subject.

The exoskeleton is designed to be used while the user is in a seated position to ensure the user does not sway from the proper usage position which causes misalignment and can lead to the user entering the hazardous operating space of the exoskeleton. The DH parameters of the 5-DOF exoskeleton are shown in Table 5.5 where the parameters for $i = 6$ represent the relationship between the coordinate system of Joint 5 and the coordinate system defined at the hand position. The angular parameters α_i and θ_i are obtained from the design optimisation of the 4R

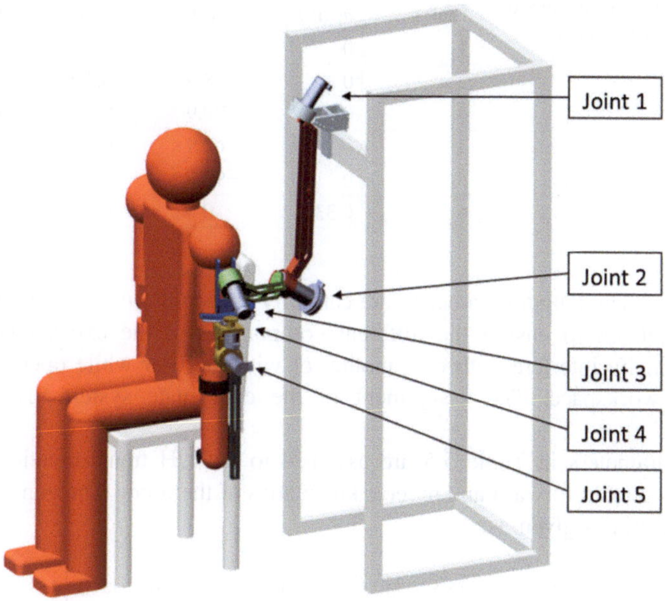

Fig. 5.15 The 5-DOF upper limb exoskeleton with a shoulder complex designed using the optimised 4R mechanism parameters. The exoskeleton structure is constructed almost entirely from aluminium plates to allow rapid prototyping and enable future modifications

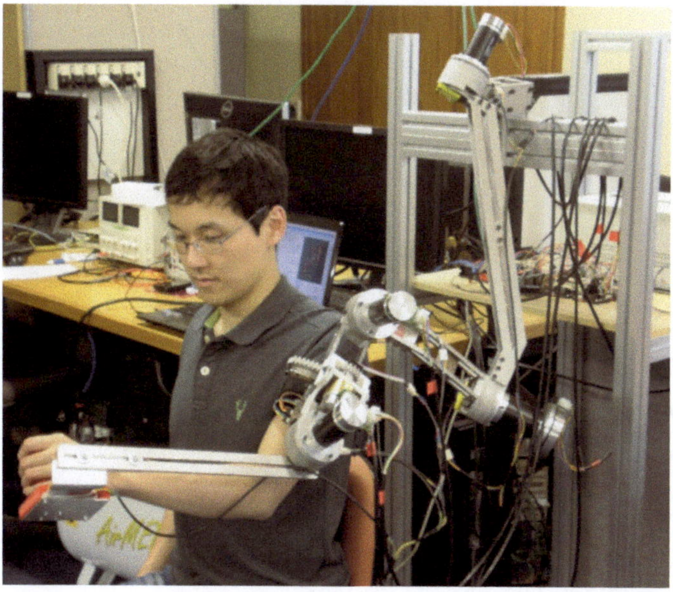

Fig. 5.16 The 5-DOF upper limb exoskeleton prototype used by a healthy subject

Table 5.5 DH parameters of the 5-DOF exoskeleton

Link i	a_i (m)	α_i (°)	d_i (m)	θ_i (°)
1	0	35.2	0	−9.0
2	0	−88.9	−0.440	θ_1
3	0	79.9	−0.247	θ_2
4	0	62.9	−0.137	θ_3
5	0	−90.0	0.126	θ_4
6	0.33	0	0	$\theta_5 - 90$

mechanism. The length parameters are carefully chosen through 3D simulations of the exoskeleton to ensure the different components of the exoskeleton do not unintentionally interfere with one another or with the user while operating in the shoulder workspace. The assignment of the coordinate systems is shown in Fig. 5.17.

The parameters in Table 5.5 are assigned to the DH transformation matrices which are used in forward and inverse kinematics of the robot. The general form of the DH matrix is given as:

$$T_i^{i-1} = \begin{bmatrix} \cos\theta_i & -\cos\alpha_i \sin\theta_i & \sin\alpha_i \sin\theta_i & a_i \cos\theta_i \\ \sin\theta_i & \cos\alpha_i \cos\theta_i & -\sin\alpha_i \cos\theta_i & a_i \sin\theta_i \\ 0 & \sin\alpha_i & \cos\alpha_i & d_i \\ 0 & 0 & 0 & 1 \end{bmatrix} \quad (5.20)$$

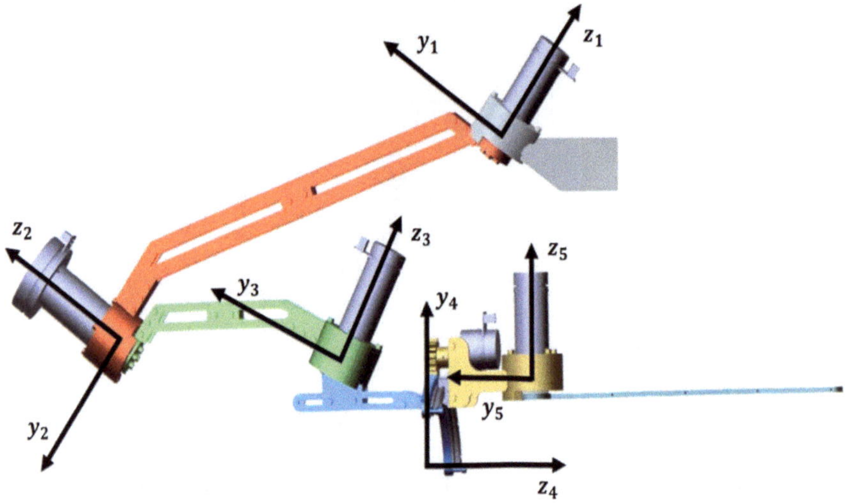

Fig. 5.17 Default configuration of the 5-DOF exoskeleton

The matrices representing the geometric relationship between each pair of adjacent coordinate systems now include the parameters d_i for the actual design which was omitted for simplicity during design optimisation:

$$T_1^0 = \begin{bmatrix} \cos\varphi_z & -\cos\varphi_x \sin\varphi_z & \sin\varphi_x \sin\varphi_z & 0 \\ \sin\varphi_z & \cos\varphi_x \cos\varphi_z & -\sin\varphi_x \cos\varphi_z & 0 \\ 0 & \sin\varphi_x & \cos\varphi_x & 0 \\ 0 & 0 & 0 & 1 \end{bmatrix} \tag{5.21}$$

$$T_2^1 = \begin{bmatrix} \cos\theta_1 & -\cos\alpha_1 \sin\theta_1 & -\sin\alpha_1 \sin\theta_1 & 0 \\ \sin\theta_1 & \cos\alpha_1 \cos\theta_1 & \sin\alpha_1 \cos\theta_1 & 0 \\ 0 & -\sin\alpha_1 & \cos\alpha_1 & d_1 \\ 0 & 0 & 0 & 1 \end{bmatrix} \tag{5.22}$$

$$T_3^2 = \begin{bmatrix} \cos\theta_2 & -\cos\alpha_2 \sin\theta_2 & \sin\alpha_2 \sin\theta_2 & 0 \\ \sin\theta_2 & \cos\alpha_2 \cos\theta_2 & -\sin\alpha_2 \cos\theta_2 & 0 \\ 0 & \sin\alpha_2 & \cos\alpha_2 & d_2 \\ 0 & 0 & 0 & 1 \end{bmatrix} \tag{5.23}$$

$$T_4^3 = \begin{bmatrix} \cos\theta_3 & -\cos\alpha_3 \sin\theta_3 & \sin\alpha_3 \sin\theta_3 & 0 \\ \sin\theta_3 & \cos\alpha_3 \cos\theta_3 & -\sin\alpha_3 \cos\theta_3 & 0 \\ 0 & \sin\alpha_3 & \cos\alpha_3 & d_3 \\ 0 & 0 & 0 & 1 \end{bmatrix} \tag{5.24}$$

$$T_5^4 = \begin{bmatrix} \cos\theta_4 & 0 & -\sin\theta_4 & 0 \\ \sin\theta_4 & 0 & \cos\theta_4 & 0 \\ 0 & -1 & 0 & d_4 \\ 0 & 0 & 0 & 1 \end{bmatrix} \tag{5.25}$$

$$T_6^5 = \begin{bmatrix} \cos(\theta_5 - 90) & -\sin(\theta_5 - 90) & 0 & a_5 \cos(\theta_5 - 90) \\ \sin(\theta_5 - 90) & \cos(\theta_5 - 90) & 0 & a_5 \sin(\theta_5 - 90) \\ 0 & 0 & 1 & 0 \\ 0 & 0 & 0 & 1 \end{bmatrix} \tag{5.26}$$

Note that the numbering of the parameters is delayed by one compared to the link number in Table 5.5 since the first line of parameters is used to define the orientation of Joint 1 with respect to the global coordinate system. Applying the geometric parameters of the exoskeleton design in (5.21)–(5.26), the following DH matrices which represent the kinematic structure of the exoskeleton are obtained:

$$T_1^0 = \begin{bmatrix} 0.9877 & 0.0902 & 0.1278 & 0 \\ -0.1564 & 0.5693 & 0.8071 & 0 \\ 0 & -0.8171 & 0.5764 & 0 \\ 0 & 0 & 0 & 1 \end{bmatrix} \tag{5.27}$$

$$T_2^1 = \begin{bmatrix} \cos\theta_1 & -0.0192\sin\theta_1 & -0.9998\sin\theta_1 & 0 \\ \sin\theta_1 & 0.0192\cos\theta_1 & 0.9998\cos\theta_1 & 0 \\ 0 & -0.9998 & 0.0192 & -0.440 \\ 0 & 0 & 0 & 1 \end{bmatrix} \tag{5.28}$$

$$T_3^2 = \begin{bmatrix} \cos\theta_2 & -0.1754\sin\theta_2 & 0.9845\sin\theta_2 & 0 \\ \sin\theta_2 & 0.1754\cos\theta_2 & -0.9845\cos\theta_2 & 0 \\ 0 & 0.9845 & 0.1754 & -0.247 \\ 0 & 0 & 0 & 1 \end{bmatrix} \tag{5.29}$$

$$T_4^3 = \begin{bmatrix} \cos\theta_3 & -0.4555\sin\theta_3 & 0.8902\sin\theta_3 & 0 \\ \sin\theta_3 & 0.4555\cos\theta_3 & -0.8902\cos\theta_3 & 0 \\ 0 & 0.8902 & 0.4555 & -0.137 \\ 0 & 0 & 0 & 1 \end{bmatrix} \tag{5.30}$$

$$T_5^4 = \begin{bmatrix} \cos\theta_4 & 0 & -\sin\theta_4 & 0 \\ \sin\theta_4 & 0 & \cos\theta_4 & 0 \\ 0 & -1 & 0 & 0.126 \\ 0 & 0 & 0 & 1 \end{bmatrix} \tag{5.31}$$

$$T_6^5 = \begin{bmatrix} \cos(\theta_5 - 90) & -\sin(\theta_5 - 90) & 0 & 0.33\cos(\theta_5 - 90) \\ \sin(\theta_5 - 90) & \cos(\theta_5 - 90) & 0 & 0.33\sin(\theta_5 - 90) \\ 0 & 0 & 1 & 0 \\ 0 & 0 & 0 & 1 \end{bmatrix} \tag{5.32}$$

5.3 Design Considerations

There are numerous important design factors that must be considered in the design of the 5-DOF exoskeleton prototype to ensure it can achieve the required performance and is user-friendly. These are discussed in the subsequent sections.

5.3.1 Mechanical Interference

The exoskeleton must not collide with other parts of its structure or with the user while operating in the human upper limb workspace. This is particularly challenging for the shoulder mechanism of the exoskeleton since the shoulder has a very large range of motion which limits the space available for the exoskeleton structure and its components. In addition, there are many joints and links that move in close proximity to one another which increases the possibility of mechanical interference. Mechanical interference is considered during the design of the links and joints as well as in the selection of actuators and sensors.

End-effector positions reaching the edge of the shoulder workspace have been found to be the most likely to cause mechanical interference and are carefully considered during the design process. Figure 5.18 shows the final exoskeleton design at key end-effector positions along the edge of the shoulder workspace. It can be seen that interference does not occur and the exoskeleton can feasibly reach these extreme shoulder positions.

Interference analysis is done by simulating a 3D CAD model of the exoskeleton in the PTC Creo Parametric software [10]. Results show that unintentional interference does not occur for the 89 optimal joint configurations obtained from the

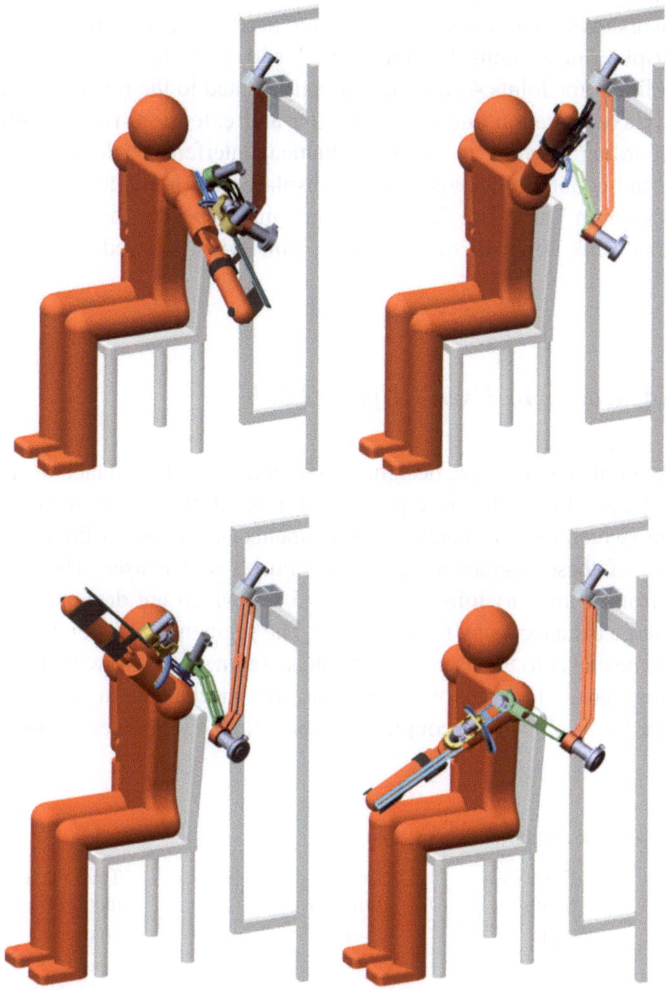

Fig. 5.18 The exoskeleton with the upper arm at four different positions along the edge of the shoulder workspace. These extreme positions can be feasibly reached by the exoskeleton without causing mechanical interference

NSGA II optimisation. These 89 configurations are presented in Appendix A. Intentional interference such as the interference between the exoskeleton's hand interface and the user's torso when the hand is moved towards the torso is not considered a problem.

5.3.2 Range of Motion of Exoskeleton Joints

The optimal configurations that the joints of the kinematically redundant 4R mechanism operate in were previously determined for 89 upper arm positions in the shoulder workspace. These configurations are used to identify the upper and lower angular displacement limits for Joints 1, 2 and 3 in the exoskeleton. The displacement limits for Joints 4 and 5 are directly related to the range of motion limits of shoulder axial rotation and elbow flexion and extension, respectively, and are chosen accordingly while ensuring mechanical interference does not occur. The clockwise and counter-clockwise angular displacement limits for each exoskeleton joint are shown in Table 5.6. The angles are with respect to the directional axis of the proximal link towards the previous joint when viewed from an external perspective.

5.3.3 Clearance to User's Upper Limb

The exoskeleton segments are designed to maintain a safe distance away from the user during operation. This is especially important for the segments of the 4R mechanism (which do not match the movements of the user's limb segments) as interference of these segments can cause injuries to the user. This includes the segments from Joint 1 to Joint 3 (see Fig. 5.15) which are designed to operate a relatively large distance away from the user. The segments from Joint 3 onwards are designed to be closer to the user's limb as these segments move with the user's limb and therefore have a low risk of causing harmful interference to the user. This also makes it easier to physically couple the user's limb to the exoskeleton segments.

Table 5.6 Range of motion of exoskeleton joints

Exoskeleton joint	Clockwise limit (°)	Counter-clockwise limit (°)	Total range of motion (°)
1	14	−89	103
2	120	−25	145
3	−57	−132	75
4	18	−78	96
5	180	55	125

The smallest distance between the axis of the user's limb and an exoskeleton link is 8 cm. This gives a clearance of approximately 4 cm for a typical user.

The exoskeleton base is supported by a mechanically grounded aluminium frame behind the user. This means that the user does not carry the weight of the exoskeleton but is instead supported by the exoskeleton during rehabilitation. Such support is important since the user's upper limb is expected to have some level of impairment. Furthermore, reaction forces from the exoskeleton due to actuation are transmitted to the ground via this frame.

This research focuses on developing an exoskeleton for the shoulder joint and the presented 5-DOF prototype does not include movements of the forearm, wrist or fingers. To allow for the inclusion of these joints in future developments, the forearm segment of the exoskeleton is designed to be easily replaceable.

5.3.4 *Joint Alignment*

An exoskeleton is designed to operate alongside the human limb with the exoskeleton joints aligned with the corresponding upper limb joints of the user. Operating the exoskeleton when there is a misalignment between the joints of the exoskeleton and the human limb causes the generation of undesirable interaction forces and limb positioning errors. Therefore, the exoskeleton structure is designed to keep all five joints aligned with the human counterpart throughout the entire upper limb workspace. Joints 1, 2, 3 and 4 correspond to the shoulder joint and are permanently aligned with the ICOR of the shoulder, whereas Joint 5 is kept aligned with the user's elbow joint.

To facilitate users with different arm lengths, links with adjustable lengths are used for the exoskeleton segments corresponding to the upper arm and forearm so that joint alignment can be maintained. In addition, the height of the exoskeleton can be adjusted at the support frame to align the shoulder joint when the user is in a seated position. These adjustments are achieved using passive linear slider mechanisms which are locked into position once they are adjusted to the correct lengths. Table 5.7 shows the typical human segment dimensions and the adjustable ranges of the corresponding exoskeleton segments. The lengths of the adult upper limb segments are obtained from average values in the literature [11].

Table 5.7 Dimensions of upper limb and exoskeleton segments

Segment	Average adult dimensions	Exoskeleton dimensions (mm)	
		Lower limit	Upper limit
Shoulder ICOR to elbow	278	255	335
Elbow to palm	349	125	365
Shoulder to ground	1000	800	1200

As a result of the optimisation, the optimised 4R mechanism can maintain a close match between the drifting angular positions of Joint 4 and shoulder axial rotation throughout the shoulder workspace. This means the range of motion requirement of Joint 4 is close to that of shoulder axial rotation. Therefore, a relatively small rail can be used which makes the exoskeleton easy to don and reduces the exoskeleton's interference with the user.

Joint 4 in the 4R mechanism of the exoskeleton is implemented using a curved rail mechanism as opposed to the simple pin joints used for the other 4-DOF. The curved rail is achieved using a pinion gear engaged on a curved rack as shown in Fig. 5.19. This mechanism converts the rotational motion of the motor into a translational motion along an arc around the upper arm. Thus, joint alignment is achieved without mechanical interference between the exoskeleton and the user.

The curved rail consists of two 60° curved rail segments (THK, Japan) [12] which gives an axial rotation range of motion close to 120°. The use of a 120° section as opposed to a 360° ring allows the user to easily don the exoskeleton without needing to make difficult manoeuvres with the limb. In addition, the 120° rail is positioned lateral to the upper arm and therefore does not interfere with the torso, whereas a 360° rail cannot avoid contact with the torso when the upper arm is lowered. A rail size of 120° is used as this size can achieve the range of motion of shoulder axial rotation without sacrificing the range of motion of other DOF due to mechanical interference of the rail with the user's body. The centre of the rail is

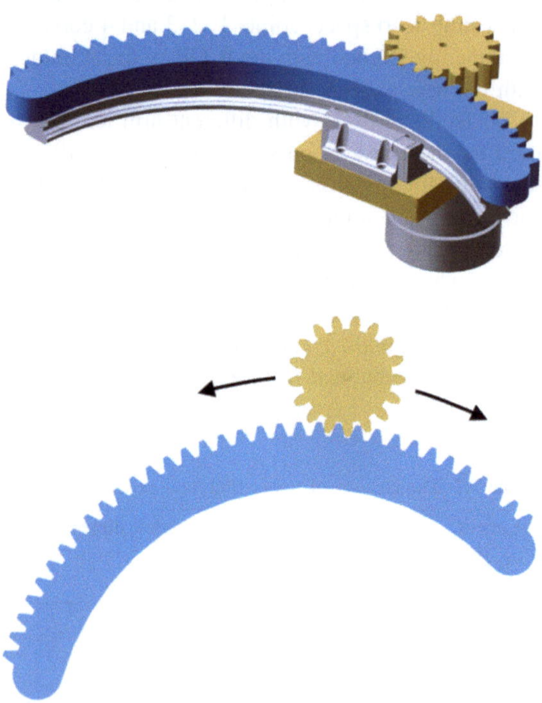

Fig. 5.19 The 120° curved rail mechanism for generating upper arm axial rotation used in Joint 4 of the 5-DOF exoskeleton

offset posteriorly by 30° to match the shoulder range of motion. This also conveniently prevents the rail from interfering with the user's head when flexing the shoulder to raise the upper arm above the horizontal plane.

5.4 System Configuration

5.4.1 Actuators and Sensors

Past upper limb exoskeletons most commonly use electromagnetic motors or PMA for actuation. The main advantages of PMAs are their high power-to-weight ratio and their mechanical compliance. However, the many drawbacks of PMAs make them not suitable for the upper limb exoskeleton. For every joint in the exoskeleton, a pair of PMA is required to enable bidirectional actuation. The 5-DOF exoskeleton has five joints in close proximity with each other, and there is no space for five pairs of PMAs on the exoskeleton links. Furthermore, PMAs have a relatively small actuation range and is not suitable for actuating the shoulder joint which has a very large range of motion. PMAs also respond slowly to command signals and have nonlinear actuation characteristics which make them difficult to control. In addition, PMAs are driven by compressed air which is noisy and inconvenient.

In the case of motors, their lower power-to-weight ratio is not a major issue since the human upper limb is mainly used for precise movements over a large range of motion rather than load support and the motors do not need to be high power. Furthermore, it is possible to produce compliant behaviour in a motor-driven exoskeleton with the appropriate control strategies. Hence, motors are used for the actuation of the 5-DOF upper limb exoskeleton.

Sensors are installed on the exoskeleton to measure rotational displacement of the five exoskeleton joints and the interaction force between the user's limb and the exoskeleton. Joint displacements are used in forward kinematics to determine the exoskeleton configuration and therefore the upper limb postures in real-time.

5.4.2 Safety Features

Safety is a major concern for any device that actively interacts with a human user. The actuated exoskeleton is physically coupled to the user's upper limb and can cause severe injuries to the user in the event of an accident or malfunction. The fact that the exoskeleton can generate larger torques than those generated by users with severe upper limb impairment further increases the need for reliable safety measures. A number of features have been included in the exoskeleton system to ensure safe and comfortable operation for the user.

Mechanical stoppers are used at each of the five actuated joints to prevent the exoskeleton joints from moving beyond their standard operating range of motion. The software also monitors the position of each joint via the magnetic encoder sensors and prevents the motor from driving the joint beyond the range of motion limits. The range of motion limits for each of the five exoskeleton joints was presented. Motor speeds are also limited by software. Emergency stop buttons are available for the exoskeleton user and external users to manually stop the exoskeleton if a problem occurs.

5.4.3 Human–Robot Interface

The human upper limb has 9-DOF which are located at the shoulder, elbow and wrist and is kinematically redundant. In other words, constraining the hand will still leave the upper arm and forearm free to move. Therefore, to kinematically resolve all 9-DOF of the entire upper limb, at least two physical HRI must be used. In the 5-DOF exoskeleton, the two HRI are located at the upper arm near the elbow and at the hand. The HRI at the upper arm consists of a platform and a strap to couple the arm to the exoskeleton between Joint 4 and Joint 5. The HRI at the hand consists of a handle and a platform to rest the hand. The two HRI are designed to allow the user to easily don the exoskeleton with minimal effort and without the need to make difficult manoeuvres with the arm. A two-axis force sensor is incorporated into the upper arm HRI to measure forces in the directions of shoulder flexion and extension and abduction and adduction. A one-axis force sensor is used in the hand HRI to measure elbow flexion and extension forces.

The exoskeleton system is controlled by a PC via USB. A microcontroller is used to communicate with each device in the exoskeleton. These include five motor controllers, five rotary encoders, one two-axis force sensor and one single-axis force sensor. A flow diagram of the exoskeleton system is presented in Fig. 5.20.

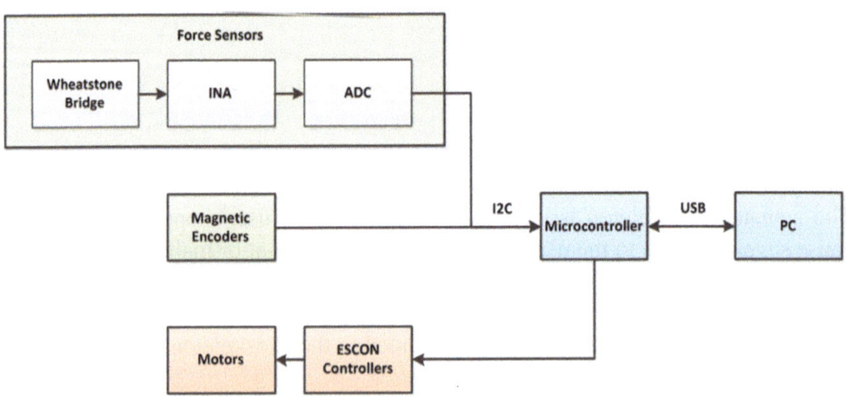

Fig. 5.20 Exoskeleton system diagram

Digital communication with the magnetic encoder sensors and force sensors is implemented using an I2C bus [13]. The I2C protocol is an elegant method of implementing communication in a system with many devices such as the exoskeleton system. Furthermore, future addition of sensors or other devices into the system can be done simply by configuring the device with a unique address and connecting it to the I2C bus. The I2C bus in the present exoskeleton system is shown in Fig. 5.21.

A graphical user interface (GUI) is developed in MATLAB for operating the 5-DOF exoskeleton (Fig. 5.22). The GUI is used to:

- Switch between admittance and impedance control modes;
- Enable and disable support of forearm and upper arm weight;
- Plan a trajectory;
- Visualise a 3D simulation of the trajectory before applying it on the exoskeleton;
- Change user limb mass and length parameters; and
- Change assistance gain and artificial stiffness, damping and inertia constants.

Admittance mode allows the user's limb to physically move the exoskeleton, whereas in impedance mode the exoskeleton moves the user's limb through a trajectory path. Under impedance mode, a trajectory point is created by setting the target position of the 4 upper limb DOF and the desired travel time to reach this position. Subsequent target points are added to the sequence to create the trajectory plan. Once the trajectory plan is prepared, a smooth trajectory is calculated and demonstrated in the 3D model for verification before performing the movements with the exoskeleton. The GUI provides an intuitive trajectory planning process by simplifying movements of the spherical shoulder into horizontal and vertical displacements.

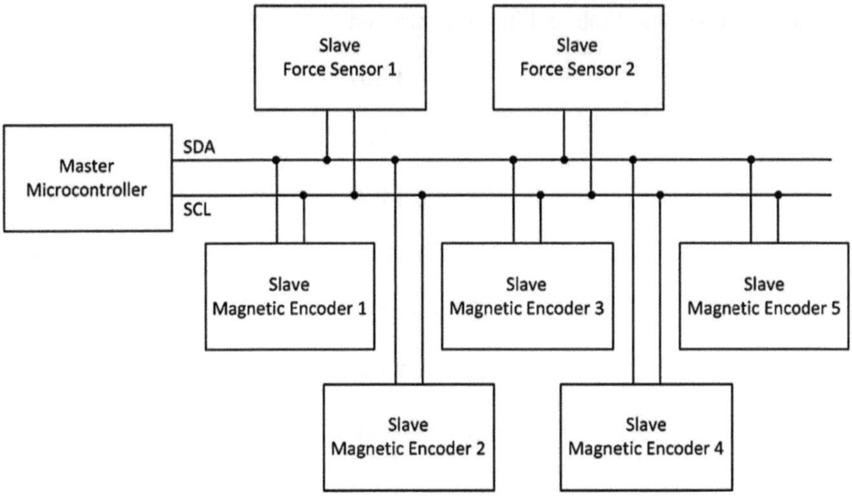

Fig. 5.21 The I2C bus in the exoskeleton system. This bus is used to communicate with five magnetic encoders and two force sensors

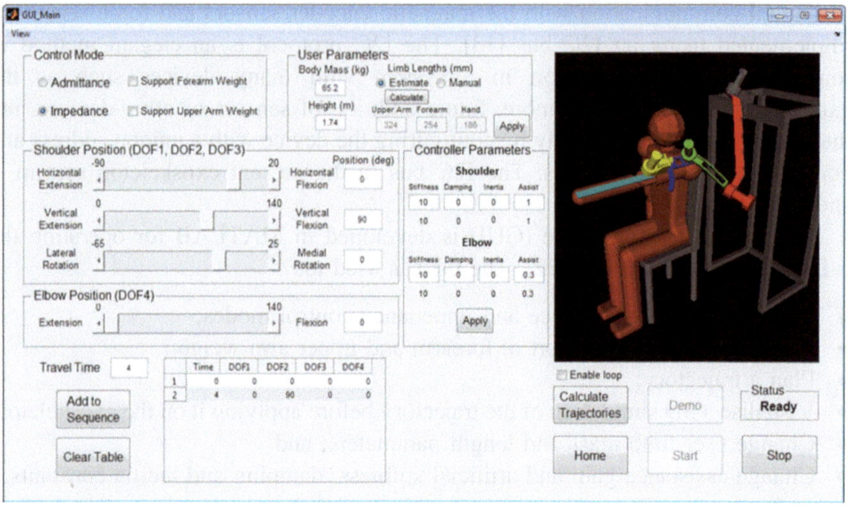

Fig. 5.22 GUI developed for operating the exoskeleton

The kinematic parameters of the user's upper limb segments can either be entered manually or estimated. The inertial and kinematic parameters of each upper limb segment are approximated using the total body mass and height of the user, respectively [11] using (5.33)–(5.44), where UA refers to the upper arm, FA refers to the forearm, HA refers to the hand, H is the height of the subject, M is the total body mass of the subject, l is the length of the segment, d is the distance to the segment's centre of mass from the proximal joint, m is the segment mass and I is the inertia tensor of the segment. These parameters are used to determine the required torque to support the limb and in the controllers.

$$l_{\text{UA}} = 0.186H \tag{5.33}$$

$$l_{\text{FA}} = 0.146H \tag{5.34}$$

$$l_{\text{HA}} = 0.146H \tag{5.35}$$

$$d_{\text{UA}} = 0.436 l_{\text{UA}} \tag{5.36}$$

$$d_{\text{FA}} = 0.43 l_{\text{FA}} \tag{5.37}$$

$$d_{\text{HA}} = 0.506 l_{\text{HA}} \tag{5.38}$$

$$m_{\text{UA}} = 0.0263M \tag{5.39}$$

$$m_{\mathrm{FA}} = 0.015M \tag{5.40}$$

$$m_{\mathrm{HA}} = 0.0059M \tag{5.41}$$

$$I_{\mathrm{UA}} = \begin{bmatrix} m_{\mathrm{UA}}(0.282 l_{\mathrm{UA}})^2 & 0 & 0 \\ 0 & m_{\mathrm{UA}}(0.265 l_{\mathrm{UA}})^2 & 0 \\ 0 & 0 & m_{\mathrm{UA}}(0.153 l_{\mathrm{UA}})^2 \end{bmatrix} \tag{5.42}$$

$$I_{\mathrm{FA}} = \begin{bmatrix} m_{\mathrm{FA}}(0.265 l_{\mathrm{FA}})^2 & 0 & 0 \\ 0 & m_{FA}(0.108 l_{\mathrm{FA}})^2 & 0 \\ 0 & 0 & m_{\mathrm{FA}}(0.261 l_{\mathrm{FA}})^2 \end{bmatrix} \tag{5.43}$$

$$I_{\mathrm{HA}} = \begin{bmatrix} m_{\mathrm{HA}}(0.266 l_{\mathrm{HA}})^2 & 0 & 0 \\ 0 & m_{\mathrm{HA}}(0.169 l_{\mathrm{HA}})^2 & 0 \\ 0 & 0 & m_{\mathrm{HA}}(0.222 l_{\mathrm{HA}})^2 \end{bmatrix} \tag{5.44}$$

5.5 Summary

The design of a 5-DOF active upper limb exoskeleton prototype is presented in this chapter. A redundant 4R spherical wrist mechanism has been proposed for a shoulder exoskeleton to solve the singularity and workspace limitations present in the 3R spherical wrist. The 4R mechanism has been optimised using the NSGA II multi-objective optimisation algorithm to achieve the entire human shoulder workspace while operating far away from singular configurations and without interfering with the user. The kinematically redundant 4R mechanism allows the exoskeleton to achieve the entire range of motion of the human shoulder while staying well away from singular configurations and with no mechanical interference. To kinematically resolve the user's upper limb, two HRI are used to constrain the user's limb at the upper arm and hand.

References

1. K. Deb, A. Pratap, S. Agarwal, T. Meyarivan, A fast and elitist multiobjective genetic algorithm: NSGA-II. IEEE Trans. Evol. Comput. **6**, 182–197 (2002)
2. J. Knowles, D. Corne, The Pareto archived evolution strategy: a new baseline algorithm for Pareto multiobjective optimisation, in Congress on Evolutionary Computation, vol. 1 (1999), p. 105
3. E. Zitzler, L. Thiele, Multiobjective evolutionary algorithms: a comparative case study and the strength Pareto approach. IEEE Trans. Evol. Comput. **3**, 257–271 (1999)
4. H.S. Lo, S.S.Q Xie, Optimization of a redundant 4R robot for a shoulder exoskeleton, in IEEE/ASME International Conference on Advanced Intelligent Mechatronics (2013), pp. 798–803

5. N.A. Teanby, An icosahedron-based method for even binning of globally distributed remote sensing data. Comput. Geosci. **32**, 1442–1450 (2006)
6. P.K. Jamwal, S. Xie, K.C. Aw, Kinematic design optimization of a parallel ankle rehabilitation robot using modified genetic algorithm. Rob. Auton. Syst. **57**, 1018–1027 (2009)
7. J.K. Salisbury, J.J. Craig, Articulated hands—force control and kinematic issues. Int. J. Rob. Res. **1**, 4–17 (1982)
8. C. Gosselin, J. Angeles, Global performance index for the kinematic optimization of robotic manipulators. J. Mech. Transmissions Autom. Des. **113**, 220–226 (1991)
9. A.A. Maciejewski, C.A. Klein, Singular value decomposition: computation and applications to robotics. Int. J. Rob. Res. **8**, 63–79 (1989)
10. PTC Creo. Available: http://creo.ptc.com/
11. P. De Leva, Adjustments to zatsiorsky-seluyanov's segment inertia parameters. J. Biomech. **29**, 1223–1230 (1996)
12. THK. Available: http://www.thk.com/
13. D. Paret, The I2C bus: from theory to practice (Wiley, New York, 1997)

Chapter 6
Motion and Interactive Control for Upper Limb Exoskeleton

This chapter presents the minimum jerk trajectory planner which is developed to generate smooth trajectories for the 5-DOF upper limb exoskeleton. The minimum jerk criterion is derived from observing normal human motion and is therefore very suitable for formulating the trajectories of a rehabilitation exoskeleton. The minimum jerk criterion is first introduced using a simple point-to-point trajectory for the 1-DOF elbow joint. For the multi-DOF shoulder joint, the minimum jerk trajectory of the shoulder movement is determined and then converted to their respective exoskeleton joint trajectories. This chapter presents force-based control strategies that allow the exoskeleton to interact with and respond to the unpredictable behaviour of the user's limb. The concept of admittance and impedance interaction method is discussed and applied to the upper limb and exoskeleton system.

6.1 Smooth Trajectory Planning

6.1.1 Minimum Jerk Trajectory

It is desirable to have the exoskeleton move with trajectories similar to the trajectories of normal human movement to ensure that the movements are comfortable and correct for rehabilitation. From observations of voluntary movement, researchers have found that normal human movements follow a trajectory that minimises the total jerk [1, 2]. Jerk is the time derivative of acceleration and is therefore the third-time derivative of position $x(t)$:

$$\text{jerk } \dddot{x}(t) = \frac{\mathrm{d}^3 x(t)}{\mathrm{d}t^3} \tag{6.1}$$

A measure of smoothness can be obtained for a trajectory x that starts at time t_i and ends at time t_f by calculating the jerk cost:

S.(S.Q.) Xie, *Advanced Robotics for Medical Rehabilitation*,
Springer Tracts in Advanced Robotics 108, DOI 10.1007/978-3-319-19896-5_6

$$\int_{t_i}^{t_f} (\dddot{x}(t))^2 \mathrm{d}t \tag{6.2}$$

To obtain the smoothest trajectory, it is necessary to optimise the trajectory function to have the minimum jerk cost. The minimum jerk trajectory of an end-effector from one point to another is obtained by minimising the integral of the squared jerk over time. This corresponds to the minimisation of the function (6.3), where T is the terminal time at which the target position x_T, velocity $\dot{x}_T$ and acceleration $\ddot{x}_T$ are to be achieved when starting with the initial position x_0, velocity $\dot{x}_0$ and acceleration $\ddot{x}_0$.

$$I(x) = \frac{1}{2}\int_0^T (\dddot{x}_t)^2 \mathrm{d}t \tag{6.3}$$

The minimum of this function is found using calculus of variations. First, a function (6.4) is defined for a trajectory x where δ is an arbitrary function such that $\delta_0 = \delta_T = 0$, $\dot{\delta}_0 = \dot{\delta}_T = 0$, $\ddot{\delta}_0 = \ddot{\delta}_T = 0$.

$$h(\epsilon, t) = x(t) + \epsilon\delta(t) \tag{6.4}$$

Let

$$F(\epsilon) = \frac{1}{2}\int_a^b (\dddot{h})^2 \mathrm{d}t \tag{6.5}$$

The condition for the trajectory x to minimise I is given as:

$$\left.\frac{\mathrm{d}F(\epsilon)}{\mathrm{d}\epsilon}\right|_{\epsilon=0} = 0 \tag{6.6}$$

Using integration by parts

$$\int_0^T \dddot{x}_t \ddot{\delta}_t \mathrm{d}t = \dddot{x}_t \ddot{\delta}_t\Big|_0^T - \int_0^T x_t^{[4]} \ddot{\delta}_t \mathrm{d}t \tag{6.7}$$

Using integration by parts again

$$-\int_0^T x_t^{[4]} \ddot{\delta}_t \mathrm{d}t = -x_t^{[4]} \dot{\delta}_t\Big|_0^T + \int_0^T x_t^{[5]} \dot{\delta}_t \mathrm{d}t \tag{6.8}$$

Thus to satisfy the condition in (6.6), it is required that

$$\int_0^T x_t^{[6]} \delta_t \mathrm{d}t = 0 \tag{6.9}$$

This must apply for arbitrary functions δ therefore for all $t \in [0, T]$

$$x_t^{[6]} = 0 \tag{6.10}$$

In other words, the minimum jerk trajectory occurs when the sixth-time derivative of the trajectory function x is equal to zero. The general solution of this equation is a fifth-order polynomial in time (6.11), where a_0, a_1, a_2, a_3, a_4 and a_5 are six constants to be determined.

$$x(t) = a_0 + a_1 t + a_2 t^2 + a_3 t^3 + a_4 t^4 + a_5 t^5 \tag{6.11}$$

$$\dot{x}(t) = a_1 + 2a_2 t + 3a_3 t^2 + 4a_4 t^3 + 5a_5 t^4 \tag{6.12}$$

$$\ddot{x}(t) = 2a_2 + 6a_3 t + 12a_4 t^2 + 20a_5 t^3 \tag{6.13}$$

The first three constants are obtained from the initial conditions $t = 0$

$$a_0 = x_0 \tag{6.14}$$

$$a_1 = \dot{x}_0 \tag{6.15}$$

$$a_2 = \frac{1}{2}\ddot{x}_0 \tag{6.16}$$

The last three constants are determined from the terminal conditions $t = T$

$$x_T = a_0 + a_1 T + a_2 T^2 + a_3 T^3 + a_4 T^4 + a_5 T^5 \tag{6.17}$$

$$\dot{x}_T = a_1 + 2a_2 T + 3a_3 T^2 + 4a_4 T^3 + 5a_5 T^4 \tag{6.18}$$

$$\ddot{x}_T = 2a_2 + 6a_3 T + 12a_4 T^2 + 20a_5 T^3 \tag{6.19}$$

In matrix form

$$\begin{bmatrix} x_T - a_0 - a_1 T - a_2 T^2 \\ \dot{x}_T - a_1 - 2a_2 T \\ \ddot{x}_T - 2a_2 \end{bmatrix} = \begin{bmatrix} T^3 & T^4 & T^5 \\ 3T^2 & 4T^4 & 5T^5 \\ 6T & 12T^2 & 20T^3 \end{bmatrix} \begin{bmatrix} a_3 \\ a_4 \\ a_5 \end{bmatrix} \tag{6.20}$$

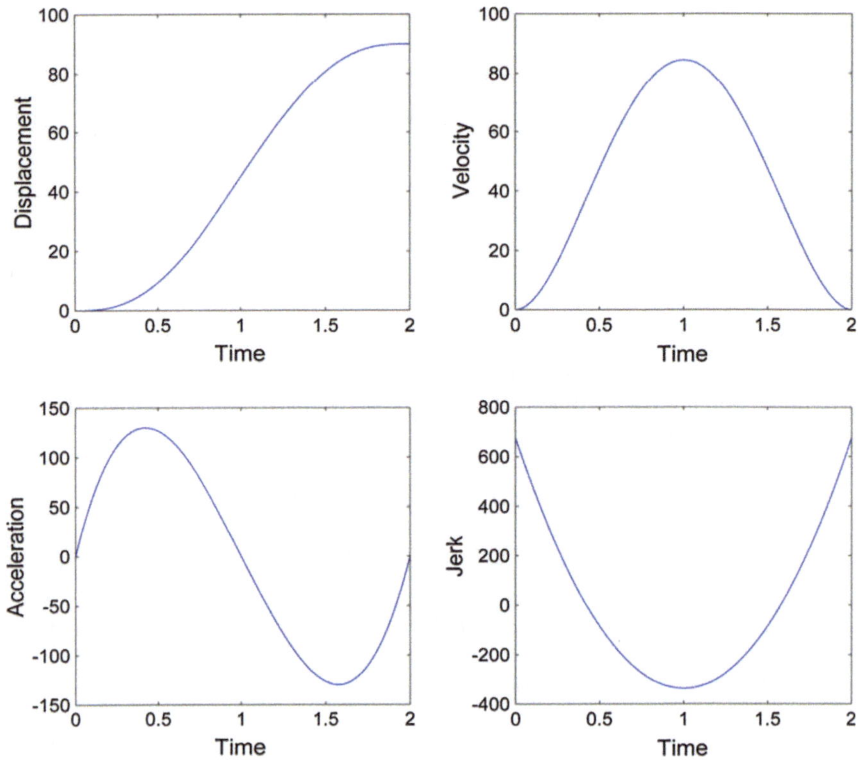

Fig. 6.1 Trajectory graphs in displacement, velocity, acceleration and jerk for the minimum jerk trajectory of the 1-DOF elbow joint moving from 0 to 90° in 2 s with a stationary start and end

$$\begin{bmatrix} a_3 \\ a_4 \\ a_5 \end{bmatrix} = \begin{bmatrix} T^3 & T^4 & T^5 \\ 3T^2 & 4T^4 & 5T^5 \\ 6T & 12T^2 & 20T^3 \end{bmatrix}^{-1} \begin{bmatrix} x_T - a_0 - a_1 T - a_2 T^2 \\ \dot{x}_T - a_1 - 2a_2 T \\ \ddot{x}_T - 2a_2 \end{bmatrix} \tag{6.21}$$

The six constants are then substituted into (6.11), (6.12) and (6.13) to obtain the minimum jerk trajectory in position, velocity and acceleration, respectively.

Figure 6.1 shows an example of the minimum jerk trajectory for the 1-DOF elbow joint. In this example, the joint starts in a stationary position and rotates for 2 s to stop at the 90° position.

6.1.2 Trajectories for the Shoulder

The minimum jerk trajectory is calculated for the human user's upper limb joints since the goal was to achieve smooth movement for the user. For the 5-DOF exoskeleton, this includes the 3-DOF shoulder joint and 1-DOF elbow joint. Deriving trajectories for the elbow joint are straightforward since the movement of the exoskeleton's Joint 5 translates directly to movements of the elbow joint. In addition, the movement of Joint 4 also translates well to movements of shoulder axial rotation. As a result, minimum jerk trajectory can be calculated directly for these two exoskeleton joints which will translate to minimum jerk trajectory movement for the respective human limb joints.

This is not the case for Joints 1, 2 and 3 in the 4R mechanism which are used to control the spherical position of the user's upper arm in 2-DOF. The nonlinear relationship between the motion of the shoulder joint and the 4R mechanism means that even if the three exoskeleton joints are moving in their minimum jerk trajectories, the user's shoulder joint will in most cases not be moving in its minimum jerk trajectory. Figures 6.2 and 6.3 illustrate this nonlinear relationship where the human shoulder is moving with constant angular velocity while Joints 1, 2 and 3 of the exoskeleton are required to follow a nonlinear trajectory in order to match the upper arm movement.

To achieve smooth movement of the shoulder, the minimum jerk trajectory must be computed for the 2-DOF shoulder movement (with axial rotation excluded) then converted to the respective trajectories of Joints 1, 2 and 3. These 2-DOF generate the spherical movement of the shoulder in 3D space and is typically described using a sequence of two Euler rotations. However, there are two problems with using Euler rotations to define a trajectory. First, singularities can occur in Euler rotations. Secondly, unlike for translations in 3D space, rotations in 3D space are not

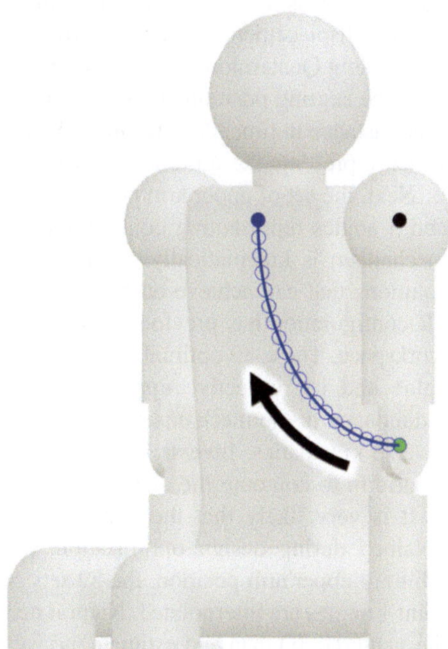

Fig. 6.2 A 90° flexion of the shoulder joint from the lowered vertical position to the horizontal forward position in 2 s with constant velocity. The solid *green* point indicates the starting position of the upper arm and the solid *blue* point indicates the ending position. Each hollow point in the trajectory path represents a 0.1-s time step

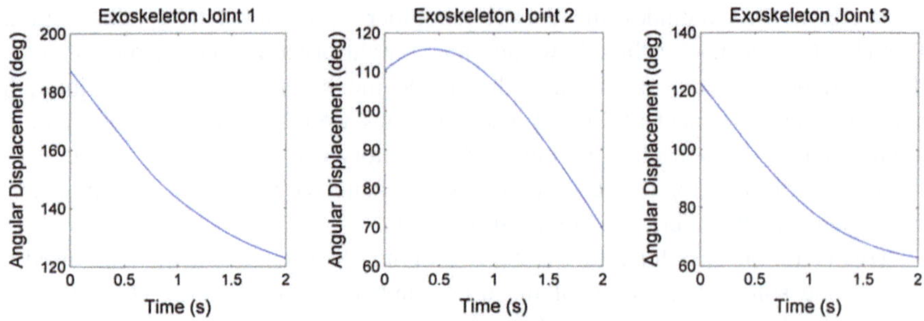

Fig. 6.3 A constant velocity flexion of the shoulder joint is shown in the top graph with the corresponding trajectories for exoskeleton Joints 1, 2 and 3 shown in the bottom three graphs. The relationship between shoulder movement and movement of exoskeleton joints is nonlinear

commutative so the order in which the two Euler rotations are applied affects the outcome. This is fine when defining a spherical coordinate in 3D space but it is not suitable for defining a spherical trajectory since information on the path of the trajectory is required. The two Euler rotations represent the target position relative to the starting position but since they are not commutative, the two rotations cannot be applied simultaneously to find a direct trajectory path between the two positions.

Instead of using Euler rotations, the minimum jerk trajectory is derived for a single rotation of the upper arm from the starting position to the target position. The travel distance of the single rotation is the angle between the two positions about the ICOR. First, the minimum jerk trajectory is computed for the one-dimensional travel angle using the given travel time. The trajectory obtained represents the angular displacement from the starting position towards the target position over time. Using Quaternion rotation, these angular displacements are then used to rotate from the starting position about the rotation axis to find the upper arm positions for each instance in time. As a result, a set of upper arm positions over time is obtained which represents the minimum jerk trajectory.

Next, the set of upper arm positions are converted to a respective set of Joint 1, 2 and 3 angles representing configurations of the 4R mechanism. However, the 4R mechanism is kinematically redundant; therefore, there are infinite configuration solutions that can achieve each upper arm position. To overcome this, an optimal 4R configuration has previously been identified for 89 upper arm positions in the workspace. These 89 optimal configurations are each represented by a Joint 1 angle value and its respective upper arm position. The Joint 1 angle eliminates the redundancy in the mechanism and enables a configuration solution to be found via inverse kinematics. Inverse kinematics is performed using the modified FABRIK algorithm to compute the angles of Joints 2 and 3.

It is very likely that the upper arm position of interest is not among the 89 obtained during design optimisation. In order to find the Joint 1 angle for an arbitrary upper arm position, the 89 sets of upper arm positions and their respective Joint 1 angles are interpolated. Natural neighbour interpolation is used to interpolate the scattered 3D data and estimate the value of Joint 1 angle for the given spherical coordinate of the upper arm position. In this interpolation method, the scattered data points are tessellated to form a network of tetrahedra using the Delaunay criterion. These tetrahedra are used to define a network of Thiessen polyhedra (3D versions of a polygon) in a 3D Voronoi diagram. The polyhedra have all surfaces equidistant to two or more neighbouring points. For a given input, natural neighbour interpolation finds the points closest to this input among the scattered data. A Thiessen polyhedra is also constructed for the input point with respect to its neighbouring points. Weights are then applied to each neighbour point based on the proportion of overlap between the volume of the new input polyhedra and the volume of each neighbour's initial polyhedra. These weights are applied to their respective neighbour points to interpolate an output value for the given input values. This ensures the interpolated output will be within the range of the neighbour points.

Now, the desired upper arm position and the interpolated Joint 1 angle are used to derive the angles of Joints 2 and 3 through inverse kinematics with the modified FABRIK algorithm. Once this is done, the angles of Joints 1, 2 and 3 are determined for a given upper arm position. This process is repeated for the upper arm positions in each time step of the minimum jerk trajectory to obtain a corresponding set of angles for Joints 1, 2 and 3. These sets of angles represent the simultaneous trajectories required from the three exoskeleton joints to achieve the minimum jerk trajectory of the upper arm in moving to the specified target position in the specified travel time. An example is shown in Figs. 6.4 and 6.5 where a minimum jerk trajectory of the upper arm is presented along with the corresponding trajectories of Joints 1, 2 and 3.

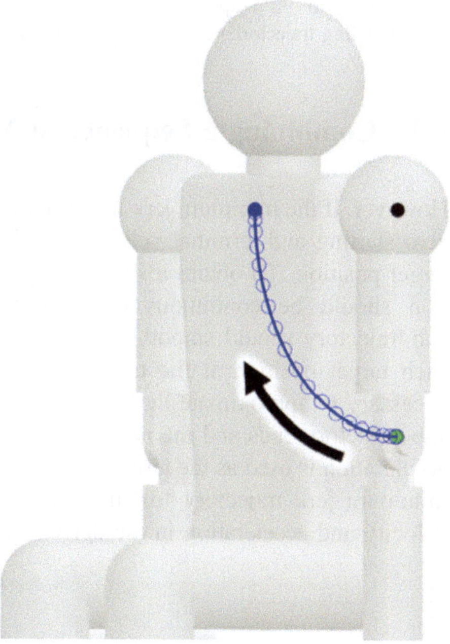

Fig. 6.4 A 90° flexion of the shoulder joint from the lowered vertical position to the horizontal forward position in 2 s with minimum jerk. Note that the points near the starting and stopping positions are denser which indicate the acceleration and deceleration of the *upper arm* in the minimum jerk trajectory

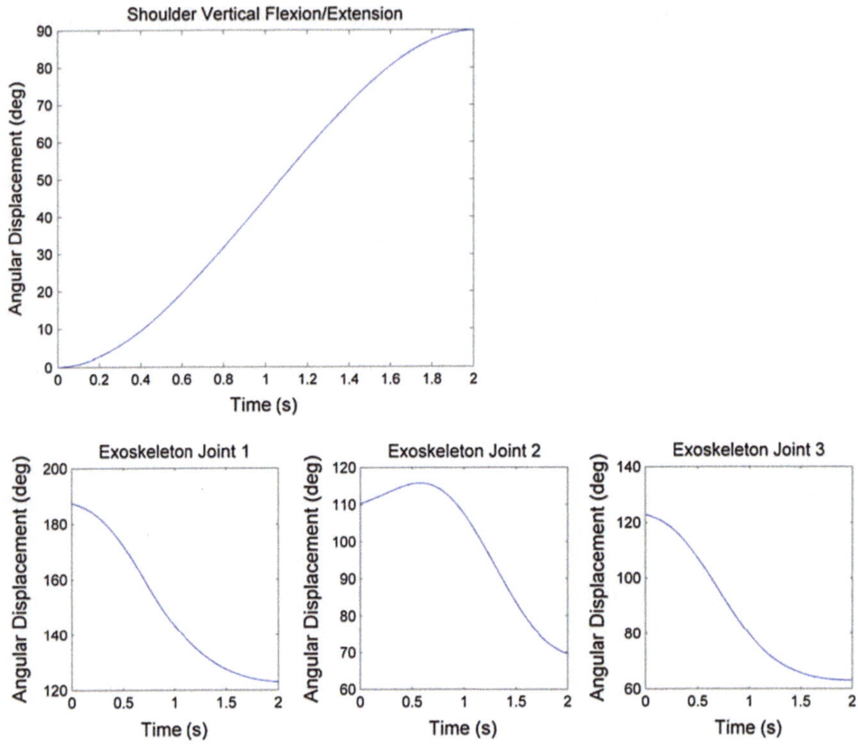

Fig. 6.5 A minimum jerk trajectory of shoulder flexion from 0° (upper arm positioned downwards) to 90° (upper arm positioned forwards) is shown in the *upper graph*. The corresponding trajectories for exoskeleton Joints 1, 2 and 3 are shown in the *lower three graphs*

6.2 Combining a Sequence of Movements

However, if the minimum jerk trajectory is found for each path independently using zero starting and terminal velocities and accelerations, the joint will stop at each target position. To obtain a smooth trajectory, the position, velocity and acceleration should be continuous throughout the entire trajectory. Therefore, each sub-trajectory should smoothly follow through to the next while passing through each target position at the target times without stopping. To achieve this, it is necessary to approximate the velocity and acceleration at the transition where one sub-trajectory ends and the next sub-trajectory begins. This transition velocity and acceleration is used as the terminal velocity and acceleration in the derivation of the minimum jerk trajectory for the initial sub-trajectory i and used as the starting velocity and acceleration in the derivation of the subsequent sub-trajectory $i+1$.

6.2.1 Cubic Spline Interpolation

The transition velocities and accelerations are obtained by approximating the entire trajectory using a cubic spline interpolation. The entire set of trajectory positions is fitted with a piecewise cubic spline that passes through all the points while minimising bending. Each point-to-point segment is approximated by a polynomial that ensures continuity between segments. Polynomials of order 3 or higher are required to achieve continuity, hence the use of a cubic spline. For n points in the trajectory, there are $n - 1$ intervals between them. A cubic polynomial is determined for each interval (6.22), where $S_i(t)$ is the polynomial segment between point i and $i+1$, and a_i, b_i, c_i and d_i are the polynomial coefficients.

$$S_i(t) = a_i(t - t_i)^3 + b_i(t - t_i)^2 + c_i(t - t_i) + d_i \tag{6.22}$$

For the spline to pass through both the desired points, the following constraints are enforced for this segment:

$$S_i(t_i) = x_i \tag{6.23}$$

$$S_i(t_{i+1}) = x_{i+1} \tag{6.24}$$

In addition, to ensure each segment continues smoothly into the next segment, each segment must satisfy the following:

$$\dot{S}_i(t_i) = \dot{S}_{i+1}(t_i) \tag{6.25}$$

$$\ddot{S}_i(t_i) = \ddot{S}_{i+1}(t_i) \tag{6.26}$$

The trajectory should have a stationary start point and end point, but this is not the case for the cubic spline generated in MATLAB. This is illustrated in the example shown in Fig. 6.6 where a joint starts at 0°, moves to the 90° position at 2 s and arrives at the 180° position at 6 s. This represents a 180° movement over 6 s with a higher velocity at the start of the trajectory followed by a lower velocity later on. The "spline" function in MATLAB creates a "natural spline" which results in a straight line at both the start and the end of the spline where $\ddot{x}$ is zero and $\dot{x}$ is constant. However, to achieve a stationary point $\dot{x}$ should be zero. To enforce this, an extra point is added slightly before the first point at the same position and another is added slightly after the final point at the same position. These additional points ensure the cubic spline will start and end with near-zero velocity. The two points are removed once the cubic spline is generated.

The velocity and acceleration at each intermediate point in the cubic spline is used as the boundary conditions for computing the minimum jerk trajectories for each interval. Figure 6.7 shows an example of a multi-point trajectory where each point-to-point segment is a minimum jerk trajectory derived using the boundary

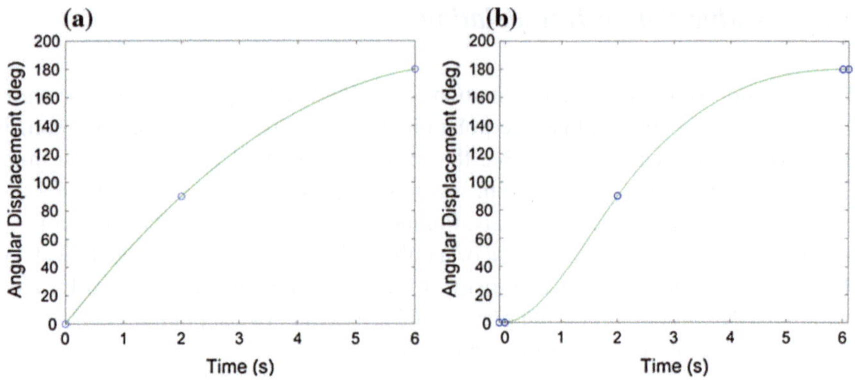

Fig. 6.6 Application of stationary end points. Trajectory plan to move the joint from 0° at 0 s to 90° at 2 s and 180° at 6 s. **a** Cubic spline interpolation of the three points. **b** Cubic spline interpolation with points added slightly before the start of the trajectory and slightly after the end of the trajectory to create stationary start and end points

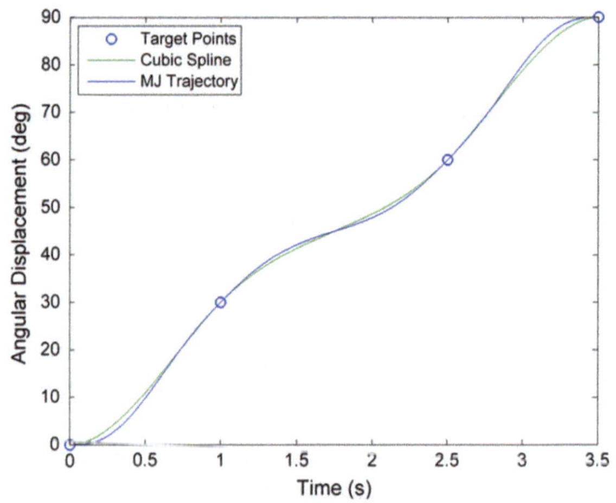

Fig. 6.7 Smooth trajectory for a multi-point trajectory plan. Plot of the target points, the cubic spline interpolation of these points with a stationary start and end, and the trajectory obtained by combining three minimum jerk trajectories (one between each pair of points) using velocity and acceleration boundary conditions obtained from the cubic spline interpolation

conditions obtained from the cubic spline interpolation. The trajectory starts at 0° and passes the 30° position at 1 s, the 60° position at 2.5 s and the 90° position at 3.5 s. This represents a 90° movement over 3.5 s with a high velocity at the start of the trajectory, followed by a decreased velocity, and then a higher velocity again before arriving at the 90° position.

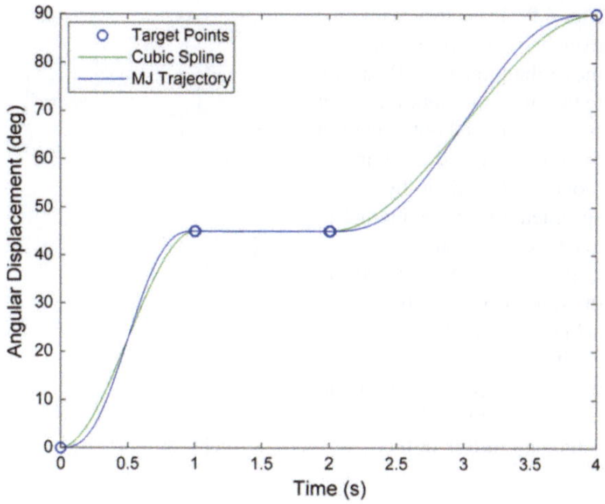

Fig. 6.8 Trajectory with a pause. Trajectory plan to move the joint from 0° at 0 s to 45° at 1 s, stay at 45° until 2 s and move to 90° at 4 s. Plot of the target points, the cubic spline interpolation and the trajectory obtained by combining three minimum jerk trajectories

A pause in the trajectory can be achieved by setting two target points in the same position with the second point delayed by the desired pause time (see Fig. 6.8). The transition velocity and acceleration are zero at the starting and ending points of the pause.

6.2.2 Trajectories with Reversing Movement

The cubic spline interpolation can cause an overshoot in the trajectory when the direction of movement is reversed. This overshoot in the cubic spline will translate to an overshoot in the final trajectory obtained using the minimum jerk criterion. An overshoot can occur either before or after an intermediate point where the target positions before and after this point are positioned in the same direction with respect to the intermediate point. A trajectory overshoot is not desirable since the joint moves further than the planned peak position. An example of an overshoot occurrence is shown in Fig. 6.9b where the trajectory plan in Fig. 6.9a is used. The joint starts at the 0° position and arrives at the 90° position at 4 s then returns to the 0° position at 6 s. This represents a movement to the 90° position followed by a faster reverse movement to return to the initial 0° position. Typically, when a trajectory that reverses upon arriving at a target position is set in the trajectory plan, the extreme target position is the furthest position the programmer wishes the joint to reach. For this reason, an overshoot should be prevented in all cases when a velocity reversal occurs.

To prevent overshoots, extra points are added slightly after each extreme point with the same position similar to how extra points were added to the start and end of

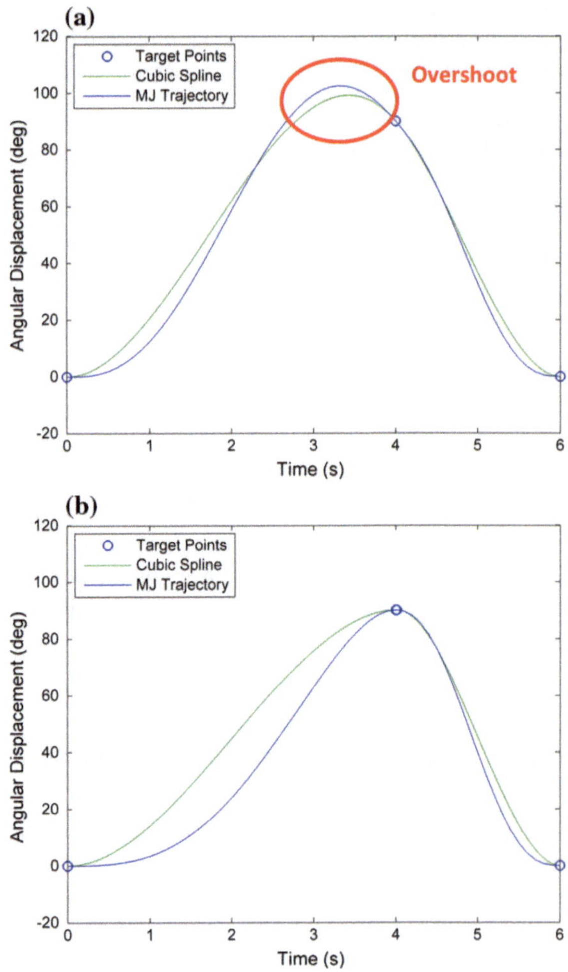

Fig. 6.9 Trajectory with overshoot. Trajectory plan to move the joint from 0° at 0 s to 90° at 4 s and return to 0° at 6 s. **a** An overshoot occurs in the trajectory and the joint moves further than the specified 90° in the attempt to generate a smoother trajectory. **b** No overshoot in the trajectory. This is achieved by including an additional point slightly after the extreme position of 90° to make the cubic spline stationary at this point

the trajectory. These extra points will ensure the cubic spline will have a maxima or minima occurring effectively at the extreme points. Then, when applying the minimum jerk criterion, the velocity at the extreme point is set to zero while the acceleration from the cubic spline is used. The improved trajectory of the example is shown in Fig. 6.9c where the overshoot no longer occurs.

6.2.3 Turning for 2-DOF Spherical Shoulder

A single point-to-point minimum jerk trajectory for the 2-DOF spherical shoulder is obtained using the displacement angle and the axis of rotation to get from the starting position to the target position. Unlike the 1-DOF case that can only move in either a clockwise or counter-clockwise direction, the 2-DOF spherical joint is two-dimensional and can turn in its trajectory path. Therefore, the target positions in the trajectory may not lie in a straight path in which case the trajectory will need to turn at the intermediate point. A sharper turn at an intermediate point will mean the trajectory should arrive at the point with a lower transition velocity.

To approximate the transition velocity, the turn angle is considered by using the angle between the two axes of rotation of the two consecutive sub-trajectories. If the turn angle is equal to or greater than 90°, the trajectory is required to stop at the intermediate point to prevent overshoot so a transition velocity of zero is used. For a turn angle between 0° and 90°, the transition velocity is maximum at 0° and decreases with a cosine function up to 90°. The turn angle is obtained using the dot product of the two rotation axes (6.27) where A and B are the two rotation axis vectors and φ is the turn angle between A and B.

$$A \cdot B = \|A\| \|B\| \cos \varphi \tag{6.27}$$

If the rotation axes are unit vectors, then the dot product becomes:

$$A \cdot B = \cos \varphi \tag{6.28}$$

Therefore, the transition velocity for a turning point, ω_T, is defined by a piecewise function (6.29) where ω_S is the transition velocity for the two sub-trajectories approximated from cubic spline interpolation while assuming they follow through in a straight path. These two cases are illustrated in Fig. 6.10. A zero transition acceleration is used for all trajectories of the 2-DOF shoulder.

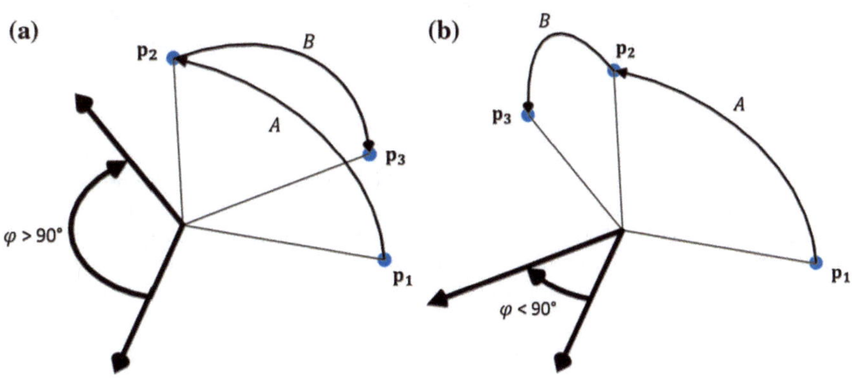

Fig. 6.10 A sequence of two consecutive spatial rotations of the upper arm (rotation $\boldsymbol{A}$ from $\mathbf{p}_1$ to $\mathbf{p}_2$ and rotation $\boldsymbol{B}$ from $\mathbf{p}_2$ to $\mathbf{p}_3$) with **a** turn angle greater than 90° (i.e. $\boldsymbol{A} \cdot \boldsymbol{B} > 0$), **b** turn angle smaller than 90° (i.e. $\boldsymbol{A} \cdot \boldsymbol{B} < 0$)

$$\omega_T = \begin{cases} \omega_S(A \cdot B) & \text{for } A \cdot B > 0 \\ 0 & \text{for } A \cdot B \leq 0 \end{cases} \tag{6.29}$$

To demonstrate turning of the 2-DOF shoulder, Figs. 6.11a, b and 6.12 show the trajectory of the upper arm along with the corresponding trajectories of Joints 1, 2 and 3 of the exoskeleton for performing shoulder circumduction where the upper arm makes a circular movement along the perimeter of the workspace. This example uses 8 points along the circular path with a roughly equal spacing between each point. This generates a smooth circular trajectory of the left upper arm in a clockwise direction from the user's perspective where the upper arm begins and ends at the vertical lowered position. A smoother curvature can be achieved by specifying more intermediate points along the curved trajectory path.

Note that condition number results indicated the 4R mechanism operates the closest to singular configurations at the edge of the shoulder workspace. Therefore, the trajectories of Joints 1, 2 and 3 in the circumduction movement is an indication of the 4R mechanism's worst performance (i.e. highest joint velocities and accelerations compared to that of the user's shoulder) the 4R operates with. It can be seen that all the joints move with reasonable velocities and accelerations and there are no issues in exoskeleton movement.

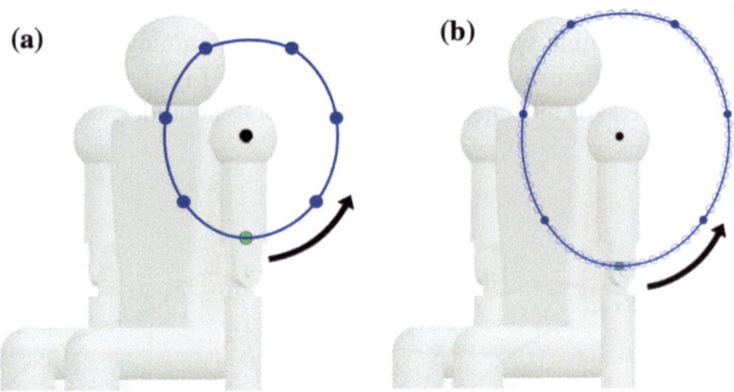

Fig. 6.11 **a** Trajectory plan for 2-DOF shoulder circumduction along the edge of the shoulder workspace which starts and ends with the *upper arm* in the lowered position. Eight points are used to generate the trajectory where the *green* point indicates the starting and ending position and the *blue* points represent the intermediate target positions. **b** Path of the smooth trajectory for the circumduction trajectory plan in **a**. Each point in the trajectory path represents a 0.1-s time step

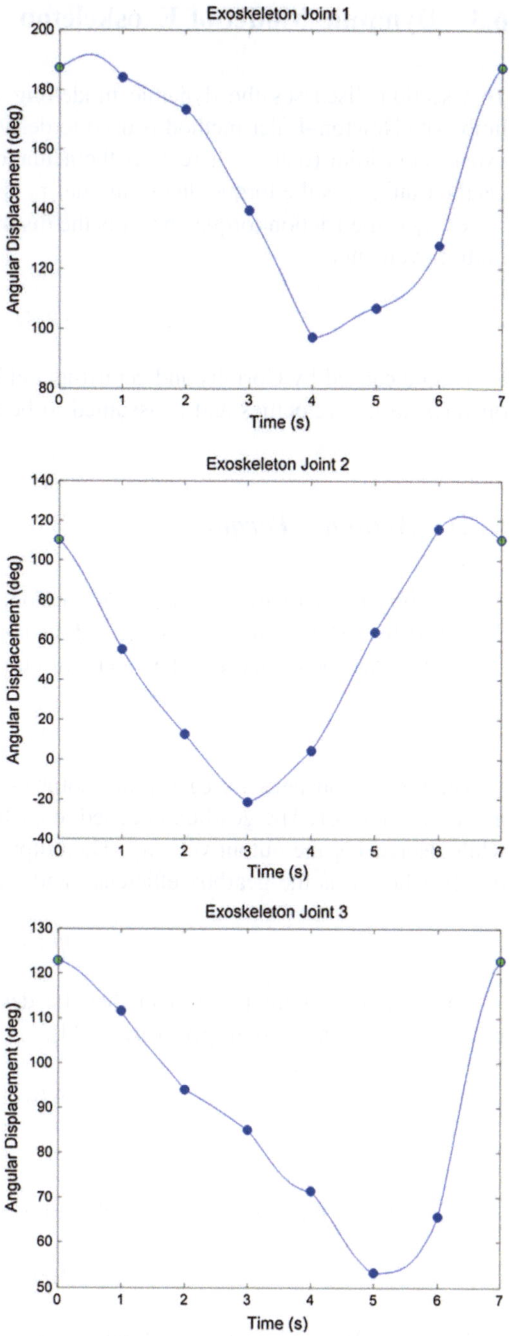

Fig. 6.12 Trajectory of exoskeleton Joints 1, 2 and 3 for achieving the shoulder circumduction trajectory shown in Fig. 6.11

6.3 Dynamic Model of Exoskeleton

This section discusses the dynamic modelling of the exoskeleton and the upper limb. The Newton–Euler method is used to derive the equations of motion for each exoskeleton joint (6.30), where τ_a is the actuation torque produced by the motor–gearbox unit, τ_i is the torque due to inertia, τ_g is the torque caused by gravitational forces, τ_f is the friction torque and τ_d is the disturbance torque caused by the user's limb movements.

$$\tau_a = \tau_i + \tau_g + \tau_f + \tau_d \tag{6.30}$$

Torque caused by Coriolis and centrifugal effects is small since the exoskeleton operates at low velocities and is assumed to be negligible.

6.3.1 *Actuator Torque*

The torque output of the brushless DC motors used in the exoskeleton joints is described by (6.31), where τ_m is the output torque of the motor, k_t is the torque constant of the motor and i is the electrical current.

$$\tau_m = k_t i \tag{6.31}$$

The torque constants for each joint motor in the present exoskeleton design are given in Table 6.1. The gearbox attached to each motor increases the output torque while decreasing the output velocity. The output torque of the gearbox is given by (6.32), where η is the gearbox efficiency and r is the gearbox reduction.

$$\tau_a = \eta r \tau_m \tag{6.32}$$

The gearbox output torque can then be described by (6.33), where k_r is the gearbox reduction constant given by (6.34).

$$\tau_a = k_r \tau_m \tag{6.33}$$

$$k_r = \eta r \tag{6.34}$$

Using (6.31), the output torque at the joint becomes:

$$\tau_a = k_r k_t i \tag{6.35}$$

The motor and gearbox combinations were carefully selected during design to ensure their reduction ratio and efficiency allows the motor to operate the joints at the required velocities and torques while their size and weight allow them to be

Table 6.1 Motor and gearbox specifications

Joint	Maxon motor	Torque constant k_t (m Nm/A)	Gear reduction r (r:1)	Efficiency η	Reduction constant k_r
1	EC 45 Flat 24V	33.5	156	0.72	132.4
2	EC 90 Flat 24V	70.5	91	0.75	78.8
3	EC 45 Flat 24V	33.5	319	0.64	255.2
4	EC 45 Flat 24V	33.5	47 (*282)	0.76	41.0 (*245.8)
5	EC 45 Flat 24V	33.5	156	0.72	132.4

*Value after a further reduction of 6:1 is applied to Joint 4 by the curved rail mechanism

mounted on the exoskeleton joints without causing interference problems. The gearbox reduction ratio of each motor is given in Table 6.1.

6.3.2 Inertial Torque

The inertial torque experienced by an exoskeleton joint is given by (6.36), where I_s is the inertia tensor of the segment s at the joint coordinate system, α is the angular acceleration of the joint and N is the total number of segments acting on the joint.

$$\tau_{\mathrm{i}} = \sum_{s}^{N} I_s \times \alpha \tag{6.36}$$

The inertial parameters for the exoskeleton and upper limb segments are presented in Table 6.2. The mass, centre of mass and inertia tensor at the centre of mass for each exoskeleton segment are obtained from a 3D model of the 5-DOF exoskeleton in Creo Parametric. For the human limb segments, inertial parameter values for an average adult are obtained from the literature [3]. The wrist joint is assumed to be fixed at the normal anatomical position in the model.

The position and orientation of the segments change during operation; therefore, the inertia tensor of these segments with respect to the exoskeleton joints will also change. To determine the inertia tensor of each segment with respect to the joint coordinate system, the centre of mass of the segment with respect to the joint coordinate system is firstly determined through forward kinematics. The inertia tensor at the segment's centre of mass is then transformed to the joint coordinate system by a rotation and a translation. The rotation of the inertia tensor is achieved using a similarity transformation (6.37), where I_R is the inertia tensor that has been rotated into the orientation of the joint coordinate system, I_m is the inertia tensor at

Table 6.2 Inertial parameters of the exoskeleton and upper limb

Segment	Mass (kg)	Centre of mass (*m* from proximal joint)	Inertia tensor at COM (kg m^2)
Link 1	2.34	(0, 0.282, −0.371)	$\begin{bmatrix} 0.0711 & 0 & 0 \\ 0 & 0.0461 & 0.0315 \\ 0 & 0.0315 & 0.0264 \end{bmatrix}$
Link 2	1.34	(0, −0.168, −0.184)	$\begin{bmatrix} 0.0140 & 0 & 0 \\ 0 & 0.0075 & -0.0057 \\ 0 & -0.0057 & 0.0070 \end{bmatrix}$
Link 3	0.80	(0.017, −0.093, −0.005)	$\begin{bmatrix} 0.0028 & 0 & 0 \\ 0 & 0.0020 & 0 \\ 0 & 0 & 0.0039 \end{bmatrix}$
Link 4	1.57	(0, 0.141, 0.070)	$\begin{bmatrix} 0.0046 & 0 & 0 \\ 0 & 0.0032 & 0 \\ 0 & 0 & 0.0021 \end{bmatrix}$
Link 5	0.18	(0.027, −0.161, 0)	$\begin{bmatrix} 0.0025 & 0 & 0 \\ 0 & 0 & 0 \\ 0 & 0 & 0.0026 \end{bmatrix}$
Upper arm	1.71	0.141	$\begin{bmatrix} 0.0143 & 0 & 0 \\ 0 & 0.0126 & 0 \\ 0 & 0 & 0.0042 \end{bmatrix}$
Forearm	0.98	0.109	$\begin{bmatrix} 0.0044 & 0 & 0 \\ 0 & 0.0007 & 0 \\ 0 & 0 & 0.0043 \end{bmatrix}$
Hand	0.38	0.095	$\begin{bmatrix} 0.0010 & 0 & 0 \\ 0 & 0.0004 & 0 \\ 0 & 0 & 0.0007 \end{bmatrix}$

the segment's centre of mass in the segment's coordinate system and R is the rotation matrix relating the segment coordinate system to the joint coordinate system.

$$I_R = RI_mR^T \tag{6.37}$$

Translation of the inertia tensor involves using the parallel axis theorem (6.38), where I_T is the inertia tensor that has been translated into the origin of the joint coordinate system, m is the segment mass, p_m is the displacement vector from the centre of mass of the segment to the origin of the joint coordinate system and I_3 is the 3×3 identity matrix.

$$I_T = I_m + m\left[\left(p_m^T p_m\right)I_3 - p_m p_m^T\right] \tag{6.38}$$

The inertia tensor of a segment with respect to the joint coordinate system can be obtained by applying the rotation followed by the translation:

$$I_s = RI_mR^T + m\left[(p_m^Tp_m)I_3 - p_mp_m^T\right] \quad (6.39)$$

Since the translation is applied after the rotation, p_m here is expressed in the joint coordinate system.

6.3.3 *Gravity Compensation*

As with inertial torque, the torque caused by gravitational effects also depends on the configuration of the exoskeleton. The gravitational torque acting on an exoskeleton joint is given by (6.40), where p_s is the displacement vector from the joint to the centre of mass of segment s, m_s is the mass of the segment, R_s is the rotation transformation matrix between the global coordinate system and the joint coordinate system and g is the gravitational constant vector in the global coordinate system.

$$\tau_g = \sum_s^N p_s \times (m_s(R_s g)) \quad (6.40)$$

6.3.4 *Friction Compensation*

Friction is a resistance to joint motion and is present in the motor, gearbox, bearings and the Joint 4 rail. In the present work, friction is modelled using a piecewise function (6.41), where k_f is the positive torque constant determined experimentally. The friction torque is assumed to act in the direction opposite to joint motion, and if the joint is stationary, then the friction torque is considered to be acting opposite to the direction of the control output.

$$\tau_f = \begin{cases} k_f & \text{if } (\dot{\theta}<0) \text{ or } (\dot{\theta}=0 \;\&\; \tau_m<0) \\ 0 & \text{if } (\dot{\theta}=0) \;\&\; (\tau_m=0) \\ -k_f & \text{if } \left(\dot{\theta}>0\right) \text{ or } (\dot{\theta}=0 \;\&\; \tau_m>0) \end{cases} \quad (6.41)$$

6.4 Interactive Control Strategies

The physical interaction between the exoskeleton and the user can be classified into two main types. One type involves the exoskeleton actively moving the user's limb and the other involves the exoskeleton moving in the direction of the force applied by the user. In both types of interaction, the impedance of the exoskeleton can be adjusted to modulate the softness of the interaction from the user's perspective. This can enable a wide variety of rehabilitation processes to be realised. For stroke patients, the first type of interaction is expected to be most beneficial as this best mimics current rehabilitation exercises which focus on motion.

6.4.1 Impedance of an Exoskeleton

Advancements in robotic technology over the past decades have mainly focused on the area of industrial robots. In industrial applications, the robot's purpose is typically for position control, and it is treated as an isolated system with little to no consideration of its dynamic interaction with the environment. However, this type of control method is not suitable for a rehabilitation robot since the robot is required to physically interact with and respond to a human user. A strategy to control the dynamic interactions between the robot and the human limb is required.

Interacting physical systems can be classified into two types, an admittance which accepts effort inputs (such as force) and produces flow outputs (such as motion) and an impedance which accepts flow inputs and produces effort outputs [4–6]. For a mechanical interaction between two physical systems, one system must physically complement the other. In other words, if one system is behaving as an impedance, then the other must behave as an admittance. For an industrial robot manipulator, the environment is a physical system that accepts forces applied to it and produces motion in response. Therefore, the robot's environment is described as an admittance. To ensure physical compatibility between the robot and its environment, the robot should assume the behaviour of an impedance.

In the case of an exoskeleton robot, both the robot and the user can behave as an impedance and impose motion. Therefore, the exoskeleton can operate in two distinct control modes. The first is admittance control in which the exoskeleton assumes the behaviour of an admittance and moves when a force is applied to it by the user's limb which is behaving as an impedance. In other words, the user's limb imposes the position of the combined system of the upper limb and exoskeleton. The second control mode is impedance control in which the exoskeleton assumes the behaviour of an impedance and applies force to the user's limb through motion of its structure. Unlike traditional position control which ignores dynamic interactions with the environment, impedance control also allows modulation of the robot's impedance behaviour. A reduction in robot impedance will allow user-generated forces to have an effect on the robot's position. In other words, the exoskeleton imposes the position but the system can deviate from this position when force is applied by the user. This allows the exoskeleton to achieve position control with an artificial compliance or softness when interacting with the user's limb.

6.4.2 Control of the Elbow Joint

Control strategies are firstly discussed for this simpler 1-DOF joint before addressing the more complex multi-DOF shoulder mechanism.

6.4.2.1 Admittance Control

In admittance control mode, the exoskeleton assumes the behaviour of an admittance and its movements are determined by the external force applied to it by the user's limb. With gravity and friction compensation, the exoskeleton joint will be stationary when there is no interaction force and moves when a light force is applied at the hand HRI. This makes the motorised joint feel like a lightweight and unconstrained joint from the user's perspective. The interaction force is perceived by the user as a small resistance to movement. Furthermore, if gravity compensation of the user's limb is enabled, then the exoskeleton will support the relaxed limb at its current position and can assist the weak movements of the impaired limb. The control scheme of admittance mode is presented in Fig. 6.13.

Admittance control of the 1-DOF elbow joint is implemented by using the force sensor readings as a control signal for the motor at Joint 5. A gain is applied to the force signal to drive the motor in the direction of the force using (6.42), where τ_{adm} is the torque output of the admittance controller, k_{adm} is the admittance gain, d_{HRI} is the displacement vector between the joint axis and the location of the interaction force and F_{HRI} is the interaction force measured by the force sensor.

$$\tau_{\text{adm}} = k_{\text{adm}}(d_{\text{HRI}} \times F_{\text{HRI}}) \tag{6.42}$$

A higher gain will cause the resistance to movement to feel smaller to the user and vice versa. However, if the gain is too high, then the exoskeleton will move faster than the user. This causes a reversal of the interaction force as the interaction switches from that of a "push" to a "pull" which in turn causes the exoskeleton joint

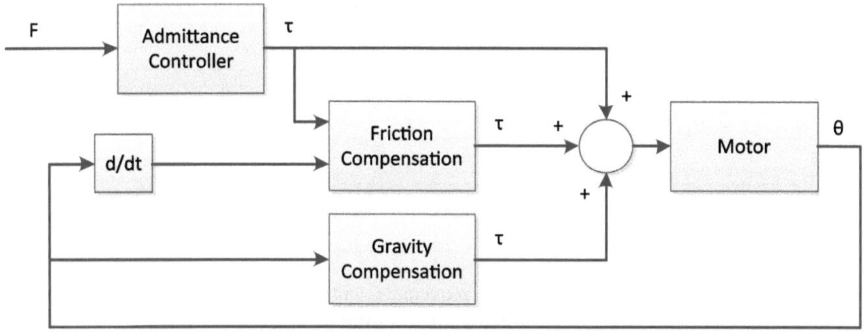

Fig. 6.13 The control scheme of admittance mode

movement to reverse. The exoskeleton movement is then opposite to that of the user's movement and the interaction switches from a "pull" back to a "push", causing another reversal of joint movement. The exoskeleton joint will produce an oscillating output. Therefore, a suitable gain is one that is high to reduce the resistance to movement but not so high that it causes the exoskeleton to move faster than user.

To demonstrate admittance control, force is applied at the hand HRI by a healthy human subject to move Joint 5 by 90° and back as shown by the graphs in Fig. 6.14. The peak force occurs only for a short instant and drops soon after due to the friction compensation. After this, force is required to keep the joint moving and the joint stops when the force is removed. For comparison, Fig. 6.15 shows the same

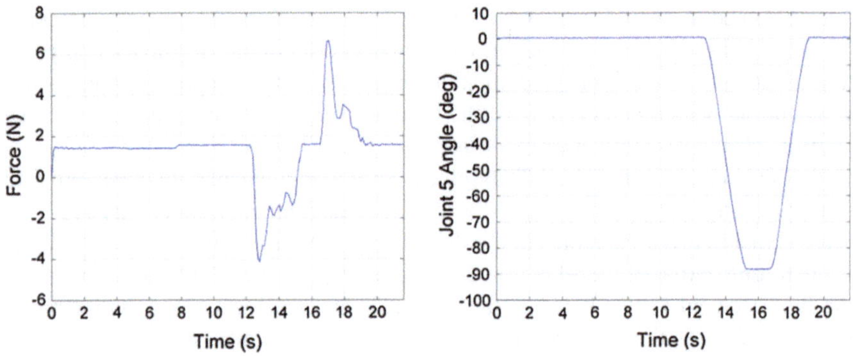

Fig. 6.14 An example of user-generated movement in admittance control. Force is applied at the hand HRI (*top graph*) to move Joint 5 from 0° to approximately the −90° position and back (*bottom graph*)

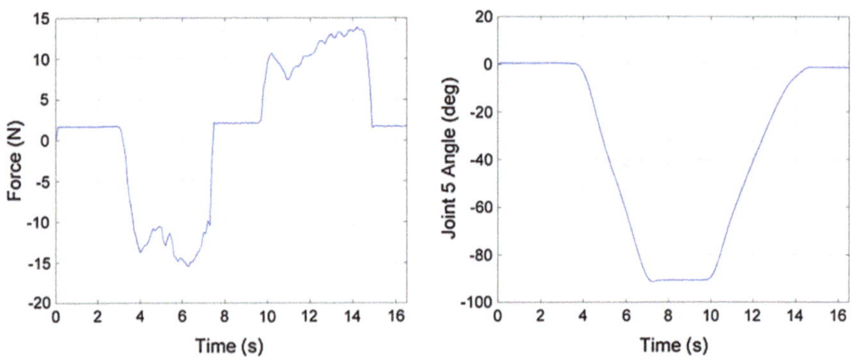

Fig. 6.15 An example of user-generated movement with no exoskeleton actuation. Force is applied at the hand HRI (*top graph*) to move Joint 5 from 0° to approximately the −90° position and back (*bottom graph*)

experiment with the back-drivable motor switched off (i.e. no admittance control). This requires approximately three times the peak force that occurred with admittance control and this high force is required throughout the entire movement.

The resistance to movement is low in full admittance mode but it is possible to increase the impedance of the exoskeleton to produce an artificial resistive behaviour. This artificial resistance can be implemented in two different forms, namely an artificial damping which is a function of joint velocity and an artificial inertia which is a function of joint acceleration. These are expressed in (6.43) and (6.44), where $\tau_{imp,c}$ and $\tau_{imp,i}$ are the resistive torques from the artificial damping and inertia, respectively; k_c is the artificial damping constant and k_i is the artificial inertia constant.

$$\tau_{\mathrm{imp,c}} = -k_c\dot{\theta} \tag{6.43}$$

$$\tau_{\mathrm{imp,i}} = -k_i\ddot{\theta} \tag{6.44}$$

This gives the controller output torque as:

$$\tau_{\mathrm{adm}} = k_{\mathrm{adm}}(d_{\mathrm{HRI}} \times F_{\mathrm{HRI}}) - k_c\dot{\theta} - k_i\ddot{\theta} \tag{6.45}$$

An example of admittance control with artificial damping is shown in Fig. 6.16 where the movement requires a constant force to be applied. Figure 6.17 shows admittance control with artificial inertia. Here, it can be seen that a peak force occurs indicating the sudden acceleration of the inertia. The joint also continues to move after the force is removed but with a decelerating velocity as expected.

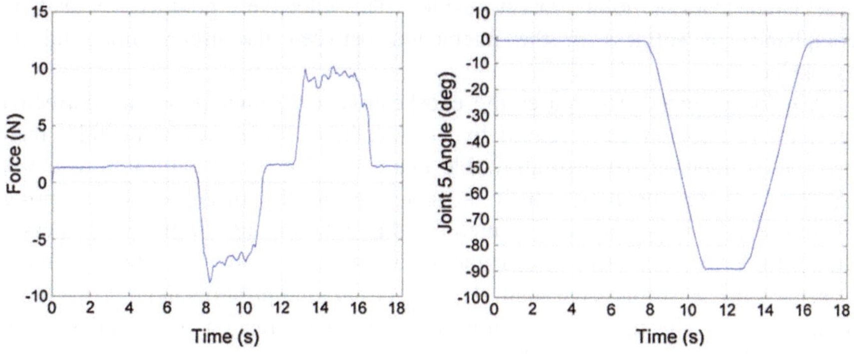

Fig. 6.16 An example of user-generated movement in admittance control with artificial damping. Force is applied at the hand HRI (*top graph*) to move Joint 5 from 0° to approximately the −90° position and back (*bottom graph*)

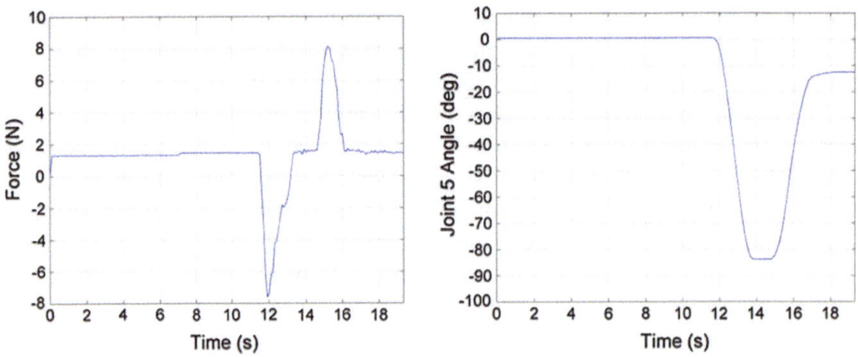

Fig. 6.17 An example of user-generated movement in admittance control with artificial inertia. Force is applied at the hand HRI (*top graph*) to move Joint 5 from 0° to approximately the −90° position and back (*bottom graph*)

6.4.2.2 Impedance Control

In impedance control mode, the exoskeleton assumes the behaviour of an impedance and moves to impose a position on the user's limb. When the use's limb is relaxed, it is behaving as an admittance and the exoskeleton acting as an impedance will achieve a performance similar to normal position control. However, when the user tries to move the limb, the limb can be seen to have an increase in impedance but if the exoskeleton is operating with high impedance it will not respond to the user's force exertions. To allow the user to interact with the exoskeleton, the exoskeleton can operate with a reduced impedance so that the limb can have some control of position. Modulation of impedance allows user-generated forces to cause a deviation from the joint's target position. This effectively produces an artificial compliance or softness in the interaction between the user's limb and the exoskeleton.

A reduced impedance causes the exoskeleton to produce a smaller corrective response to position error caused by user-generated forces. Consequently, there becomes a trade-off between allowable interaction force and allowable deviation from the desired position which is analogous to the behaviour of a spring. Therefore, joint impedance can be modulated by introducing an artificial stiffness in the controller (6.46), where $\tau_{\text{imp},k}$ is the opposing torque from the artificial stiffness, k_k is the artificial stiffness constant, θ is the current joint position and θ_t is the target joint position. The trade-off relationship between interaction force and position error can then be adjusted by changing the artificial stiffness constant.

$$\tau_{\text{imp},k} = -k_k(\theta - \theta_t) \tag{6.46}$$

Unfortunately, if joint stiffness is reduced, then the position-tracking performance will degrade. This is fine for a stationary target position but the joint will be unable to accurately follow a specified trajectory even when there is no interaction with the user's limb. To overcome this, the admittance controller is used to amplify the influence of the user-generated forces. As a result, the artificial stiffness will be high enough to accurately track a target trajectory and only the amplified user-generated force can cause the joint to significantly deviate from its trajectory.

The control scheme of impedance mode is shown in Fig. 6.18. Examples of impedance control are also provided. Figure 6.19 shows the behaviour of Joint 5 at a stationary target position when force is applied at the hand HRI.

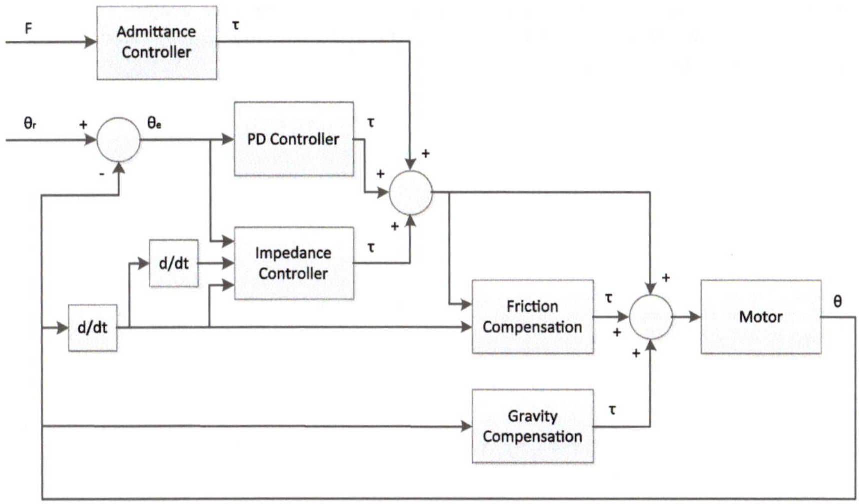

Fig. 6.18 The control scheme of impedance mode

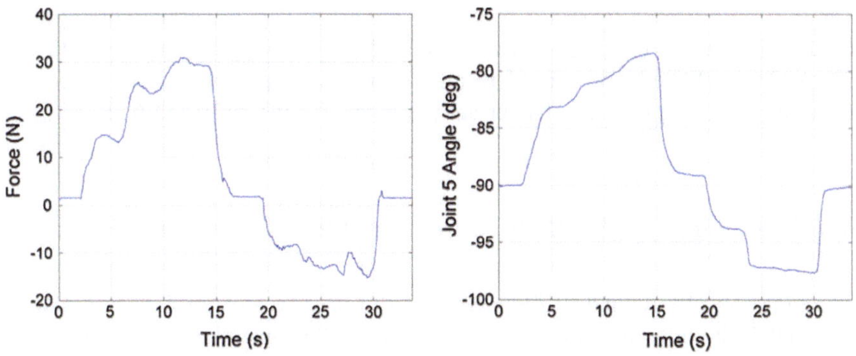

Fig. 6.19 An example of user-generated force applied in impedance control with a stationary target position. Force is applied at the hand HRI (*top graph*) which causes Joint 5 to deviate from its stationary target position (*bottom graph*)

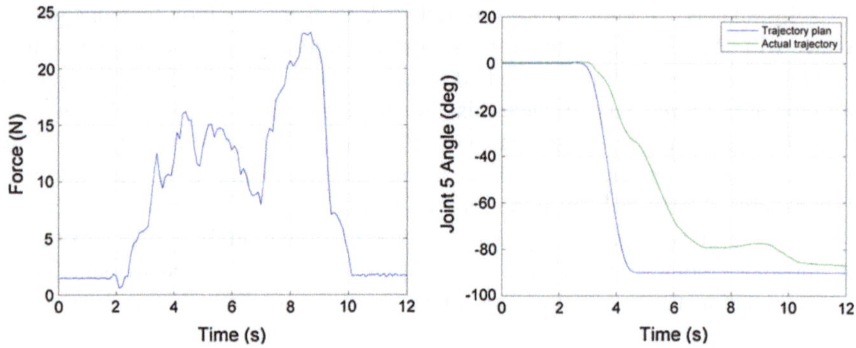

Fig. 6.20 An example of user-generated force applied while impedance control is following a trajectory with low stiffness. The force applied at the hand HRI (*top graph*) causes Joint 5 to deviate from its path (*bottom graph*)

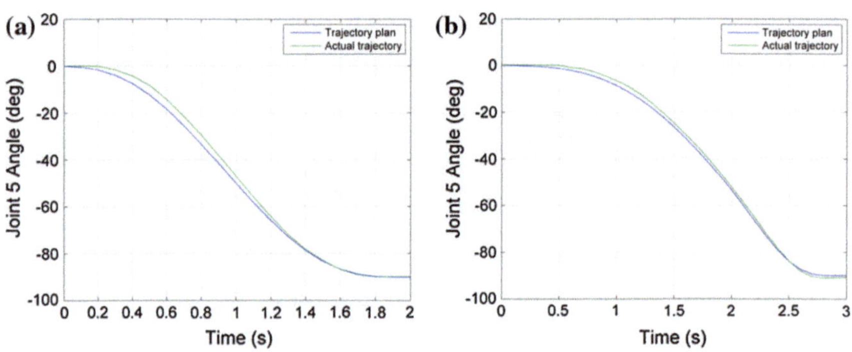

Fig. 6.21 **a** An example of impedance control following a smooth point-to-point trajectory with a target at −90° in 2 s. **b** An example of impedance control following a smooth trajectory with acceleration. Trajectory targets are set at −45° in 2 s and −90° in 3 s

Figure 6.20 shows force applied while Joint 5 is following a trajectory path with low stiffness. Impedance control results for various types of trajectories derived from the smooth trajectory planner are presented in Figs. 6.21 and 6.22.

6.4.3 Control of the Redundant Shoulder Mechanism

The kinematically redundant 4R mechanism in the exoskeleton is used to control the 3-DOF shoulder movements, namely shoulder flexion and extension, abduction and adduction and axial rotation. In the 5-DOF exoskeleton prototype, Joint 4 in the exoskeleton can independently control shoulder axial rotation. However, measuring interaction force for this DOF at the upper arm HRI is not reliable since slipping can

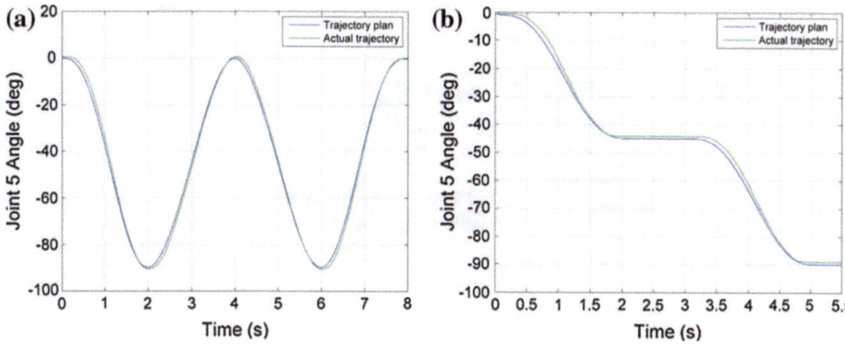

Fig. 6.22 **a** An example of impedance control following a smooth trajectory with reversing direction of motion. Trajectory targets are set at −90° in 2 s, 0° in 4 s, −90° in 6 s and 0° in 8 s. **b** An example of impedance control following a smooth trajectory with a pause during motion. Trajectory targets are set at −45° in 2 s, −45° in 3 s and −90° in 5 s

occur between the upper arm and the HRI during axial rotation. Alternatively, force can be measured at the hand HRI but it becomes challenging to distinguish the force caused by shoulder axial rotation from forces caused by other upper limb DOF. Therefore, in the present exoskeleton only position control is implemented for Joint 4 and force-based control methods are not used.

A 2-axis force sensor has been integrated into the upper arm HRI to measure forces generated by the 2-DOF spherical movements of the upper arm, namely shoulder flexion and extension and abduction and adduction. However, the measured two-dimensional force does not translate linearly to the exoskeleton joints as was the case with the 1-DOF elbow. Furthermore, the 4R shoulder mechanism is kinematically redundant and there are infinite inverse kinematics and inverse dynamics solutions. To overcome these issues, the measured two-dimensional force is used to shift the target position of the upper arm rather than derive the exoskeleton joint outputs. The target upper arm position is then used to determine the corresponding optimal Joint 1, 2 and 3 positions by using the inverse kinematics process. This allows the use of interaction forces to move the exoskeleton shoulder mechanism while maintaining the optimal 4R configurations.

6.4.3.1 Admittance Control

When the exoskeleton behaves as an admittance, it moves in the direction of the user-generated force. This behaviour is achieved by moving the target position of the upper arm in the direction of the force vector measured at the upper arm HRI. The magnitude of the measured force is used in the control gain to reduce the position error of each joint and move them to the new target position. Figure 6.23 shows an example of admittance control where force is applied at the upper arm HRI by a healthy human subject to move the upper arm in a circular path.

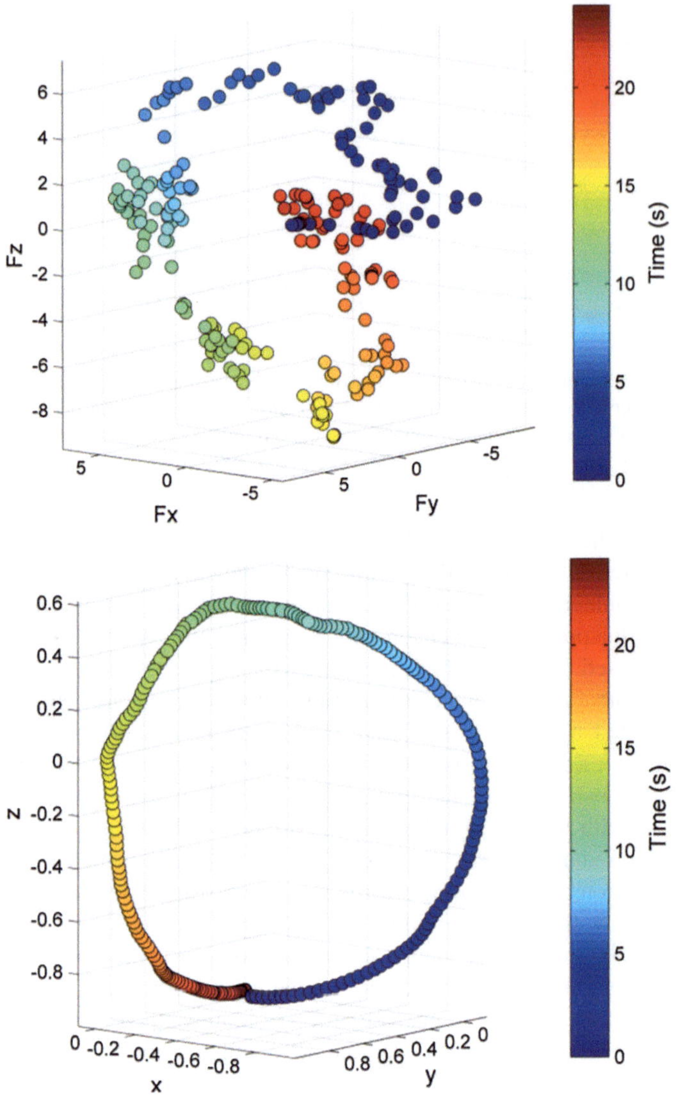

Fig. 6.23 An example of user-generated force applied in admittance control of the 2-DOF spherical shoulder. Force is applied at the upper arm HRI to move the upper arm in a circular path. The top plot shows the measured force vector with respect to the global coordinate system and the bottom plot shows the unit position of the upper arm relative to the ICOR

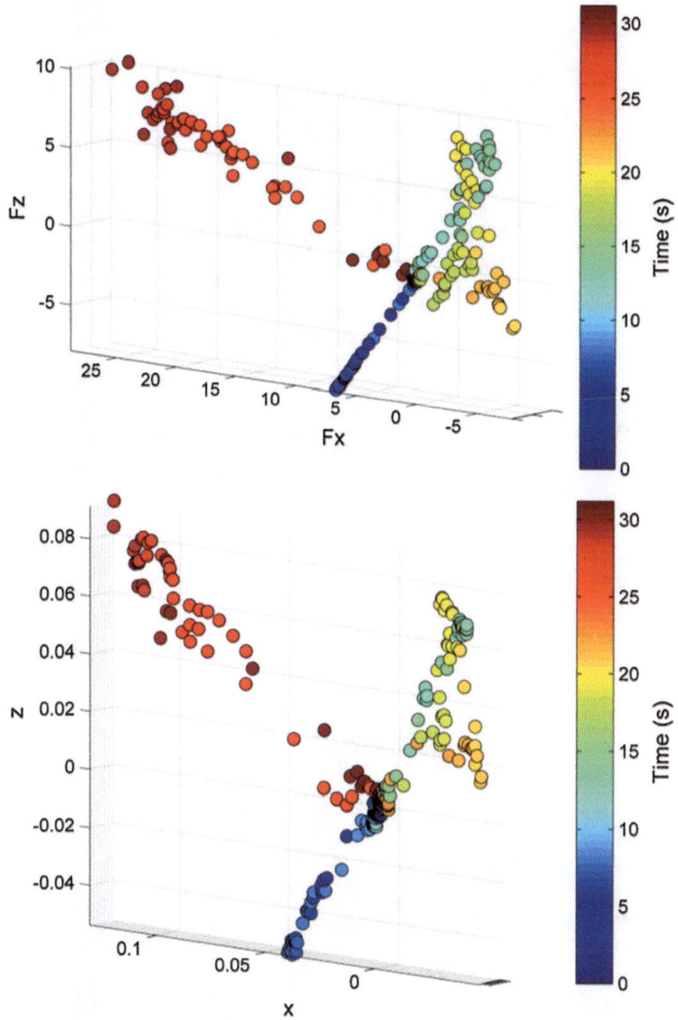

Fig. 6.24 An example of user-generated force applied in impedance control of the 2-DOF shoulder with a stationary target position. A force is applied at the upper arm HRI and then released. This is repeated for multiple arbitrary directions. The *top plot* shows the measured force vector with respect to the global coordinate system and the *bottom plot* shows the unit position of the upper arm relative to the ICOR

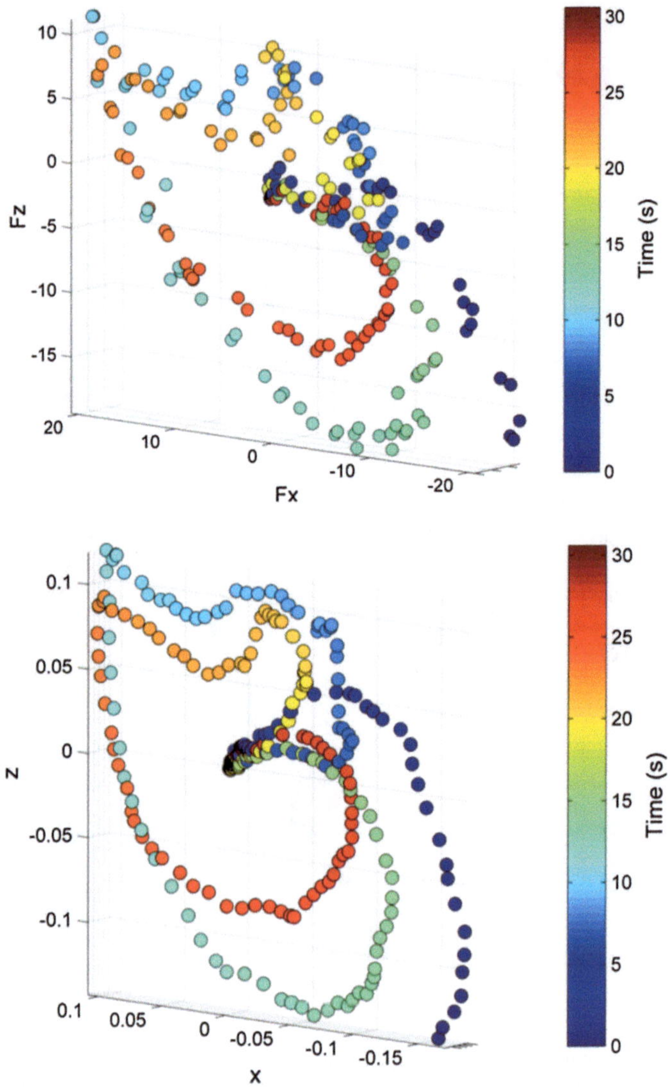

Fig. 6.25 An example of user-generated force applied in impedance control of the 2-DOF shoulder with a stationary target position. Force is applied at the upper arm HRI in a circular motion and then released. This is repeated multiple times. The *top plot* shows the measured force vector with respect to the global coordinate system and the *bottom plot* shows the unit position of the upper arm relative to the ICOR

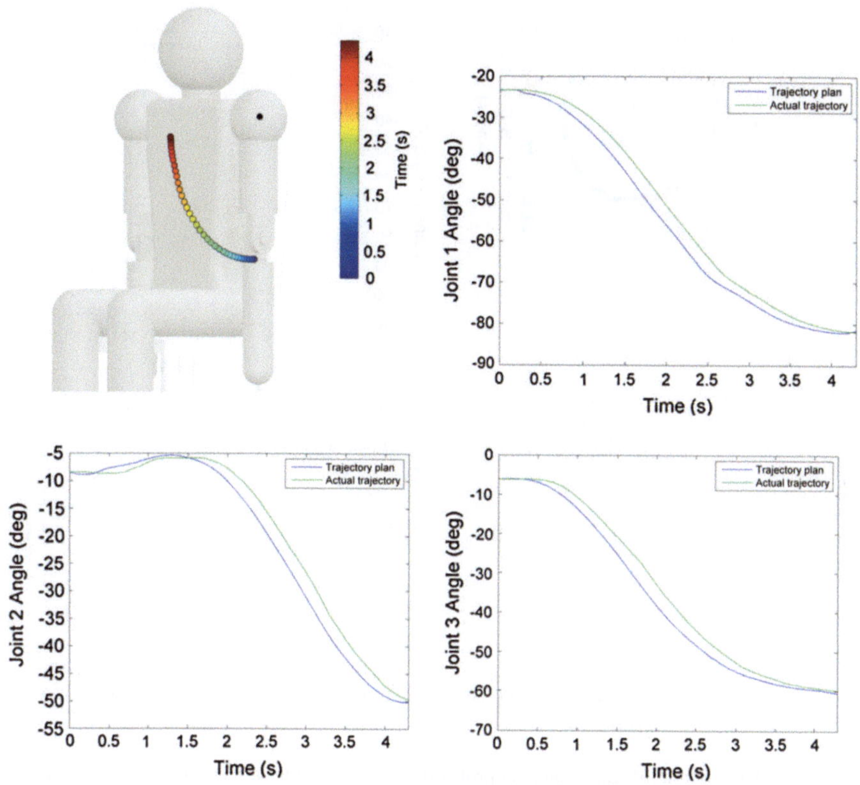

Fig. 6.26 An example of impedance control following a 90° shoulder flexion trajectory

6.4.3.2 Impedance Control

Impedance control for the 2-DOF shoulder movements is implemented using the same approach as that for the 1-DOF elbow. An artificial stiffness is used which allows the joints to deviate from their target positions according to the admittance controller output. Two examples of applying force during impedance control with a stationary upper arm target position are shown in Figs. 6.24 and 6.25. In Figs. 6.26 and 6.27, the impedance controller is applied to generate two different trajectories obtained from the smooth trajectory planner.

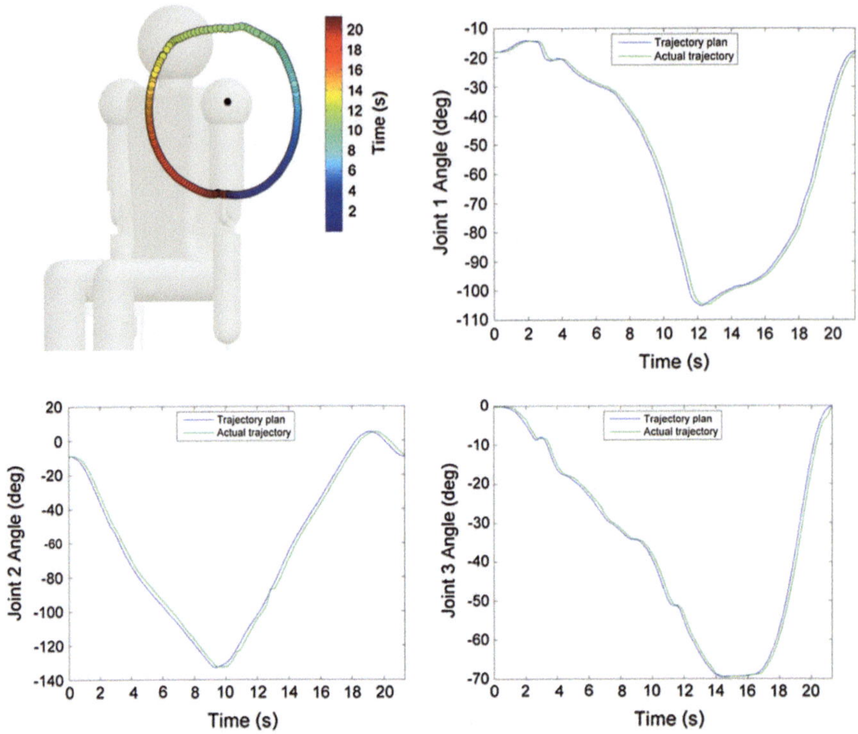

Fig. 6.27 An example of impedance control following a shoulder circumduction trajectory

6.5 Summary

Minimum jerk trajectory planning is used with the exoskeleton to generate a smooth trajectory profile for the user's upper limb joints while passing through specified target positions at target times. A trajectory that minimises the minimum jerk criterion is considered the smoothest trajectory that can be obtained for achieving the target goals. A method is proposed to generate a single smooth trajectory from a sequence of target positions by using a series of minimum jerk trajectories derived for every point-to-point path. Two main control modes, admittance and impedance control, are developed to allow the 5-DOF exoskeleton prototype to interact and respond to user-generated limb movements. In admittance mode, the position of the exoskeleton is unconstrained and the user can physically move the exoskeleton. Interaction force is measured by the force sensors at the HRI and used to drive the exoskeleton in the direction of the user-generated force. In this mode, the exoskeleton can generate either resistive or assistive forces in response to the user's movement. Experimental results are presented throughout this chapter to demonstrate various implementations of admittance and impedance control for both the elbow joint and the shoulder joint.

References

1. N. Hogan, An organizing principle for a class of voluntary movements. J. Neurosci. **4**, 2745–2754 (1984)
2. T. Flash, N. Hogan, The coordination of arm movements: an experimentally confirmed mathematical model. J. Neurosci. **5**, 1688–1703 (1985)
3. P. De Leva, Adjustments to zatsiorsky-seluyanov's segment inertia parameters. J. Biomech. **29**, 1223–1230 (1996)
4. N. Hogan, Impedance control: an approach to manipulation: part I—theory. J. Dyn. Syst. Meas. Control Trans. ASME **107**, 1–7 (1985)
5. N. Hogan, Impedance control: an approach to manipulation: part II—implementation. J. Dyn. Syst. Meas. Control Trans. ASME **107**, 8–16 (1985)
6. N. Hogan, Impedance control: an approach to manipulation: part III—applications. J. Dyn. Syst. Meas. Control Trans. ASME **107**, 17–24 (1985)

Chapter 7
Kinematic and Computational Model of Human Ankle

Knowledge of ankle kinematics is a fundamental requirement when constructing a dynamic model of the human ankle since the kinematic constraints at the ankle–foot complex can be used to select suitable generalised coordinates to describe ankle–foot motion. A recursive algorithm was therefore developed in this research for the online identification of ankle kinematic parameters. This chapter presents a computational ankle model developed to facilitate controller development of the ankle rehabilitation robot and provides a description of the ankle mechanical characteristics through considerations of forces applied along anatomical elements around the ankle joint, which include ligaments and muscle–tendon units. The dynamics of the ankle–foot structure and its surrounding ligaments and muscle–tendon units were formulated into a state space model to facilitate simulation of the robot. Finally, based on observations from preliminary testing, a modified recursive least square (RLS) algorithm was proposed and tested on experimental data.

7.1 Mathematical Description of the Biaxial Ankle Model

The kinematics of a biaxial ankle model with fixed relative orientations can be easily described using homogeneous transformation matrices. The resulting representation may not be the minimal parameterisation, but it can more intuitively depict the location and orientation of different coordinate frames used in the model. The homogeneous transformation matrix is commonly used to describe rigid body position and orientation. It uses the orientation and translation of frame B relative to frame A to transform a point expressed in frame B coordinates to its equivalent representation in frame A. This operation is described in (7.1), where $T_{AB} \in \mathbb{R}^{4\times4}$ (7.2) is the homogeneous transformation matrix, $R_{AB} \in \mathbb{R}^{3\times3}$ is the orthonormal matrix that describes the orientation of frame B with respect to frame A and $t_{AB} \in \mathbb{R}^3$ is the translation from origin of frame A to frame B (expressed in frame A). $x_A \in \mathbb{R}^3$ is the location of the point relative to the origin of frame A, expressed in frame A coordinates. Similarly, $x_B \in \mathbb{R}^3$ is the location of the point relative to the

S.(S.Q.) Xie, *Advanced Robotics for Medical Rehabilitation*,
Springer Tracts in Advanced Robotics 108, DOI 10.1007/978-3-319-19896-5_7

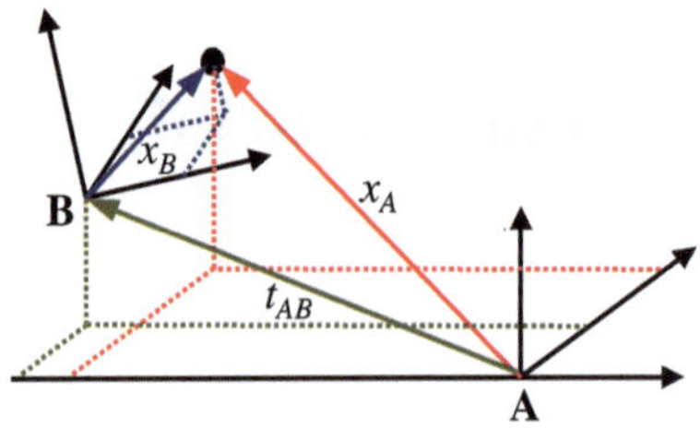

Fig. 7.1 Graphical representation of variables used

origin of frame *B*, expressed in frame *B* coordinates. *A* diagram depicting these is shown in Fig. 7.1. It is also useful to note that the inverse of a homogeneous transformation matrix can be represented by (4.3).

$$\begin{bmatrix} x_A \\ 1 \end{bmatrix} = T_{AB} \begin{bmatrix} x_B \\ 1 \end{bmatrix} \tag{7.1}$$

$$T_{AB}{}^{-1} = T_{BA} = \begin{bmatrix} R_{AB}{}^{\mathrm{T}} & -R_{AB}{}^{\mathrm{T}} t_{AB} \\ 0_{1\times 3} & 1 \end{bmatrix} \tag{7.2}$$

Using the homogeneous transformation matrices, the ankle, subtalar and foot coordinate frames can be defined with respect to a fixed global frame. These frames are shown in Fig. 7.2. For the purpose of this research, all foot bones from the calcaneus to the phalanges were considered as one single rigid body and its orientation and translation were represented by the foot coordinate frame. The subtalar frame was taken to be located on the talus, where its position is fixed and its orientation can change via rotation about the subtalar joint (red axis in the subtalar frame).

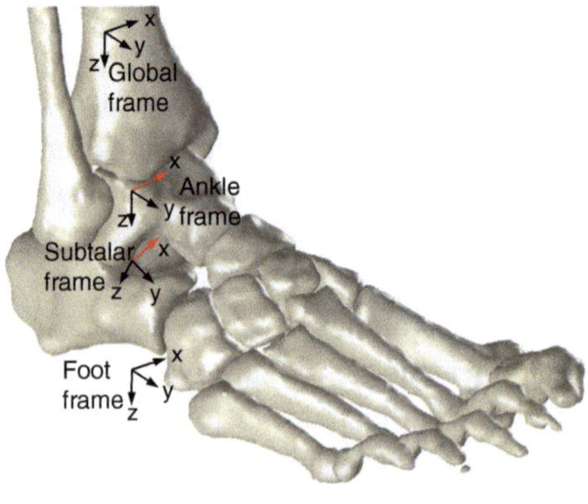

Fig. 7.2 The superposition of indicative ankle, subtalar, foot and global coordinate frames on a three-dimensional surface model of the foot–ankle structure. *Red axes* represent the axes about which rotations occur

Similarly, the ankle frame was considered to be fixed on the tibia in terms of location and free to rotate about the ankle joint axis (red axis of the ankle frame). Since the axes of revolution are denoted as the x-axes of the coordinate frames, the orientation of the ankle frame with respect to the global coordinates can be represented by consecutively applying rotations about the y- and z-axes of the global frame, while the subtalar frame can be obtained by applying y- and z-rotations about the ankle frame. Each of these frames also uses three translations to reposition its origin at designated points in the global frame. A total of five parameters were therefore required to define each of the ankle and subtalar frames at the foot's neutral position. For convenience, the orientation of the foot coordinate frame was taken to be identical to that of the global frame and three parameters were used to determine the origin of the foot frame.

The homogeneous transformation matrices representing the ankle, subtalar and foot coordinate frames at the neutral foot position are given by (7.3)–(7.5), where R_z and R_y are, respectively, the rotational transformation matrices about the z- and y-axes, and subscripts a, s and f are used to represent quantities related to the ankle, subtalar and foot coordinate frames. It should also be noted that subscript i is used to indicate a variable's correspondence to the neutral foot position.

$$T_{0a,i} = \begin{bmatrix} R_{0a,i} & t_{0a} \\ 0_{1\times3} & 1 \end{bmatrix} = \begin{bmatrix} R_{z,a}R_{y,a} & t_{0a} \\ 0_{1\times3} & 1 \end{bmatrix} \tag{7.3}$$

$$T_{0s,i} = T_{0a,i}T_{as,i} = T_{0a,i}\begin{bmatrix} R_{as,i} & t_{as,i} \\ 0_{1\times3} & 1 \end{bmatrix} = T_{0a,i}\begin{bmatrix} R_{z,s}R_{y,s} & t_{as,i} \\ 0_{1\times3} & 1 \end{bmatrix} \tag{7.4}$$

$$T_{0f,i} = \begin{bmatrix} R_{0f,i} & t_{0a} \\ 0_{1\times3} & 1 \end{bmatrix} = \begin{bmatrix} I_3 & t_{0f,i} \\ 0_{1\times3} & 1 \end{bmatrix} \tag{7.5}$$

Since x-axis rotations are permissible at the ankle and subtalar joints, the final homogeneous transformation matrix associated with the foot frame can be obtained by including the angular displacements at the ankle and subtalar joints as shown in (7.6), where R_x is used to represent the transformation matrix for an x-axis rotation. It can be seen that the foot coordinate frame at the neutral position is recovered when both the ankle and subtalar displacements are zero.

$$T_{0f} = T_{0a,i}\begin{bmatrix} R_{x,a} & 0_{3\times1} \\ 0_{1\times3} & 1 \end{bmatrix} T_{0a,i}^{-1}T_{0s,i}\begin{bmatrix} R_{x,s} & 0_{3\times1} \\ 0_{1\times3} & 1 \end{bmatrix} T_{0s,i}^{-1}T_{0f,i} \tag{7.6}$$

It is worth noting that the model formulated above will generally have 16 parameters. This is because six parameters will be required to define $T_{0f,i}$ if the orientation of the neutral foot frame is left arbitrary. As the models proposed by van den Bogert et al. [1] and Lewis et al. [2] only use 12 parameters, the model presented above is not a minimal realisation of the biaxial model. Two of the four additional parameters can be viewed as the angular offsets needed at each revolute

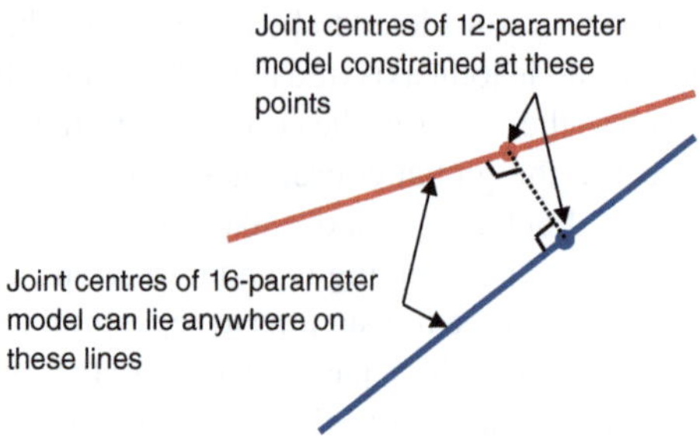

Fig. 7.3 Diagram showing additional degrees of freedom available in the 16-parameter kinematic model when compared with the 12-parameter model

joint to zero the ankle and subtalar joint displacements at the neutral foot orientation. The presence of the remaining two parameters is related to the fact that the origins for the ankle and subtalar frame can be placed anywhere along the corresponding revolute axis (as illustrated in Fig. 7.3). This means an additional degree of freedom is used for the location of each of these origins. While the 16-parameter model allows arbitrary combinations of origins along these two axes, the location of these origins is constrained in the 12-parameter model to lie on points where the distance between lines representing the two axes is at its minimum. For the purpose of simulation, the added number of parameters will not make any difference to the resulting foot motion as these models describe identical kinematic constraints.

7.1.1 Identification of the Reduced Biaxial Model

Where parameter identification is concerned, additional parameters will introduce redundancy in the system to be identified and this may lead to problems in estimation results. Models with no redundancy are therefore preferred in the formulation of system identification problems. However, while algorithms used in [1, 2] are designed to identify both orientation and location of the ankle and subtalar revolute joints, the emphasis of the identification algorithm in this research is mainly on the orientations of the ankle and subtalar joint axes, which are required for controller parameter adaptation strategies, the translations of the foot rigid bodies are therefore not considered in the proposed parameter identification scheme and the redundant parameters used to describe the joint centres in the kinematic formulation presented above were not of any interest in this work. It is also important in this application that the neutral foot position corresponds with zero ankle and subtalar joint displacements, and it can be seen that this condition is inherently satisfied in the kinematic model defined above, hence justifying the inclusion of the two additional axis orientation parameters in the proposed estimation problem.

The foot orientation as obtained from the kinematic model, $\widehat{R}_{0f}$, is represented by the rotational transformation matrix and it takes the form of (7.7) when the initial orientation of the foot is taken to be identical to that of the global reference frame.

$$\widehat{R}_{0f} = R_{0a,i}R_{x,a}R_{as,i}R_{x,s}R_{as,i}{}^{\mathrm{T}}R_{0a,i}{}^{\mathrm{T}} \tag{7.7}$$

As previously discussed, $R_{0a,i}$ and $R_{0s,i}$ can each be defined using two rotations. A biaxial kinematic model with fixed revolute joints therefore has four parameters governing its final orientation. Since these are the only parameters of interest for this work, the identification problem used in this application can be made simpler than that described in [1, 2], thus making it more feasible for online implementation.

Formally, the kinematic model considered in this study is represented by (7.8). It can be seen that this model outputs the model foot orientations in terms of Euler angles $\widehat{\Theta}$ and uses the model parameters, ρ, and joint displacements, θ_{as}, as inputs. Here, $\rho = [\,\theta_{z,a} \quad \theta_{y,a} \quad \theta_{z,s} \quad \theta_{y,s}\,]^{\mathrm{T}}$, where $\theta_{z,a}$ is the z-rotation angle for the ankle axis, $\theta_{y,a}$ is the y-rotation angle for the ankle axis, $\theta_{z,s}$ is the z-rotation angle for the subtalar axis, and $\theta_{y,s}$ is the y-rotation angle for the subtalar axis. These parameters will be collectively referred to as the axis tilt angles hereafter.

$$\widehat{\Theta} = f(\rho, \theta_{as}) = g(\rho, \Theta) \tag{7.8}$$

Since the ankle and subtalar joint angles cannot be readily measured, they have to be estimated from the Euler angles used to describe the observed foot orientation, Θ. By keeping this in mind, it can be seen that $\widehat{\Theta}$ is in fact a function of ρ and Θ. The parameter identification problem in this study is therefore one which seeks to minimise the differences between Euler angles estimated from the kinematic model and those obtained via measurement of the foot orientation. The desired model parameters are therefore the solution to (7.9), where k is the observation number and N the total number of observations.

$$\underset{\rho \in \mathbb{R}^{\ntrianglerighteq}}{\arg\min} \sum_{k=1}^{k=N} [\Theta_k - g(\rho, \Theta_k)]^{\mathrm{T}} [\Theta_k - g(\rho, \Theta_k)] \tag{7.9}$$

7.1.2 Gradient Computation of the Kinematic Model

The parameter identification of the ankle kinematic model is basically an optimisation problem, and the ability to compute the parameter gradient of the model will facilitate this process by permitting the use of line search optimisation routines. Despite the model being nonlinear in parameter, knowledge of its parameter gradient will still make the system amenable to application of online parameter identification algorithms such as the Kalman filter, the RLS and the least mean squares. This section will therefore describe the procedures required to compute this parameter gradient.

It can be seen that the output of the model is given in terms of Euler angles, while the foot orientation is presented in the form of a rotational matrix. An appropriate Euler angle convention must therefore be used to describe this orientation matrix. In this chapter, the *ZXY* Euler angles are used since this is the convention in which the measured pitch(*X*) and roll(*Y*) measurements are supplied by the inclinometer used in the prototype ankle rehabilitation robot. As the yaw component is not readily available from the inclinometer, it is computed by considering the forward kinematics of the robot. For completeness, the relationship between a rotational matrix and its corresponding *ZXY* Euler angles is given in (7.10), where R_x is the matrix describing rotation about the *x*-axis by θ_x, C_x is short for $\cos\theta_x$, and S_x is short for $\sin\theta_x$. This notation extends to the *y*- and *z*-axes, where they are, respectively, indicated by the *y* and *z* subscripts. By representing the *ZXY* Euler angles in a column vector, it can be expressed as (7.11) when the foot orientation is known.

$$R_{0f} = R_z R_x R_y = \begin{bmatrix} C_zC_y - S_zS_xS_y & -S_zC_x & C_zS_y + S_zS_xC_y \\ S_zC_y + C_zS_xS_y & C_zC_x & S_zS_y - C_zS_xC_y \\ -C_xS_y & S_x & C_xC_y \end{bmatrix} \tag{7.10}$$

$$\Theta = \begin{bmatrix} \theta_x \\ \theta_y \\ \theta_z \end{bmatrix} = \begin{bmatrix} \sin^{-1} R_{0f32} & \tan^{-1}\left(\frac{-R_{0f31}}{R_{0f33}}\right) & \tan^{-1}\left(\frac{-R_{0f12}}{R_{0f22}}\right) \end{bmatrix}^{\mathrm{T}} \tag{7.11}$$

It is also clear from the previous discussion that ankle and subtalar joint displacements are a function of ρ and Θ (7.12). As a result, the parameter gradient of the *ZXY* Euler angles in the ankle kinematic model can be obtained by considering (7.13).

$$\theta_{as} = h(\rho, \Theta) \tag{7.12}$$

$$\frac{\partial \widehat{\Theta}}{\partial \rho} = \frac{\partial f(\rho, \theta_{as})}{\partial \rho} + \frac{\partial f(\rho, \theta_{as})}{\partial \theta_{as}} \frac{\partial \theta_{as}}{\partial \rho} \tag{7.13}$$

7.2 Online Identification of a Biaxial Ankle Model

The main objective of this work on ankle kinematic parameter estimation is to extract information of the orientations of the ankle and subtalar joint axes, while the ankle rehabilitation robot is in operation. An online parameter identification algorithm is therefore crucial for the realisation of this goal. This section will discuss the application of different online parameter identification algorithms to the kinematic parameter estimation problem in this research.

7.2.1 Online Identification Algorithms

7.2.1.1 Extended Kalman Filter/Recursive Least Square

The extended Kalman filter (EKF) is an algorithm for state estimation of nonlinear dynamic systems. It predicts system states by considering the measured system outputs, a state space model of the system dynamics and covariance matrices related to the uncertainties found in the measurements and system model. Kalman filters can also be used to simultaneously estimate both states and parameters of a system [3]. This can generally be achieved by augmentation of the parameters of interest to the system state vector. In this particular application, the emphasis is on obtaining an estimate of the system's kinematic parameters. The dynamic model of the ankle and foot motion is therefore not considered.

The algorithm involved in the EKF has the same form as that of a conventional Kalman filter except for the use of linearised state transition and observation matrices. It should be noted, however, that while the Kalman filter is an optimal state estimator, the EKF is not optimal due to the linearisation of the output function. In this problem, the state transition matrix is simply an identity matrix, while the observation matrix is given by the gradient matrix computed from (7.19). The process and measurement noise covariance matrices will control the extent to which the filter will modify the model parameters to fit the measured data. The algorithm of the EKF for this application is given in Table 7.1.

The RLS algorithm is another common approach for online identification of linear models and is related to the Kalman filter. The RLS adaptive filter works by "memorising" previous measurements in the form of a cross-correlation matrix and the current estimated parameters. The correlation matrix is then used together with the estimation error of the current iteration to further adjust the model parameters. Even though the RLS algorithm will not produce the optimal estimates for

Table 7.1 The EKF algorithm

Prediction step	$\hat{\rho}_{k\|k-1} = \hat{\rho}_{k-1\|k-1}$ $P_{k\|k-1} = P_{k-1\|k-1} + Q_k$
Update step	$\widetilde{\Theta}_k = \Theta_k - g\left(\hat{\rho}_{k\|k-1}, \Theta_k\right)$ $\hat{\rho}_{k\|k} = \hat{\rho}_{k\|k-1} + P_{k\|k-1}H_k^T\left(H_kP_{k\|k-1}H_k^T + R_k\right)^{-1}\widetilde{\Theta}_k$ $P_{k\|k} = \left[I - P_{k\|k-1}H_k^T\left(H_kP_{k\|k-1}H_k^T + R_k\right)^{-1}H_k\right]P_{k\|k-1}$ where $H_k = \frac{\partial\widehat{\Theta}}{\partial\rho}$ and I is an identity matrix

nonlinear systems, its simplicity has warranted an investigation into its effectiveness for this application. Since the RLS algorithm works with linear systems, the linearised ankle kinematic model shown in (7.14) has to be used. It can be seen that the model is linearised about the set of parameters denoted by ρ_{lin} and the measured *ZXY* Euler angles given by Θ. H is the gradient of the nonlinear model about its linearisation point and is used to relate changes in Euler angles to changes to the model parameters, with $\Delta\Theta = \widehat{\Theta} - \widehat{\Theta}_{\text{lin}}$, $\Delta\hat{\rho} = \hat{\rho} - \rho_{\text{lin}}$ and $\widehat{\Theta}_{\text{lin}} = g(\rho_{\text{lin}}, \Theta)$.

$$\widehat{\Theta} \approx g(\rho_{\text{lin}}, \Theta) + \left.\frac{\partial\widehat{\Theta}}{\partial\rho}\right|_{\rho_{\text{lin}},\Theta} (\hat{\rho} - \rho_{\text{lin}}) \Rightarrow \Delta\Theta \approx H\Delta\rho \tag{7.14}$$

Using this linear model, the RLS algorithm is given by (7.15), where $\Delta\hat{\rho}$ is the deviation in model parameter needed to reduce estimation error, $\hat{\rho}$ is the estimated parameter, P is the inverse cross-correlation matrix, λ is a geometric forgetting factor where a value of 1 will lead to all historical data being considered, k is the iteration number, and I is an identity matrix.

$$P_k = \frac{1}{\lambda}\left[P_{k-1} - P_{k-1}H_k{}^{\mathrm{T}}\left(\lambda I + H_k P_{k-1} H_k{}^{\mathrm{T}}\right)^{-1} H_k P_{k-1}\right] \tag{7.15}$$

$$\rho_k = \rho_{\text{lin},k} + \Delta\hat{\rho}_k \tag{7.16}$$

A comparison of the RLS and EKF algorithm reveals that they are equivalent if:

1. The process noise covariance, Q, in the EKF is zero and the measurement noise covariance, R, is an identity matrix.
2. The geometric forgetting factor in the RLS algorithm is unity.
3. The parameters about which the model is linearised are the same as their estimates obtained from the previous iteration ($\rho_{\text{lin},k} = \hat{\rho}_{k-1}$).
4. Estimate of the parameter deviation vector brought forward from the previous iteration is always zero ($\Delta\hat{\rho}_{k-1} = \mathbf{0}$).

Condition 1 above implies that the RLS algorithm is essentially an EKF which assumes that the model is perfect while allowing large uncertainties in the measurements. A look at conditions 3 and 4 also suggests that recurrent update of ρ_{lin} and persistent reset of $\Delta\hat{\rho}$ will align the behaviour of the RLS algorithm with that of the EKF. Since the estimated gradient will become less accurate as the parameters deviate further from ρ_{lin}, this frequent update should be able to improve on the accuracy of the RLS algorithm.

7.2.1.2 Least Mean Square

In addition to the EKF, the parameters of the kinematic model can also be estimated through the use of the least mean square algorithm. This algorithm uses the idea of steepest descent for parameter identification and therefore also requires information on the parameter gradient of the kinematic model. However, it does not explicitly store the previous measurements in memory as with the case of EKF or RLS and is therefore more efficient in terms of memory usage. It is also less complex as computation of the inverse cross-correlation matrix is not required.

The overall concept of this iterative method is to modify the model parameters so that a step would be made in the direction which will reduce the estimation error according to the information available in the current iteration. If the parameter gradient is readily available, this can be accomplished by changing the parameter estimates in the manner shown in (7.17), where η is a vector that is dependent on the estimation error.

$$\Delta\hat{\rho}_k = \Delta\hat{\rho}_{k-1} + {H_k}^{\mathrm{T}}\eta \tag{7.17}$$

In order to obtain a suitable expression for η, one can first consider the case where the model is linear in parameter. The convergence of the above algorithm can be determined by examining the behaviour of the function (7.18), where V_k is a positive function and ρ^* is the true parameter vector of the system.

$$V_k = (\hat{\rho}_k - \rho^*)^{\mathrm{T}}(\hat{\rho}_k - \rho^*) \tag{7.18}$$

Substitution of the linearised version (where Δ is removed) of (7.17) into (7.18) will then result in (7.19). It can also be seen that the parameters will converge to the optimal parameters if (7.20) holds. The minimisation of ΔV_k with respect to η then produces the optimal expression for η shown in (7.21). Since $d = H_k\rho^*$ holds for a linear system (with d being the noise-free system output), η can finally be represented as (7.22).

$$V_k = \left(\hat{\rho}_{k-1} + {H_k}^{\mathrm{T}}\eta - \rho^*\right)^{\mathrm{T}}\left(\hat{\rho}_{k-1} + {H_k}^{\mathrm{T}}\eta - \rho^*\right) \tag{7.19}$$

$$\Delta V_k = V_k - V_{k-1} < 0 \tag{7.20}$$

$$\eta = -\left(H_k{H_k}^{\mathrm{T}}\right)^{-1}H_k(\hat{\rho}_{k-1} - \rho^*) \tag{7.21}$$

$$\eta = \left(H_k{H_k}^{\mathrm{T}}\right)^{-1}(d - H_k\hat{\rho}_{k-1}) \tag{7.22}$$

Incorporation of η as given in (7.22) into the parameter update algorithm will then lead to (7.23). If the nominal parameters were to be constantly updated as with the case of the RLS algorithm described above (i.e. $\Delta\hat{\rho}_{k-1}$ is perpetually reset to 0), the resulting parameter estimate at iteration k is given by (7.24), which is basically the normalised least mean square filter. A closer look at (7.24) will suggest that this update rule is somewhat similar to the update rule used in the Gauss–Newton method. Since the ankle kinematic model is nonlinear in parameter system, the optimality and convergence properties of the correction step shown in (7.24) are no longer guaranteed and the use of the $(H_k H_k^{\mathrm{T}})^{-1}$ term may lead to divergence of the estimated parameters, particularly when the parameter gradient is badly conditioned or when it has a large maximum singular value. The parameter update in (7.24) is therefore reformulated as (7.25) to include a term similar to that used in the Levenberg–Marquardt algorithm [4], where the parameter ε can be used to control magnitude and direction of the step size. The use of a large ε will lead to smaller parameter updates along the direction of steepest descent for the estimation error, while a small value of ε will revert the algorithm back to (7.24).

$$\Delta\hat{\rho}_k = \Delta\hat{\rho}_{k-1} + H_k^{\mathrm{T}}\left(H_k H_k^{\mathrm{T}}\right)^{-1}\left(\Delta\Theta - H_k\Delta\hat{\rho}_{k-1}\right) \tag{7.23}$$

$$\hat{\rho}_k = \hat{\rho}_{k-1} + H_k^{\mathrm{T}}\left(H_k H_k^{\mathrm{T}}\right)^{-1}\left[\Theta_k - g(\hat{\rho}_{k-1}, \Theta_k)\right] \tag{7.24}$$

$$\hat{\rho}_k = \hat{\rho}_{k-1} + H_k^{\mathrm{T}}\left(\varepsilon I + H_k H_k^{\mathrm{T}}\right)^{-1}\left[\Theta_k - g(\hat{\rho}_{k-1}, \Theta_k)\right] \tag{7.25}$$

7.2.2 Variation of Axis Tilt Angles with Joint Displacements

A simple extension of the constant axis model is to allow the axis tilt angles to vary linearly with the ankle and subtalar joint displacements. A linear relationship had been chosen as it does not introduce significant computational complexity. Additionally, while the actual dependency may not be perfectly linear, the choice of a model with linear dependency should still be applicable as a local approximation of more complex nonlinear relationships. The new parameters involved in this modified kinematic model can therefore be represented as (7.26), where parameters of the original biaxial ankle model with constant axis tilt angles can be expressed as (7.27), with $\otimes$ as the operator for the Kronecker product. It is straightforward that the original biaxial model is a subset of this extended model where all α and β terms have the value of zero. As this configuration-dependent model utilises a different parameter vector, the gradient matrix required in the estimation algorithms is also different. However, due to the similarity in the models, the required gradient matrix (7.28) can be easily obtained by considering (7.27).

$$\begin{bmatrix} \alpha_{z,a} & \beta_{z,a} & \gamma_{z,a} & \alpha_{y,a} & \beta_{y,a} & \gamma_{y,a} & \alpha_{z,s} & \beta_{z,s} & \gamma_{z,s} & \alpha_{y,s} & \beta_{y,s} & \gamma_{y,s} \end{bmatrix}^{\mathrm{T}} \tag{7.26}$$

$$\rho = \{I_4 \otimes [\theta_a \quad \theta_s \quad 1]\}\rho' \tag{7.27}$$

$$\frac{\partial\widehat{\Theta}}{\partial\rho'} = \frac{\partial\widehat{\Theta}}{\partial\rho}\frac{\partial\rho}{\partial\rho'} = \frac{\partial\widehat{\Theta}}{\partial\rho}\{I_4 \otimes [\theta_a \quad \theta_s \quad 1]\} \tag{7.28}$$

The major problem associated with this new parameterisation is that the ankle and subtalar joint displacements can no longer be easily expressed as an explicit function of the measured *ZXY* Euler angles and the model parameters. Due to the increased complexity of the relationship between the model parameters, joint displacements and measured Euler angles, a numerical algorithm had been employed to resolve the joint displacements that will minimise the discrepancies between the elements of the matrix being considered in the MEM approach. Naturally, the solution of the parameter gradient of the ankle and subtalar displacements is also made more complicated. The formulation of the kinematic model is therefore not ideal for the purpose of online parameter identification.

7.2.3 Variation of Axis Tilt Angles with Measured Euler Angles

An alternative approach that can be used is to allow the ankle and subtalar axis orientations to vary according to the Euler angles. Since only two degrees of freedom is available in the kinematic model, it follows that only two of the three Euler angles are required to establish the configuration dependency. For simplicity, a linear variation can also be used. However, it should be noted that due to the nonlinear relationship between the joint displacements and Euler angles, the linear dependencies of axis tilt angles on the joint displacements will not be retained if these tilt angles are described as a linear function of the Euler angles. Since there is no conclusive evidence in the literature that suggests a linear relationship between the axis tilt angles and the joint displacements, variation from this original assumption should be tolerable. A matter of greater importance, however, is the existence of a one-to-one mapping between the Euler angle pair and the joint displacement. For this reason, different conventions and combinations of the Euler angles should be examined to select suitable angle pairs that can be used as substitutes for the ankle and subtalar joint displacements.

As an illustrative example, Fig. 7.4 shows the relationship between the joint displacements and the *X* and *Y* components of the *XYZ* Euler angles when the axis tilt angles are configuration independent and have the same values as those given by Inman [5]. The relationships shown here were obtained by first computing the *XYZ* Euler angles corresponding to the foot orientation at various ankle and subtalar joint displacements and then reorganising the resulting data so that the ankle and subtalar joints are plotted against the *X* and *Y* Euler angles. A visual inspection of these relationships suggests that linear planes may be able to provide an adequate approximation to these surfaces. Clearly, these surfaces would vary when the model parameter changes. The selection of the Euler angle pair must therefore be based on consideration of a larger variety of model parameters. This had led to the computation of the relationships shown in Fig. 7.4 across model parameters which were varied randomly about those given by Inman [5]. The result of such an analysis is presented in Fig. 7.5, where 500 randomly selected sets of model parameters (all within ±0.5 rad of the nominal parameters) were used to establish the joint displacement–foot orientation relationships. In this analysis, the mappings between different pairs of Euler angles (in both the *XYZ* and *ZXY* conventions) to the ankle

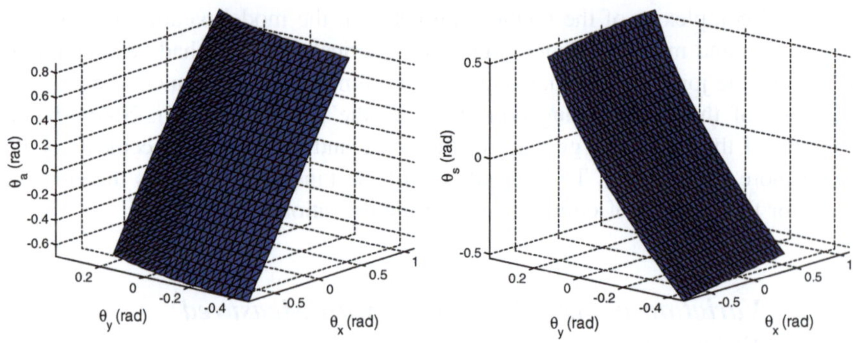

Fig. 7.4 The relationships between the *X* and *Y* components of the *XYZ* Euler angles and the ankle and subtalar joint displacements when the axis tilt angles of the ankle kinematic model are identical to those presented in the literature

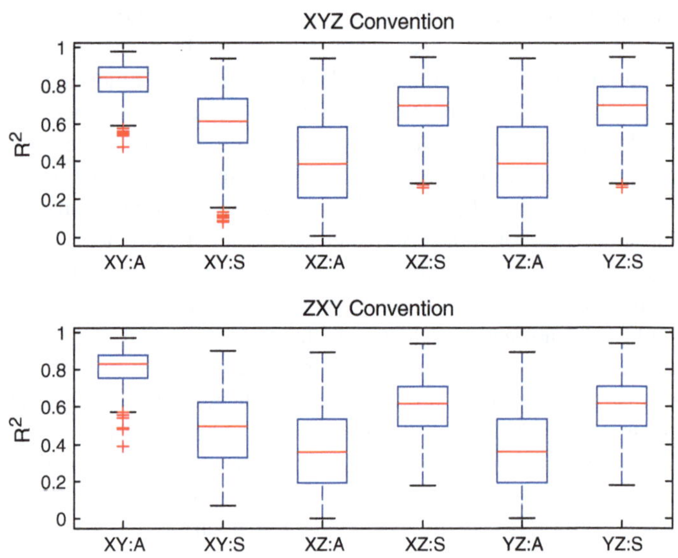

Fig. 7.5 Box plots for R^2 values found by fitting a linear model through the Euler angle–joint displacement relationships over 500 randomly generated model parameters. The *top plot* shows the R^2 values for relationships obtained using various pairwise combinations of the *XYZ* Euler angles, while the *bottom plot* shows the same obtained using different pairwise combinations of the *ZXY* Euler angles. Note that the notation of *P*:*Q* is used to identify results relating to the angle pairing *P* and displacement output *Q*, with *A* and *S* denoting the ankle and subtalar joint displacements, respectively

and subtalar joints were obtained and fitted with a linear plane. The coefficients of determination (R^2 values) of these linear planes were then computed and plotted in the box plots as shown in Fig. 7.5.

As it is difficult to establish whether the joint displacements are proper functions of the Euler angle pairs, the goodness of fit of the linear planes as given by the R^2 values was used as a measure of suitability for the different Euler angle pairs. This is because while a large R^2 value does not guarantee a one-to-one mapping between the Euler angles and the joint displacements, it does give an indication that this relationship can be well approximated by a linear model. Based on these results, the pairing of the X and Y components of the XYZ Euler angles was determined to be the best candidate to represent the ankle joint displacement. The subtalar joint displacements on the other hand seem to be better represented by the X and Z components of the XYZ Euler angles. To reduce the number of parameters involved in the extended kinematic model, the X and Y components of the XYZ Euler angles were used to represent the configuration dependency in the model, since it provides the best R^2 values for the ankle displacement and a reasonable R^2 value for the subtalar displacement.

Another issue is that the XYZ Euler angles used in this approach should be those computed from the corresponding model foot orientation, which brings back the initial dilemma of a non-explicit solution for the joint displacements. However, by accepting an approximate solution for this parameter identification problem, the measured XYZ Euler angles that are readily available from sensor measurements and forward kinematics of the robot can be used as an estimate instead to limit the increase in complexity of the estimation algorithm. The parameters of the extended kinematic model used in the final online estimation algorithm can therefore be rewritten as (7.29) where (7.30) is the relationship that links these parameters back to the axis tilt angles in the original ankle kinematic model. Also, $\theta_{x,XYZ}$ and $\theta_{y,XYZ}$ are, respectively, used to represent the X and Y components of the XYZ Euler angles relating to the measured foot orientation. The gradient matrix for the model proposed in this section can be shown in (7.31).

$$\begin{bmatrix} \alpha'_{z,a} & \beta'_{z,a} & \gamma'_{z,a} & \alpha'_{y,a} & \beta'_{y,a} & \gamma'_{y,a} & \alpha'_{z,s} & \beta'_{z,s} & \gamma'_{z,s} & \alpha'_{y,s} & \beta'_{y,s} & \gamma'_{y,s} \end{bmatrix} \tag{7.29}$$

$$\rho = \{I_4 \otimes [\,\theta_{x,XYZ} \quad \theta_{y,XYZ} \quad 1\,]\}\rho'' \tag{7.30}$$

$$\frac{\partial\widehat{\Theta}}{\partial\rho'} = \frac{\partial\widehat{\Theta}}{\partial\rho}\frac{\partial\rho}{\partial\rho''} = \frac{\partial\widehat{\Theta}}{\partial\rho}\{I_4 \otimes [\,\theta_{x,XYZ} \quad \theta_{y,XYZ} \quad 1\,]\} \tag{7.31}$$

7.3 Computational Model of the Human Ankle

7.3.1 Determination of Model Complexity

Information regarding the mechanical properties of the human ankle is important for the development and evaluation of interaction control strategies for the ankle rehabilitation robot. In addition to describing the end point mechanical behaviour of the human ankle, a model with sufficient detail can also be used to estimate the forces applied to different tissues around the ankle and the reaction moments and forces exerted on the joints. This information is particularly applicable for ankle rehabilitation as injuries are typically a result of overstretching and excessive tensioning of fibrous tissues such as ligaments and tendons. The availability of these forces can therefore facilitate the evaluation of different rehabilitation strategies. With the above in mind, the ankle model required in this research is one which can be used in controller simulations and development while also capable of providing estimates of the forces and moments acting on various ankle anatomical elements.

From the review on existing computational biomechanical ankle–foot models, it can be seen that a range of computational ankle models with varying levels of complexities had been developed by researchers to advance the understanding of foot biomechanics and to study foot-related pathologies. Models belonging to the lower end of the complexity spectrum mainly involve the treatment of the foot and lower limb as rigid bodies, while more advanced models typically utilise finite element analysis to study stresses and strains within the soft tissues [6–8], as well as three-dimensional contacts to describe the ankle kinematic behaviour [9]. While finite element models can give more accurate and realistic results, they are also more computationally intensive. The same holds for the use of three-dimensional contacts to describe the kinematics between foot bones. Since this research aims to incorporate the ankle–foot dynamics into an overall robot controller model, the use of such advanced methods will result in a system which may not be suitable for dynamic simulation over longer timescales. A three-dimensional rigid body-based model with relatively simple kinematic constraints is therefore considered to be a more appropriate choice for this application. The model proposed by Wright et al. [10, 11] and the lower limb model available in OpenSim [12] appear to be the most fitting for this application due to their lower complexity and hence lighter computational demand. However, it should be noted that since knowledge of the forces along the ankle ligaments is important for this work and the above models do not offer such information, a computational model had been developed specifically for this research.

7.3.2 Modelling of Force Elements

7.3.2.1 Modelling of Ligaments

The ligaments considered in the model are fibrous tissues that connect bones to bones. Ligaments are viscoelastic and can be found at various joints in the body. The main role of ligaments is to keep the articulating bones in place during motion. A ligament can be modelled as a piece of elastic string which can only apply a resistive force while in tension. The instantaneous force–length relationship of ligaments can be represented by a piecewise function shown in (7.32) [13], where F_{lig} is the tension force along the ligament and ε is the strain of the ligament.

Additionally, A and B are, respectively, parameters used to control the magnitude and shape the exponential relationship.

$$F_{\mathrm{lig}}(\varepsilon) = \begin{cases} 0 & \varepsilon < 0 \\ A(e^{B\varepsilon} - 1) & \varepsilon \geq 0 \end{cases} \tag{7.32}$$

The ligament force–length relationship shown above can produce unrealistically high tensions when the strain becomes too large. Typically, the ligaments will be damaged before they reach large forces. The use of this exponential relationship in simulation can result in an excessive increase of force for a minute increase in strain. To avoid the rapid increase of ligament forces in simulation, the exponential growth of this force is arrested when a certain force threshold is reached and replaced with a linear relationship. In this work, this threshold is set at 500 N, a value that is close to the largest of the ligament failure loads reported in [13]. The actual ligament force–length relationship used in the developed model is therefore given by (5.33), where F_{thres} is the ligament force threshold (500 N in this case) and $\varepsilon_{\mathrm{crit}}$ (7.34) is the strain required to produce F_{thres}.

$$F_{\mathrm{lig}}(\varepsilon) = \begin{cases} 0 & \varepsilon < 0 \\ A(e^{B\varepsilon} - 1) & 0 \leq \varepsilon < \varepsilon_{\mathrm{crit}} \\ F_{\mathrm{thres}} + B(F_{\mathrm{thres}} + A)(\varepsilon - \varepsilon_{\mathrm{crit}}) & \varepsilon \geq \varepsilon_{\mathrm{crit}} \end{cases} \tag{7.33}$$

$$\varepsilon_{\mathrm{crit}} = \frac{1}{B} \ln\left(\frac{F_{\mathrm{thres}}}{A} + 1\right) \tag{7.34}$$

It was also reported in the literature that ligaments exhibit viscoelastic behaviour where it undergoes force relaxation after application of an initial strain. This behaviour can be modelled using a single spring in parallel with an array of serial spring–damper units. This arrangement is shown in Fig. 7.6. In the case of a linear system, the sum of all the spring stiffness would yield the instantaneous stiffness, while the single spring in parallel, k_3, determines the force found at steady state. The dampers therefore govern the transition between the initial and steady-state forces over time.

The work by Funk et al. [13] has modelled the viscoelasticity of ankle ligaments using three serial spring–damper units in parallel with another spring. In their formulation, three states were required to describe the ligament model. However, since many ligaments are present around the ankle and subtalar joints, the use of four state variables for each of these ligaments will lead to a large state space model. As a result, only one serial spring–damper unit is incorporated in the ligament model in this work to reduce model complexity. Using this viscoelastic model structure, the forces along the force element can be decomposed into two components, a steady-state force along the single spring and a transient force along the serial spring–damper unit. The total force is then merely the sum of these two forces. The relationships between these forces are shown diagrammatically in Fig. 7.7. In the diagram, f_{tot} is the total force along the force element, δ_1 is the

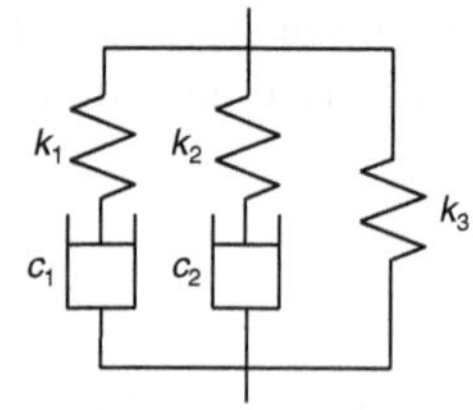

Fig. 7.6 Spring–damper system to model viscoelasticity of ligaments

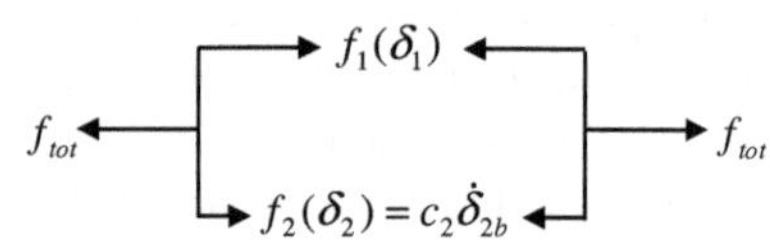

Fig. 7.7 Forces found in the ligament model

elongation along the single spring element, and δ_2 is the elongation of the spring element in the serial spring–damper unit. The forces along these spring elements are, respectively, given by the nonlinear functions $f_1(\delta_1)$ and $f_2(\delta_2)$. The damper element is assumed to be linear with a damping coefficient of c_2, while the elongation of the damper unit is represented by δ_{2b}.

Using the above formulation, the relationships shown in (7.35) and (7.36) can be established. The state space model that describes the viscoelastic ligament force is therefore given by (7.37). It should be noted that f_1 and f_2 used in the model are simply a linearly scaled version. Specifically, these functions can be represented as (7.38)–(7.39), with l_0 being the relaxed length of the ligament. λ_1 and λ_2 on the other hand are scaling factors that sum to unity, where a value of 0.75 has been used as the λ_1 parameter for all ligaments considered in this model.

$$f_{\text{tot}} = f_1(\delta_1) + f_2(\delta_2) = f_1(\delta_1) + c_2\dot{\delta}_{2b} \tag{7.35}$$

$$\delta_1 = \delta_2 + \delta_{2b} \tag{7.36}$$

$$\dot{\delta}_2 = \dot{\delta}_1 - \frac{1}{c_2} f_2(\delta_2) \tag{7.37}$$

$$f_1(\delta_1) = \lambda_1 F_{\text{lig}}\left(\frac{\delta_1}{l_0}\right) \tag{7.38}$$

$$f_2(\delta_2) = \lambda_2 F_{\text{lig}}\left(\frac{\delta_2}{l_0}\right) \tag{7.39}$$

7.3.2.2 Modelling of Muscle–Tendon Units

The Hill-based muscle model has been widely used in the literature [10, 11, 14, 15] to model muscle behaviour and was also adopted in this work. The structure of the

Hill-based model used to describe the muscle–tendon unit is shown in Fig. 7.8. The muscle–tendon unit considered in this model consists of two components (tendon and the muscle), with the tendon component modelled as a nonlinear spring K_{SE}. The muscle component on the other hand is considered to be made up of the contractile element (CE) that governs the muscle's active force characteristics and the parallel element (PE) that determines the passive muscle behaviour. The parallel element is in turn represented as a nonlinear spring K_{PE} in series with a linear damper C_{PE}. The linear damper has been included to incorporate damping in the passive muscle behaviour and to ensure that a feasible solution is obtained in the state space model during simulation.

The mathematical description of the force along the contractile element of the Hill-based muscle model is typically represented as (7.40). The variable A is used to denote the extent of muscle activation and can take on values between zero and unity, while the variable $F_{\max}$ is the maximum active force that can be exerted by the muscle. These variables are used to scale the product of normalised tension–length relationship, $f_{\mathrm{ce}}(l_{\mathrm{ce}})$, and the force–velocity relationship, $f_v(\dot{l}_{\mathrm{ce}})$, where l_{ce} is the length of the contractile element.

$$F_{\mathrm{CE}} = AF_{\max} f_v(\dot{l}_{\mathrm{ce}}) f_{\mathrm{ce}}(l_{\mathrm{ce}}) \tag{7.40}$$

Additionally, the normalised tendon and parallel element force–length relationships can also be, respectively, represented by the functions $f_t(l_t)$ and $f_{\mathrm{pe}}(l_{\mathrm{ce}})$, where l_t is the tendon length. In this work, all the force–length relationships were taken to be the same as those used by default in the OpenSim software package. These functions are shown in Fig. 7.9a–c and are defined through cubic spline interpolation of several known data points. In these functions, the length of the muscle/contractile element is normalised against the optimal muscle fibre length (length at which maximum active force can be produced). Although the force–length relationships used may not be exactly identical to those of the specific patient/user, the general shapes of these relationships are in line with what is typically reported in the literature [14, 15]. Consequently, they should be able to provide at least a qualitative description of the actual muscle behaviour. As the scope of this work is not to provide a patient-specific ankle model, the use of these relationships can be considered acceptable. Of course, large discrepancies between the actual and model force–length relationships can still lead to significant differences in the predicted muscle forces and hence ankle motion and this is a limitation of this approach.

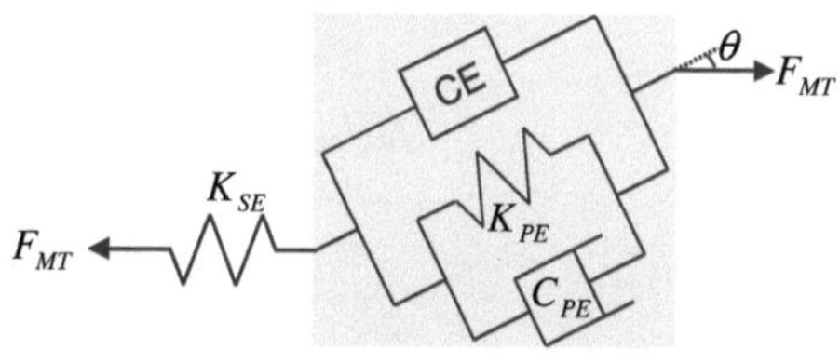

Fig. 7.8 Model structure of the muscle–tendon unit

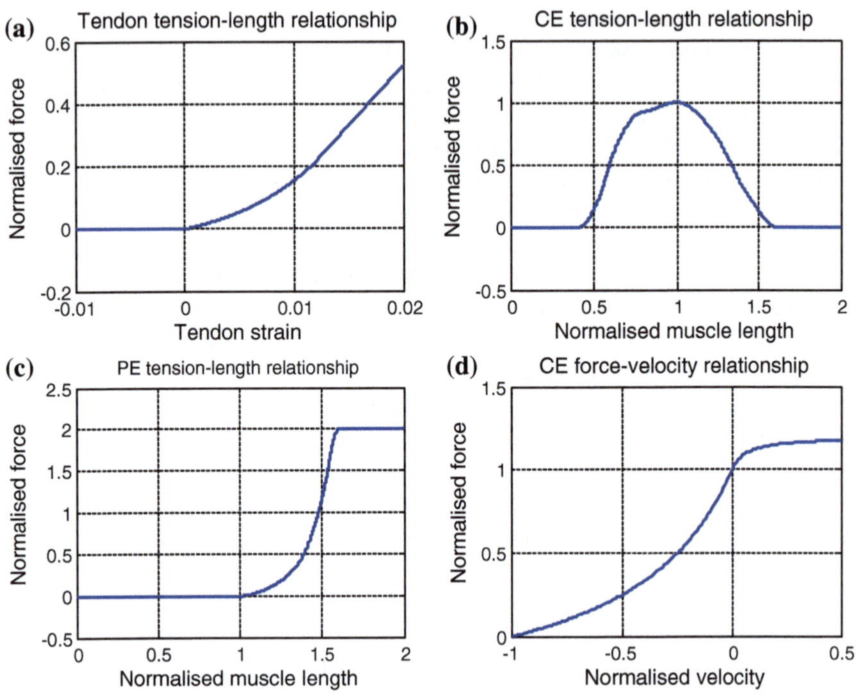

Fig. 7.9 **a** Normalised tension–length relationship for the tendon. **b** Normalised tension–length relationship for the contractile element. **c** Normalised tension–length relationship for the parallel element. **d** Normalised force–velocity relationship for the contractile element (note that negative velocity signifies contraction)

The force–velocity relationship of the contractile element, on the other hand, is given in the form of a piecewise function shown in (7.41) [14, 15], where a_f is a parameter that is dependent on the composition of slow and fast muscle fibres in the muscle and $v_{\max}$ is the maximum contraction speed of the muscle being considered. Also, α and β are parameters used to define the force–velocity relationship when the muscle stretch velocity is positive. These parameters were chosen so that a smooth transition is possible between the two piecewise segments. They have also been selected to provide a desired limiting value for $f_v(\dot{l}_{\text{ce}})$ as the muscle velocity approaches infinity. This relationship is shown in Fig. 7.9d in terms of the normalised contractile element velocity, $\dot{l}_{\text{ce}} v_{\max}^{-1}$.

$$f_v(\dot{l}_{\text{ce}}) = \begin{cases} \dfrac{1 + \dot{l}_{\text{ce}} v_{\max}{}^{-1}}{1 - \dot{l}_{\text{ce}} (a_f v_{\max})^{-1}} & \dot{l}_{\text{ce}} < 0 \\ \dfrac{1 + \alpha \dot{l}_{\text{ce}} v_{\max}{}^{-1}}{1 + \beta \dot{l}_{\text{ce}} v_{\max}{}^{-1}} & \dot{l}_{\text{ce}} \geq 0 \end{cases} \tag{7.41}$$

Using the above formulation, a state space model governing the dynamics of the muscle–tendon unit was established in this work, with the length of the contractile element as the state variable. This model can be derived by first considering the relationships between the lengths and forces of different components as shown in (7.42) and (7.43), where l_{mt} is the total length of the muscle–tendon unit and F_{MT} is the force along the muscle–tendon unit. Additionally, the force along the tendon, F_T, and the force along the parallel element, F_{PE}, can be represented by (7.44) and (7.45), respectively.

$$l_{mt} = l_t + l_{ce}\cos\theta \tag{7.42}$$

$$F_{MT} = F_T = (F_{CE} + F_{PE})\cos\theta \tag{7.43}$$

$$F_T = F_{max} f_t(l_t) \tag{7.44}$$

$$F_{PE} = F_{max} f_{pe}(l_{ce}) + c_{pe}\dot{l}_{ce} \tag{7.45}$$

Although $\dot{l}_{ce}$ is not explicitly given in (7.46), unique solutions for it can be found by first expanding (7.46) into a piecewise quadratic function (7.47). The roots of the function can then be found, and $\dot{l}_{ce}$ can be determined by selecting the solution with the appropriate sign. A first look at (7.46) suggests that the computation of $\dot{l}_{ce}$ will not be straightforward as this quantity is also used to determine the active segment of the piecewise function. A solution to this problem was devised in this work by taking into account the fact that $f_v(\dot{l}_{ce})$ is greater than unity for all positive contractile element velocities and less than unity when the muscle is contracting. Additionally, since A, F_{max}, f_{pe} and f_{ce} are all positive by definition, the difference between the tendon force and the static component of the muscle force as shown in (7.48) can only be positive if $\dot{l}_{ce}$ is positive and vice versa.

$$F_{max} f_t(l_{mt} - l_{ce}\cos\theta) = AF_{max} f_v(\dot{l}_{ce}) f_{ce}(l_{ce}) + F_{max} f_{pe}(l_{ce}) \tag{7.46}$$

$$F_{max} f_t(l_t) - \left[F_{max} f_{pe}(l_{ce}) + c_{pe}\dot{l}_{ce}\right]\cos\theta$$

$$= \begin{cases} AF_{max}\cos\theta \dfrac{1 + \dot{l}_{ce} v_{max}^{-1}}{1 - \dot{l}_{ce}\left(a_f v_{max}\right)^{-1}} & \widetilde{F} < 0 \\ AF_{max}\cos\theta \dfrac{1 + \alpha\dot{l}_{ce} v_{max}^{-1}}{1 + \beta\dot{l}_{ce} v_{max}^{-1}} & \widetilde{F} \geq 0 \end{cases} \tag{7.47}$$

$$\widetilde{F} = F_{max} f_t(l_t) - F_{max}\left[A f_{ce}(l_{ce}) + f_{pe}(l_{ce})\right]\cos\theta \tag{7.48}$$

7.3.3 Definition of Force Element Parameters

The lengths of ligaments and muscle–tendon units are governed by the paths that connect the origin and insertion points of force elements. Two main factors that influence the length of such a path are the displacements of joints and locations of the insertion and origin points of the force element. While the ankle and subtalar joint displacements can be viewed as state variables in the overall ankle model, the insertion and origin points of force elements represent parameters that are specific to the anatomy of an individual. Since it is clear from the previous sections that force along a ligament/muscle–tendon unit is highly dependent on its length, the definition of locations for origins and insertions of force elements is a prerequisite to the construction of a biomechanical model of the ankle.

Since all the foot bones from the calcaneus to the phalanges are treated as one rigid body in this biomechanical model, the only articulations of concern are the ankle and subtalar joints. As a result, only the main ligaments and muscle–tendon units that span these joints are considered in this model. The ligaments considered in this model are shown in Fig. 7.10, while the muscles considered are similar to those used in the OpenSim software package [12] and are shown in Fig. 7.11. The sites where ligaments and muscle–tendon units are attached to their respective bones can be found by referring to resources on human anatomy which provide information on the area of attachment for the force elements. In the model, the attachment sites are treated as points and the force elements are modelled as lines.

Since the anatomical information above is typically presented through a visual medium, it must be converted to quantitative coordinates before it can be included in the model. A graphical user interface (GUI) had been developed in this research to facilitate this process. The developed GUI is capable of presenting the bone

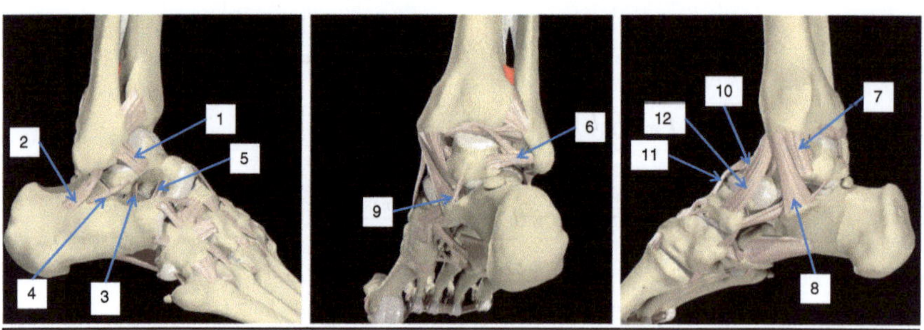

1: Anterior talofibular ligament	5: Anterior talocalcaneal ligament	9: Medial talocalcaneal ligament
2: Calcaneofibular ligament	6: Posterior talofibular ligament	10: Anterior tibiotalar ligament
3: Interosseous talocalcaneal ligament	7: Posterior tibiotalar ligament	11: Talonavicular ligament
4: Lateral talocalcaneal ligament	8: Tibiocalcaneal ligament	12: Tibionavicular ligament

Fig. 7.10 Ligaments of the ankle and subtalar joints considered in the ankle model (adapted from [16])

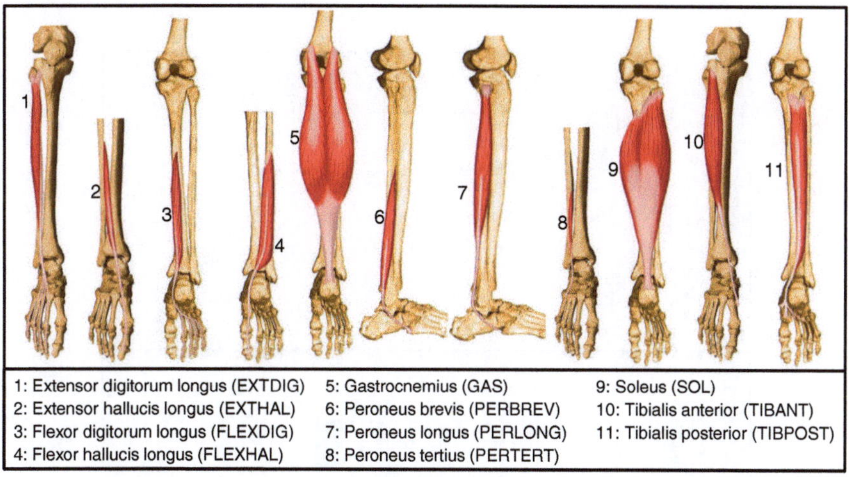

Fig. 7.11 Foot muscles considered in the ankle model (adapted from [17])

surface geometry in a graphical form and allows easy definition of the force element attachment points. In addition to the definition of the force element attachment points, the GUI developed can also be used to specify force relationship parameters of these elements. The ligament force–strain parameters used in this work are similar to those obtained from [13], while the muscle parameters used were similar to those in [12, 18]. These location and force parameters can then be stored in data files for use in the ankle model. The developed GUI therefore served as a tool to define and/or modify the force element parameters used in the biomechanical model. Screenshots of this GUI are shown in Fig. 7.12.

The GUI in this work was developed in MATLAB and utilises a three-dimensional surface model of the lower limb skeleton [19] to provide the surface geometries for various bones around the ankle and subtalar joints. These data are given as a three-dimensional point cloud with a connectivity matrix that designates the interconnection between these points to form the bone surface. Prior to the determination of the force element attachment points, the axes representing the ankle and subtalar joints were first defined. These axes were then used to define the joint coordinate frames. The ankle joint coordinate frame is fixed on the talus, while the subtalar joint coordinate frame is anchored on the calcaneus.

Once the joint coordinate frames were established, the attachment points of the ligaments and tendons were determined by selecting points on the bone surface that corresponds to the attachment sites of force elements shown in the anatomical resources [12, 17]. This is done with the aid of a rendered bone surface plot, and the points collected were expressed in the coordinate frame of the data set. The local coordinates of these points in their respective joint coordinate frames were subsequently computed and stored for use in the biomechanical model. Naturally, points located on the talus were expressed in the ankle joint coordinate frame, and points

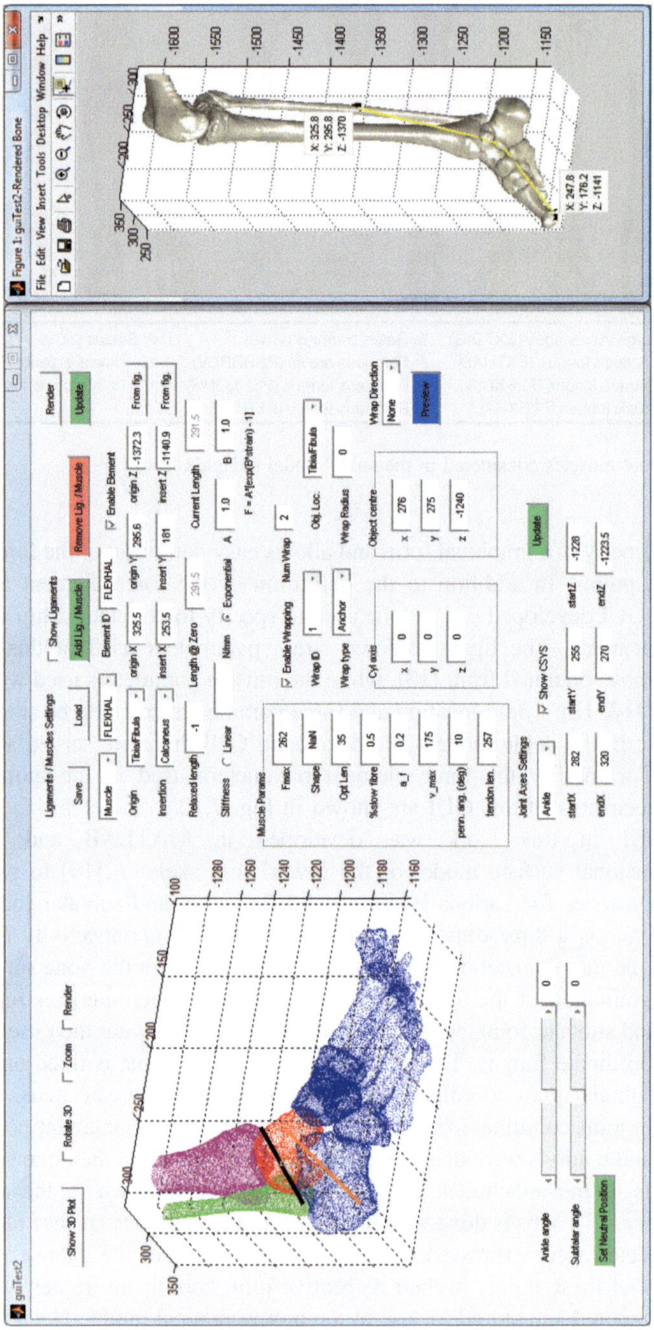

Fig. 7.12 GUI developed to facilitate definition of force element parameters

on the remaining foot bones were given in the subtalar joint coordinates. As the tibia and fibula are assumed to be stationary, all points connected to these bones are expressed in the original data set coordinate frame.

While it is convenient to consider the path of the force element to be a straight line connecting its origin to insertion points, this assumption can be inaccurate for longer force elements such as the muscle–tendon units since they typically wrap around other anatomical structures such as bones and ligaments. The incorporation of the wrapping characteristics of muscle–tendon units are therefore important to produce more realistic simulation results. In this work, muscle wrapping is represented by requiring that the muscle path passes through certain intermediate points before ending at the insertion point. The locations of these intermediate points were again determined with reference to the anatomical resources, and their local coordinates were also computed.

Using the defined local coordinates of the origin, insertion and intermediate points, the length of each force element can be computed using (7.49) and (7.50), where l_k is the length of the force element, n_k is the total number of attachment points, i is an index representing the attachment point being considered, $F_i = O, A, S$ is an identifier for the joint coordinate frame that corresponds to the ith attachment point (where O, A and S are, respectively, used to denote the data set frame, the ankle frame and the subtalar frame), T_{0F_i} is the homogeneous transformation matrix that transforms the data set coordinate frame to the corresponding joint coordinate frame and $P_{k,F_i,i}$ is the position vector of the attachment point i for the kth force element, expressed in the local coordinates of the F_i frame.

$$l_k = \sum_{i=1}^{i=n_k-1} \left\| v_{i,i+1} \right\| \tag{7.49}$$

$$v_{i,i+1} = \begin{bmatrix} I_3 & 0_{3\times1} \end{bmatrix} \left(T_{0F_{i+1}} P_{k,F_{i+1},i+1} - T_{0F_i} P_{k,F_i,i} \right) \tag{7.50}$$

7.4 Validation and Application of Ankle Model

7.4.1 Simulations Involving Constant Axis Tilt Angles

This section presents several simulation results using the previously discussed online parameter identification algorithms. System identification based on data generated from the kinematic model with constant revolute joint orientation was first considered to investigate the effectiveness of the algorithms in handling nonlinear systems and to identify suitable tuning parameters for the identification algorithms. Both the EKF and LMS algorithms were tested, and the algorithm

Table 7.2 Results' summary of different kinematic parameter estimation algorithms on a kinematic model with constant axis tilt angles

	(A) EKF: $Q = 0_{4\times4}, R = I_3$	(B) EKF: $Q = 0.1I_4, R = I_3$	(C) EKF: $Q = 0.1I_4, R = 0.1I_3$	(D) LMS: $\varepsilon = 10$	(E) LMS: $\varepsilon = 1000$
$\lvert\tilde{\theta}_{x,ZXY}\rvert_{\max}$	0.0352	0.0358	0.0493	0.0374	0.0566
$\lvert\tilde{\theta}_{y,ZXY}\rvert_{\max}$	0.0356	0.0401	0.0606	0.0488	0.0793
$\lvert\tilde{\theta}_{z,ZXY}\rvert_{\max}$	0.0355	0.0411	0.1123	0.0462	0.0599
$\tilde{\theta}_{z,a}$	0.1031	0.0991	−0.0285	0.1037	0.1384
$\tilde{\theta}_{y,a}$	0.0169	0.0099	−0.1681	0.0115	0.0243
$\hat{\theta}_{z,s}$	1.0454	1.0657	1.3352	1.0021	0.8772
$\hat{\theta}_{y,s}$	0.6647	0.6765	0.7249	0.6497	0.6472

Actual model parameters: $\theta_{z,a} = 0.1047, \theta_{y,a} = 0.0185, \theta_{z,s} = 1.0519, \theta_{y,s} = 0.6658$. All units in radians

parameters and results are summarised in Table 7.2. The EKF algorithm was tested with three different combinations of Q and R matrices, while the LMS algorithm was tested with different values of ε. A random noise of $\pm 1°$ is added to the measured *ZXY* Euler angles computed from the kinematic model. The *ZXY* Euler angles were generated periodically by computing the model foot orientation that corresponds to the ankle and subtalar joint displacements given by:

$$\theta_a = \frac{2\pi}{9}\sin\left(\frac{2\pi}{10}t\right) \quad \theta_s = \frac{\pi}{6}\sin\left(\frac{2\pi}{11}t\right)$$

A smooth time-dependent relationship was selected so that the simulation can better represent the case where the algorithms are acting on data obtained from actual motion trajectories. The difference in periods for the sine functions was used to allow greater coverage in the $\theta_a - \theta_s$ plane. The evolution of model parameters for different trials of the EKF algorithm with constant tilt angles is shown in Fig. 7.13, while that for the LMS algorithm is shown in Fig. 7.14.

From these results, it can be seen that the EKF algorithm in trial A (which is equivalent to the RLS algorithm with no forgetting factor) had provided the best performance as it gives small errors in terms of the difference between measured and observed *ZXY* Euler angles, while also allowing the estimated model parameters to converge quickly to values close to the true parameters. An inspection of other variants of the EKF shows that the estimated parameters in trial B had drifted around their actual values, while much larger parameter variations were observed for trial C. For the LMS algorithm, it was observed that the trial with $\varepsilon = 10$ performed relatively well, but with some small oscillations in the estimated parameters. On the other hand, the trial with a large ε was found to cause significantly slower convergence.

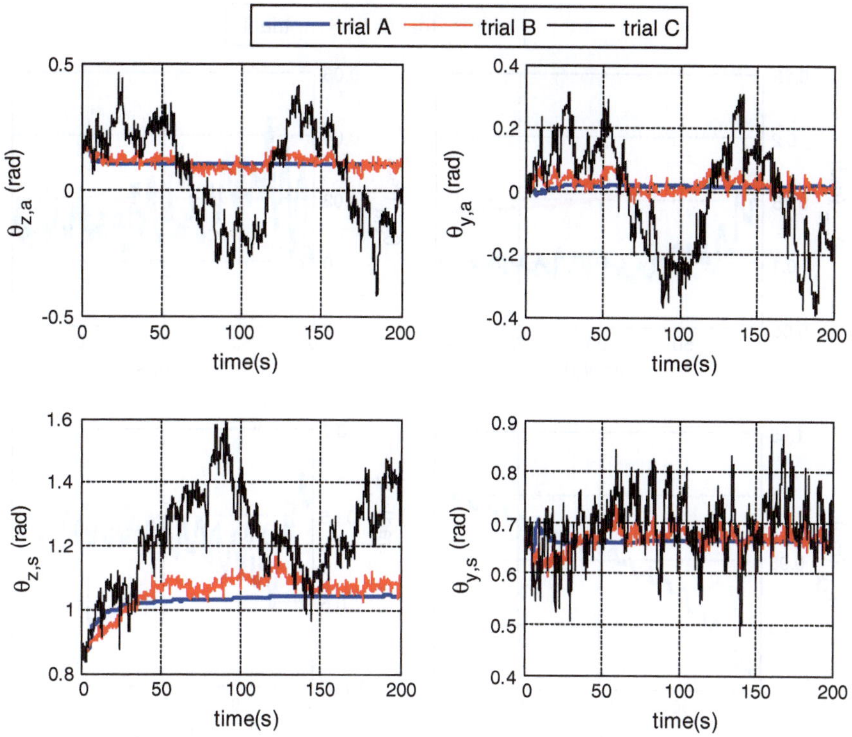

Fig. 7.13 A time history of estimated parameters for EKF algorithms with different process and measurement noise covariance matrices. The *blue*, *red* and *black lines* represent parameters obtained from trials *A*, *B* and *C*, respectively

7.4.2 *Validation of Passive Moment–Displacement Characteristics*

It is important that the developed computational ankle model be compared against real clinical data to validate its ability to approximate the behaviour of the system of interest. As the ankle–foot properties are likely to vary considerably between individuals, accurate quantitative agreement of experimental and model simulation outputs should not be expected for non-subject-specific models. However, since the model is based on the biomechanical properties of the joints under consideration, the general trends of the model outputs should still follow those obtained from experimental studies. The focus of this section is therefore to evaluate whether the behaviour of the developed model is qualitatively comparable to observations on real human ankle–foot structures.

Several simulations involving the developed model have been carried out to allow its comparison with data available in the literature and data collected from

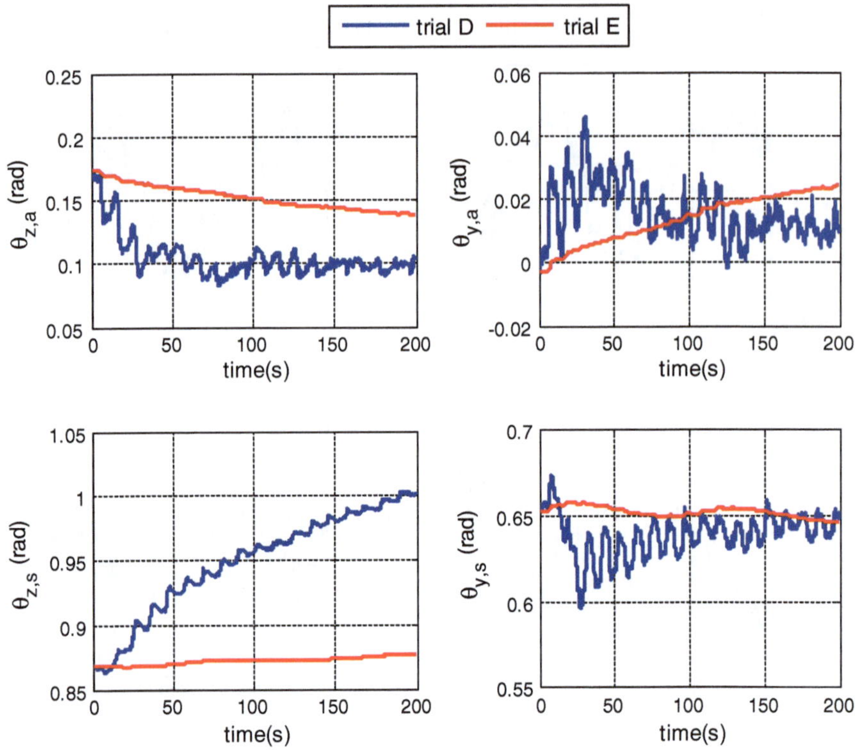

Fig. 7.14 A time history of estimated parameters for the LMS algorithm with different ε values. The *blue* and *red lines* represent trials *D* and *E*, respectively

experiments. Since an abundance of information is available on the passive moment–angular displacement relationship of the ankle, the model had been used in a "virtual experiment" to obtain this relationship. Additionally, to test the active muscle behaviour in the model, the response of the ankle–foot model was recorded when certain muscle activation profiles were inputted to emulate application of flexion and inversion–eversion moments. Finally, the model was also compared with data obtained from the ankle rehabilitation robot. In this final validation trial, the forces measured by the robot were converted to appropriate moments and applied to the ankle model. The resulting motion of the ankle–foot model was then compared against the actual recorded foot motion.

To approximate the passive moment–displacement relationships of the ankle under static conditions, a ramp input of external moment is applied along the *x*-axis of the global frame to simulate the scenario where external moments are being applied in the flexion direction. To minimise the contribution of damping, the ramp profile was chosen to have a small gradient. The results are shown in Fig. 7.15a, while a typical ankle moment–displacement found in the literature is given in

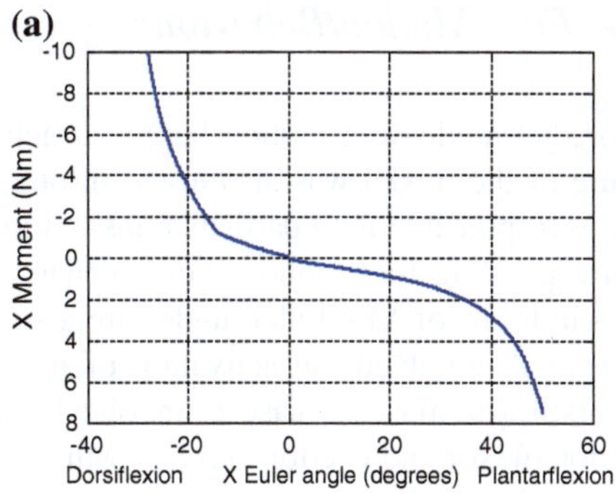

Fig. 7.15 The moment–angular displacement relationship generated by applying a slow moment ramp input to the developed ankle model. Plot **a** shows the relationship for the flexion direction, while plot **b** shows that for the inversion–eversion direction

Fig. 7.16. A comparison of both these graphs shows that the model does indeed produce a passive moment–displacement relationship similar to that found from experimental studies. Small moments were observed around the neutral foot orientation and these increased more rapidly as the foot moved further away from its neutral position. Another key feature of the simulated response is the higher stiffness and smaller motion range in the dorsiflexion direction when compared with those in the plantarflexion direction. This feature is also consistent with what is observed in the literature. The model was also simulated with moments being applied about the *Y* Euler angle axis, and the results of this are shown in Fig. 7.15b. This plot suggests that the range of motion of the ankle model is in reasonable agreement with that observed in real ankles, with a greater range of motion in the inversion direction compared to the eversion direction.

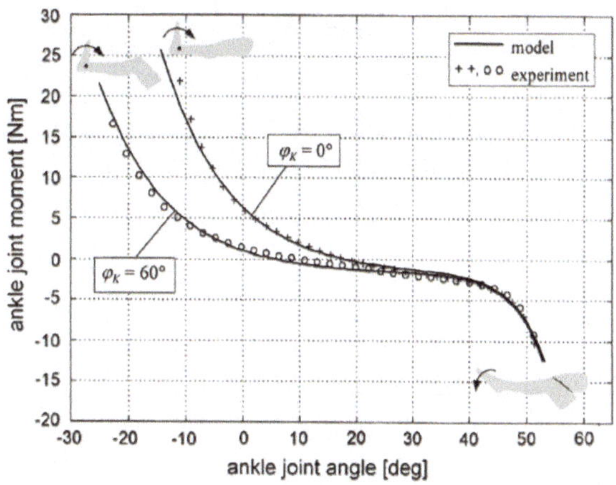

Fig. 7.16 Typical moment–angular displacement relationship in the flexion direction (reproduced from [20])

7.4.3 Simulation of Active Ankle–Foot Motion/Behaviour

The developed model has the ability to predict ankle–foot motion based on activation of different leg muscles. This feature of the model was also tested through simulations where a certain group of muscles responsible for a particular ankle–foot motion were activated to produce the corresponding foot motion. Four scenarios were considered, and the resulting motions in terms of *XYZ* Euler angles are given in Fig. 7.17. Among these simulations, case A involved the activation of plantarflexor muscles, case B involved the dorsiflexor muscles, case C involved the invertor muscles and case D involved the dorsiflexor and evertor muscles. Muscles recruited for each of these cases are shown in Table 7.3.

The muscle activation signals were defined in such a way that a step activation is passed through a low-pass filter prior to it being applied in the dynamic equations of the muscle–tendon units. In these simulations, the muscles were either fully activated or fully relaxed. The simulation results show that the model responses largely agreed with the expected foot behaviour, in the sense that activation of the muscles had produced the desired foot motion. For example, the steady-state foot orientation observed in case A that involved the activation of plantarflexor muscles had

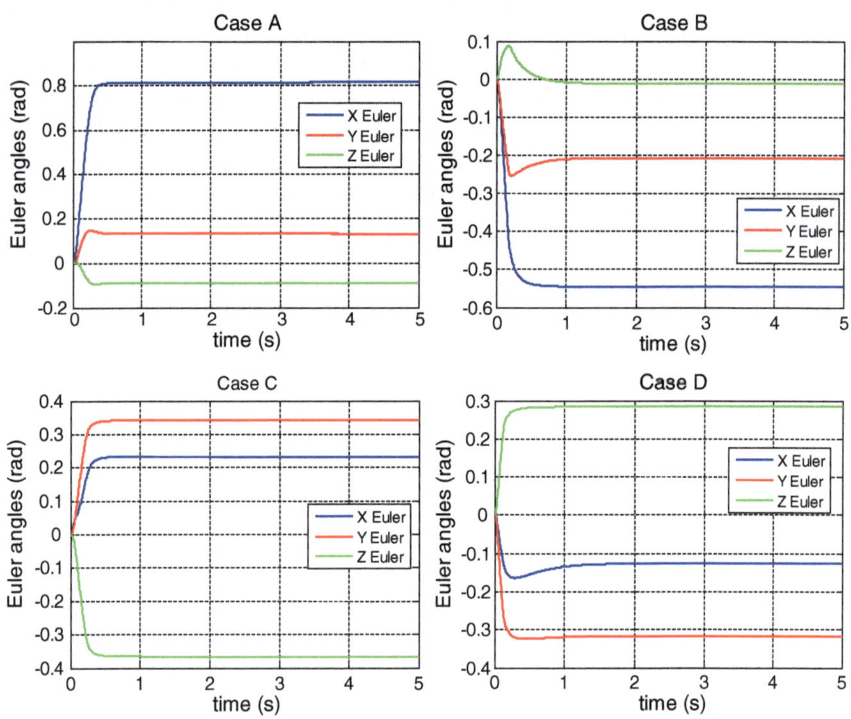

Fig. 7.17 Time histories of the foot orientation in *XYZ* Euler angles obtained from simulations of the developed ankle model with muscle activations

Table 7.3 Muscles recruited for different cases considered in simulation

	Case A (PF)	Case B (DF)	Case C (INV and PF)	Case D (EV and DF)
Activated muscles	FLEXDIG	EXTDIG	TIBANT	EXTDIG
	FLEXHAL	EXTHAL	TIBPOST	EXTHAL
	GAS	PERTERT		PERBREV
	PERBREV	TIBANT		PERLONG
	PERLONG			PERTERT
	SOL			
	TIBPOST			

PF = plantarflexion, DF = dorsiflexion, INV = inversion, EV = eversion

resulted in foot motion in predominantly the positive X Euler angle direction, which is equivalent to plantarflexion movement. Similar observations can also be made in the remaining three scenarios considered. Additionally, the extent of foot motion achieved with the different muscle activation patterns considered was also determined to be within the natural ankle range of motion.

7.4.4 *Rehabilitation Trajectory Generation*

Reference trajectory in rehabilitation robots is typically that of a predefined motion path which corresponds to limb trajectories encountered during activities of daily living. This motion trajectory is then altered during the operation of the robot through the application of impedance or compliance control strategies to maintain a certain relationship between the user–robot interaction forces and the motion tracking error. More advanced trajectory generation strategies also utilise behaviour learnt from observing the interaction between therapists and patients [21], or from consideration of healthy limb movements in hemiplegic patients [22]. However, it appears that little work had been done to generate rehabilitation trajectories from biomechanical models of the musculoskeletal system, particularly in the area of ankle rehabilitation.

One of the main motivations for developing a biomechanical model of the ankle that takes into account actions of individual ligaments and muscle–tendon units instead of lumping these into a single resistive moment–joint displacement relationship is that it can be used to provide an indication of the forces along such force elements. This information can be used to analyse how different motion trajectories influence tensions in the force elements. Since the tibia and fibula are held together by ligaments instead of being rigidly fused, the assumption that the ankle joint can be treated as a rigidly fixed revolute joint may become invalid when large moments are applied in directions perpendicular to the joint axis.

To simplify the optimisation problem, the rehabilitation trajectory was defined using cubic splines rather than allowing the trajectory to take the form of an arbitrary function. This means that the trajectories considered in this work are parameterised by several key points on the trajectory. Instead of specifying the ankle or subtalar displacement as a function of the other, a common independent variable λ is used to define the cubic splines representing each of the ankle and subtalar displacements. The advantage of this approach is that there is no restriction on the trajectory so that there is only a one-to-one mapping between the ankle and subtalar joints. This formulation is shown in more detail in (7.51)–(7.58), where $f_{ij}(\lambda)$ are cubic functions used to represent the value of the ankle or subtalar displacements at a given value of λ, $i = a, s$ is used to denote the ankle or subtalar trajectory and $j = 1, \ldots, N$ is an index of the cubic spline segment used to define the trajectory. Also, c_{ijk} are constant scalar coefficients of the kth power term in the cubic functions that can be obtained by solving (7.55)–(7.58) simultaneously for the corresponding $f_{ij}(\lambda)$. These conditions basically require that the trajectory be continuous up to its first derivative. Additionally, it is also required that the gradient at any data point located between two other data points be parallel to a straight line connecting these two outer data points. The reason for this is to ensure that the trajectory will not deviate too far from the general direction of travel.

$$\theta_a = f_a(\lambda) \tag{7.51}$$

$$\theta_s = f_s(\lambda) \tag{7.52}$$

$$f_i(\lambda) = \begin{cases} f_{i1}(\lambda) & \lambda_0 \leq \lambda < \lambda_1 \\ \vdots & \\ f_{ij}(\lambda) & \lambda_{j-1} \leq \lambda < \lambda_j \\ \vdots & \\ f_{iN}(\lambda) & \lambda_{N-1} \leq \lambda < \lambda_N \end{cases} \tag{7.53}$$

$$f_{ij}(\lambda) = c_{ij0} + c_{ij1}\lambda + c_{ij2}\lambda^2 + c_{ij3}\lambda^3 \tag{7.54}$$

where

$$f_{ij}(\lambda_{j-1}) = p_{i,j-1} \tag{7.55}$$

$$f_{ij}(\lambda_j) = p_{i,j} \tag{7.56}$$

$$\frac{\mathrm{d}f_{ij}(\lambda_{j-1})}{\mathrm{d}\lambda} = \begin{cases} \dfrac{p_{i,N} - p_{i,0}}{\lambda_N - \lambda_0} & j = 1 \\ \dfrac{p_{i,j} - p_{i,j-2}}{\lambda_j - \lambda_{j-2}} & 1 < j \leq N \end{cases} \tag{7.57}$$

$$\frac{\mathrm{d}f_{ij}(\lambda_j)}{\mathrm{d}\lambda} = \begin{cases} \dfrac{p_{i,j+1} - p_{i,j-1}}{\lambda_{j+1} - \lambda_{j-1}} & 1 \leq j < N \\ \dfrac{p_{i,N} - p_{i,0}}{\lambda_N - \lambda_0} & j = N \end{cases} \tag{7.58}$$

The parameters used to form the above ankle and subtalar trajectories are therefore the key points of the ankle and subtalar trajectories given by p_{ij}. The exact set of parameters, however, are dependent on the specific scenario being considered. For instance, if the start and end points of the trajectory are fixed, then the parameters will simply be the points between the initial and final trajectory points. Alternatively, one may wish to vary one or both of the displacement values at the end point. Under this condition, the parameters would include the displacement values being varied. Upon definition of the trajectory points, the independent variables λ_j were computed automatically by considering the cumulative and normalised Euclidean distance between two adjacent key points on the $\theta_a - \theta_s$ plane (normalisation was done with respect to the total Euclidean distance). This means that λ_0 will always be zero and λ_N will always be unity.

Since the quantities to be minimised are the force element tensions and the joint reaction forces, a cost function can be defined in a rather straightforward manner as (7.59), where t_{fe} is a vector of the steady-state force element tensions at a given set of joint displacements, μ_{AS} is a vector of the magnitudes for the ankle and subtalar joint reaction moments and γ is a variable used to denote the Euclidean distance traversed along the prescribed trajectory. The steady-state tensions can be computed by ignoring the dynamic components of the ligament and muscle–tendon models, while the magnitude of the reaction moments can be obtained by first computing the minimal norm external wrench required to maintain the ankle–foot dynamic model in steady state and then substituting the resulting wrench in the moment equations to calculate the reaction moment vector.

$$C = \int \begin{bmatrix} t_{\mathrm{fe}}^{\mathrm{T}} & \mu_{\mathrm{AS}}^{\mathrm{T}} \end{bmatrix} W \begin{bmatrix} t_{\mathrm{fe}} \\ \mu_{\mathrm{AS}} \end{bmatrix} \mathrm{d}\gamma \tag{7.59}$$

By taking into consideration the relationship between γ and λ given in (7.60), the cost function can be rewritten as (7.61). The value for the cost function can then be obtained by numerical integration of (7.61). However, this could be computationally intensive if the integral step size is too small as the ligament and muscle–tendon tensions will have to be solved repeatedly at each integration step. A simpler alternative is to obtain an approximation of this cost function by assuming that the tensions and reaction moments are constant over a small segment of the trajectory. These segments can be prescribed to be of a fixed and uniform length, where the segmental length can be computed by numerical integration of (7.60) with respect to λ.

$$\frac{\mathrm{d}\gamma}{\mathrm{d}\lambda} = \sqrt{\left(\frac{\mathrm{d}\theta_a}{\mathrm{d}\lambda}\right)^2 + \left(\frac{\mathrm{d}\theta_s}{\mathrm{d}\lambda}\right)^2} = \sqrt{\left(\frac{\mathrm{d}f_a(\lambda)}{\mathrm{d}\lambda}\right)^2 + \left(\frac{\mathrm{d}f_s(\lambda)}{\mathrm{d}\lambda}\right)^2} \tag{7.60}$$

$$C = \int \begin{bmatrix} t_{\mathrm{fe}}^{\mathrm{T}} & \mu_{\mathrm{AS}}^{\mathrm{T}} \end{bmatrix} W \begin{bmatrix} t_{\mathrm{fe}} \\ \mu_{\mathrm{AS}} \end{bmatrix} \sqrt{\left(\frac{\mathrm{d}f_a(\lambda)}{\mathrm{d}\lambda}\right)^2 + \left(\frac{\mathrm{d}f_s(\lambda)}{\mathrm{d}\lambda}\right)^2} \mathrm{d}\lambda \tag{7.61}$$

In addition to the cost function to be minimised, definition of parameter constraints is also important to complete the formulation of the optimisation problem. At the basic level, these constraints take the form of upper and lower bounds of the trajectory parameters as shown in (7.62). Other possible constraints include:

(1) The straight-line distance between a key point at λ_j and the end point of the trajectory at λ_N must be shorter than that computed using the previous key point at λ_{j-1}. This constraint can be expressed as (6.24).
(2) A trajectory point must be within the certain distance of the nominal point. This constraint can be expressed as (7.64), where δ is the proximity within which the parameters are constrained.

$$lb_i \leq p_{i,j} \leq ub_i \tag{7.62}$$

$$\sqrt{\left(p_{a,N} - p_{a,j}\right)^2 + \left(p_{s,N} - p_{s,j}\right)^2} < \sqrt{\left(p_{a,N} - p_{a,j-1}\right)^2 + \left(p_{s,N} - p_{s,j-1}\right)^2} \quad \text{where } 1 < j \leq N-1 \tag{7.63}$$

$$\sqrt{\left(p_{a,j,\text{nom}} - p_{a,j}\right)^2 + \left(p_{s,j,\text{nom}} - p_{s,j}\right)^2} \leq \delta_j \quad 1 \leq j \leq N \tag{7.64}$$

It can be seen that constraint 1 will only be appropriate for trajectories that resemble straight-line paths. For paths that involve significant deviation from straight lines such as elliptic or circular paths, constraint 1 can be applied on points located between several critical points upon which constraint 2 is imposed.

Using the above formulation, an optimisation of a test problem was carried out using the `fmincon` function in MATLAB to improve a trajectory that moves the foot from its neutral position ($\theta_a = 0°$, $\theta_s = 0°$) to a more supinated position ($\theta_a = 40°$, $\theta_s = 25°$). The initial trajectory was selected so that the entire set of trajectory points are located on a straight line passing through the start and end positions on the $\theta_a - \theta_s$ displacement plane. The trajectory was defined with a total of four segments, where in addition to the intermediate points, the subtalar displacement of the trajectory end point was also allowed to vary within 5° of its initial value. The weights in the cost function used in this test problem were selected so that only the forces along some of the lateral ankle ligaments were considered together with the reaction moment magnitudes of the ankle and subtalar joints. The weighting for all other force elements was set to be zero. This had been done to focus on minimisation of forces along the lateral ligaments that are more prone to injuries. The cost weightings used for this test problem and the values of the initial and optimised trajectories are presented in Table 7.4, where w is used to denote the weights along the diagonal of the weighting matrix W (note that weights are set to zero unless otherwise specified). Also, C_0 and C_f are used to represent the cost of the initial and improved trajectories.

The initial and improved trajectories are shown in Fig. 7.18a where the circular markers denote the key points used to define the trajectories. The values of the

Table 7.4 Weightings for ligament tensions/joint reaction moments and the cost of initial and final trajectories

w_{ATaFL}	w_{CFL}	w_{LTaCL}	w_{PTaFL}	w_{μ_A}	w_{μ_S}	C_0	C_f
$(1/300)^2$	$(1/600)^2$	$(1/300)^2$	$(1/550)^2$	$(1/10)^2$	$(1/10)^2$	0.7846	0.6180

ATaFL = anterior talofibular ligament; CFL = calcaneofibular ligament; LTaCL = lateral talocalcaneal ligament; PTaFL = posterior talofibular ligament

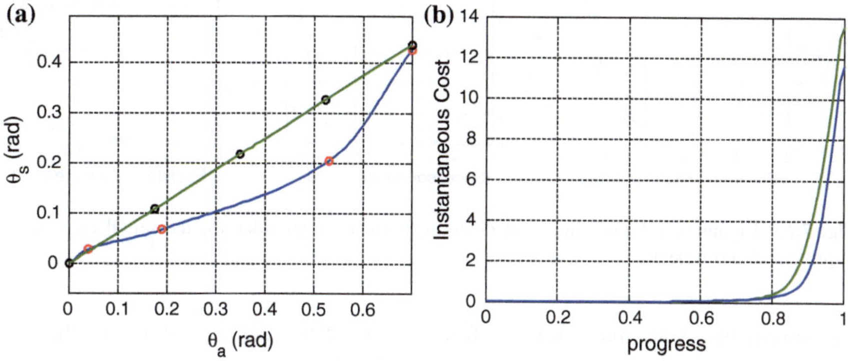

Fig. 7.18 **a** Initial (*green*) and improved (*blue*) rehabilitation trajectories. **b** Instantaneous costs related to the initial (*green*) and improved (*blue*) trajectories

instantaneous cost function to be integrated for both trajectories are also shown in Fig. 7.18b. Additionally, a comparison of the ligament forces and reaction moments is provided in Fig. 7.19.

It is shown in Table 7.4 that the use of the optimised trajectory can lead to approximately 20 % reduction in the cost function when compared with the nominal straight-line trajectory. Figure 7.18a shows that the improved trajectory had deviated considerably from the initial trajectory. It should also be noted that the subtalar displacement of the end point had decreased slightly to reduce the peak ligament tensions and joint reaction moments. It is shown in Fig. 7.19 that although the trajectory produced from the optimisation is longer in terms of path length, it still has a cost function which is about 20 % lower than that of the shortest path. Since the cost function indirectly penalises longer trajectories, this shows that an appreciable reduction in ligament tensions and joint reaction moments can be achieved by deviation from the path of minimal distance.

7.4.5 Experimental Results

In the experiment, the robot was commanded to move the user's foot along certain desired path under impedance control, while the user's foot is relaxed.

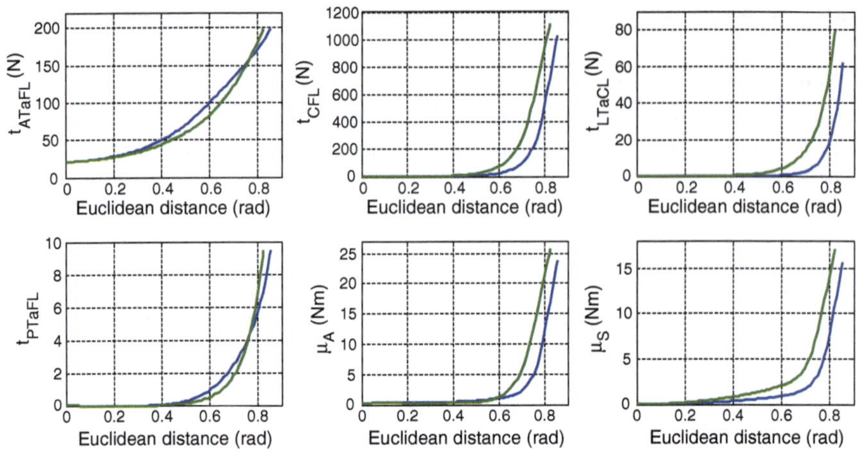

Fig. 7.19 Ligament tensions and joint reaction moment magnitudes for the initial (*green*) and improved (*blue*) trajectories

Measurements were made on the forces applied in each actuator and the foot orientation throughout the experimental trial. The obtained data were then processed to extract the approximate moments that were applied to the ankle–foot structure. These moments were subsequently applied to the developed foot model.

The dynamic model can be considered to be made up of two parts, one which describes the rigid body dynamics of the shank and foot bones and the other which describes the dynamic behaviour of force elements. Any externally applied forces and moments at the base of the foot will only directly affect the ankle and subtalar joint accelerations but not the force element states, while the time derivatives of the force element states also have no instantaneous effects on the ankle and subtalar joint accelerations. Using this system characteristic, the external force and moment vector that are required to maintain zero joint acceleration can be easily computed from the rigid body dynamics of the ankle–foot model. In the developed model, this force and moment vector are applied at a point located at the base of the foot, which is referred to as the interaction point.

The ankle–foot model was simulated with the moments obtained via the procedures described in the previous section as inputs. The results of this simulation are shown in Fig. 7.20. A comparison of the *XYZ* Euler angles obtained from measurement (blue lines) and simulation (red lines) is shown in Fig. 7.20a, while the pure moments applied to the system are shown in Fig. 7.20b.

It is shown in Fig. 7.20a that rather large differences can be found between the two sets of Euler angles. The largest discrepancies in the *X* and *Y* Euler angles are observed at the start of the simulation, and this could be caused by frictions in the 3-DOF rotary joints located at the end of each robot actuator. The main indication for this is the fact that the measured *X* and *Y* Euler angles stayed rather constant in the measured data even as the *X* and *Y* moments increased gently from their initial

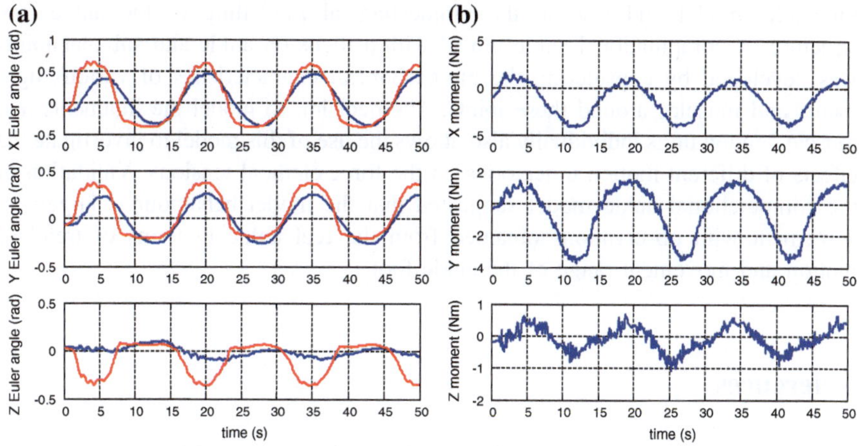

Fig. 7.20 **a** Comparison of actual (*blue*) and simulated (*red*) foot orientations in terms of *XYZ* Euler angles. **b** Moments applied at the interaction point

levels. This suggests that frictions in the joints must had been impeding motion of the end effector and hence the user's foot. Additionally, the peaks of the measured Euler angles also appear to lag behind those of the applied moment, and this could once again be caused by the presence of friction as the direction of motion changes. Another notable difference in the measured and simulated data was the *Z* Euler angle displacement, where the simulated values were far larger in the internal rotation direction. This could be caused by differences in kinematic constraints between the user and the model, as well as the larger magnitude of simulated inversion motion, which also influences internal rotation due to their coupling at the subtalar joint. Certainly, some of the errors can also be attributed to the fact that the model used was not customised to the user's ankle characteristics such as ankle and subtalar joint orientations and attachment points and properties of ligaments/tendons. Furthermore, parasitic motion between the foot and the end effector could also lead to variations in the modelled and measured data. Despite the presence of experimental errors and non-subject-specific nature of the model, qualitative agreement between the model and experimental data can still be observed. As a result, the developed model does appear to be able to give a reasonable description of ankle behaviour.

7.5 Summary

Motion of the ankle–foot structure had been modelled in this research as a series of rotations about two revolute joints (the ankle and subtalar joints). The main reason for the adoption of such a model is to obtain a relatively simple representation of ankle kinematics that can be used in the online parameter estimation of the kinematic model and also in the biomechanical modelling of the ankle–foot structure. A computational ankle model with a focus on ankle and subtalar joints was developed by considering the biomechanical characteristics of various ligaments and muscles around these joints. The decision to model the ligaments and muscle–tendon units individually also allows the use of this model to investigate the effects of different motion trajectories on the force element tensions. Validation of the computational ankle model suggested that the model behaviour is largely in agreement with observations obtained from the real ankle in terms of trend of motion and movement range of the ankle foot.

References

1. A.J. van den Bogert, G.D. Smith, B.M. Nigg, In vivo determination of the anatomical axes of the ankle joint complex: an optimization approach. J. Biomech. **27**, 1477–1488 (1994)
2. G.S. Lewis, H.J. Sommer, S.J. Piazza, In vitro assessment of a motion-based optimization method for locating the talocrural and subtalar joint axes. J. Biomech. Eng. **128**, 596–603 (2006)
3. J.R. Raol, G. Girija, J. Singh, *Modelling and parameter estimation of dynamic systems* (Institution of Electrical Engineers, London, 2004)
4. K. Madsen, H.B. Nielsen, O. Tingleff, Methods for non-linear least squares problems (2004). Available http://www2.imm.dtu.dk/pubdb/views/edoc_download.php/3215/pdf/imm3215.pdf
5. V.T. Inman, *The joints of the ankle* (Williams and Wilkins, Baltimore, 1976)
6. J.T.-M. Cheung, B.M. Nigg, Clinical applications of computational simulation of foot and ankle. Sports Orthop. Traumatol. **23**, 264–271 (2008)
7. J.T.-M. Cheung, M. Zhang, K.-N. An, Effects of plantar fascia stiffness on the biomechanical responses of the ankle-foot complex. Clin. Biomech. **19**, 839–846 (2004)
8. J.T.-M. Cheung, M. Zhang, A.K.-L. Leung, Y.-B. Fan, Three dimensional finite element analysis of the foot during standing—A material sensitivity study. J. Biomech. **38**, 1045–1054 (2005)
9. P.C. Liacouras, J.S. Wayne, Computational modeling to predict mechanical function of joints: application to the lower leg with simulation of two cadaver studies. J. Biomech. Eng. **129**, 811–817 (2007)
10. I.C. Wright, R.R. Neptune, A.J. Van den Bogert, B.M. Nigg, The influence of foot positioning on ankle sprains. J. Biomech. **33**, 513–519 (2000)
11. I.C. Wright, R.R. Neptune, A.J. Van den Bogert, B.M. Nigg, The effects of ankle compliance and flexibility on ankle sprains. Med. Sci. Sports Exerc. **32**, 260–265 (2000)
12. S.L. Delp, F.C. Anderson, A.S. Arnold, P. Loan, A. Habib, C.T. John, E. Guendelman, D.G. Thelen, OpenSim: open-source software to create and analyze dynamic simulations of movement. IEEE Trans. Biomed. Eng. **54**, 1940–1950 (2007)
13. J.R. Funk, G.W. Hall, J.R. Crandall, W.D. Pilkey, Linear and quasi-linear viscoelastic characterization of ankle ligaments. J. Biomech. Eng. **122**, 15–22 (2000)
14. J.M. Winters, Hill-based muscle models: a system engineering perspective, in *Multiple Muscle Systems: Biomechanics and Movement Organization*, eds. by J.M. Winters, S.L.-Y. Woo (Springer, New York, 1990), pp. 69–91
15. H. Yamada, J. Kajzer, A mathematical model of skeletal muscle and numerical simulations of its response under stretching. JSME Int. J. Ser. C **42**, 508–513 (1999)
16. Primal Pictures Ltd. www.anatomy.tv
17. Department of Radiology, University of Washington. http://www.rad.washington.edu/academics/academic-sections/msk/muscle-atlas/lower-body/

18. G.T. Yamaguchi, A.G.U. Sawa, D.W. Moran, M.J. Fessler, J.M. Winters, A survey of human musculotendon actuator parameters, in *Multiple Muscle Systems: Biomechanics and Movement Organization*, eds. by J.M. Winters, S.L.-Y. Woo (Springer, New York, 1990)
19. VAKHUM public dataset. http://www.ulb.ac.be/project/vakhum/public_dataset/public-data.htm
20. R. Riener, T. Edrich, Identification of passive elastic joint moments in the lower extremities. J. Biomech. **32**, 539–544 (1999)
21. P. Martin, M.R. Emami, Real-time fuzzy trajectory generation for robotic rehabilitation therapy, in IEEE International Conference on Rehabilitation Robotics (2009), pp. 354–359
22. H. Vallery, E.H.F. van Asseldonk, M. Buss, H. van der Kooij, Reference trajectory generation for rehabilitation robots: complementary limb motion estimation. IEEE Trans. Neural Syst. Rehabil. Eng. **17**, 23–30 (2009)

Chapter 8
Development of the Ankle Rehabilitation Robot

This chapter begins with an overview of the design requirements of an ankle rehabilitation robot. A suitable kinematic structure of the robot is then proposed. Workspace, singularity and force analyses of mechanisms having this structure are then presented. This is followed by a description of the robot hardware and interface. Operation of the developed rehabilitation robot relies on implementation of a suitable interaction controller, and a force-based impedance control approach had been taken in this research, whereby the desired robot impedance is realised through actuator-level force control. This chapter details the development of the multi-input multi-output (MIMO) actuator force controller devised in this work.

8.1 Determination of a Suitable Robot Kinematic Structure

The ankle–foot motion is primarily rotational and is often described by rotations on three mutually perpendicular anatomical planes. These rotations are illustrated in Fig. 8.1. The plane which distinguishes the left and right sides of the body is termed the sagittal plane. The frontal plane as its name suggests, divides the body into front and back halves. Rotational motion of the foot on the sagittal plane is termed plantarflexion when the toes are pushed further away from the head and dorsiflexion in the opposing direction. Inversion is used to describe the rotation of the foot on the frontal plane where the inner or medial side of the foot is raised upwards, with eversion being its complementary motion. Lastly, internal rotation or adduction is used to describe rotational motion on the transverse plane which moves the toes towards the centre of the body while movement in the contrary direction is termed external rotation or abduction. The typical motion limits along these different directions as determined in an in vitro study by Siegler et al. [1] are shown in Table 8.1.

For the purpose of this section, the quantification of different rotations of the foot is made through the use of Euler angles. The *XYZ* Euler angle convention had been adopted whereby the orientation of the foot is described by a rotation about an

S.(S.Q.) Xie, *Advanced Robotics for Medical Rehabilitation*,
Springer Tracts in Advanced Robotics 108, DOI 10.1007/978-3-319-19896-5_8

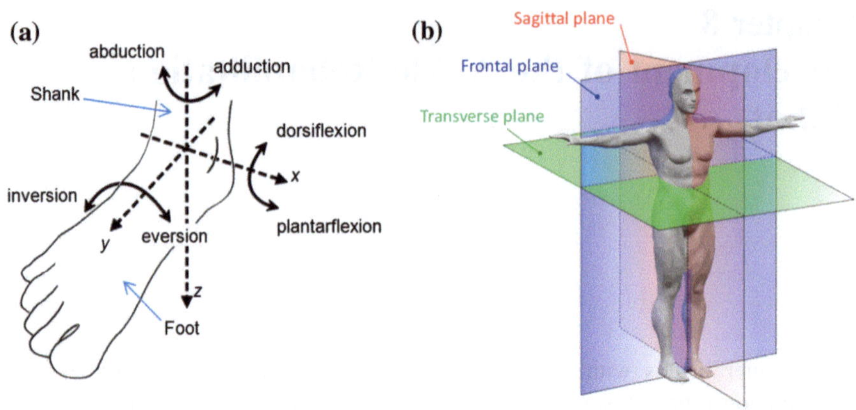

Fig. 8.1 **a** Rotational motions of the human ankle. **b** Anatomical planes of the human body (adapted from [2])

Table 8.1 Typical range of motion at the human ankle

Type of motion	Maximum allowable motion Range	Mean	Standard deviation
Dorsiflexion	20.3°–29.8°	24.68°	3.25°
Plantarflexion	37.6°–45.75°	40.92°	4.32°
Inversion	14.5°–22°	16.29°	3.88°
Eversion	10°–17°	15.87°	4.45°
Internal rotation	22°–36°	29.83°	7.56°
External rotation	15.4°–25.9°	22.03°	5.99°

Data reproduced from [1]

x-axis, followed by a rotation about the resulting *y*-axis and then finally a rotation about the resulting *z*-axis. The angular displacements about these axes are referred to as the *X*, *Y* and *Z* Euler angles, respectively. The arrangement of the axes (see Fig. 8.1a) was selected in such a way that in the absence of rotations about other axes, the plantar/dorsiflexion movement is described by the *X* Euler angle; the inversion/eversion movement is described by the *Y* Euler angle, and the abduction/adduction movement is described using the *Z* Euler angle.

It can be seen that the extent of motion available in different directions are quite different and that the overall ankle range of motion is rather small. It should be noted that since the robot should be able to cater for both the left and right legs, the different motion limits in the inversion–eversion and internal–external rotation directions will be inverted in the robot coordinate frame when a foot from the different side of the body is placed on the robot. The limits of the required robot rotational workspace on the frontal and transverse planes are therefore symmetric.

Another quantity that has a significant influence on the design of the ankle rehabilitation robot is the level of moment that the ankle–foot structure is expected to experience during rehabilitation. In terms of maximum moment required at the plantar/dorsiflexion motion, results from an in vivo study in [3] have found that a maximum range of 71.7 Nm is required to move the foot of the subject passively from maximum plantarflexion to maximum dorsiflexion. The same study also evaluated the torques produced by maximum voluntary contraction of the subjects, and the corresponding values for dorsiflexion and plantarflexion are 54.4 and 126.0 Nm, respectively. Similar results in terms of passive ankle moments were also observed in an in vitro study by Parenteau et al. [4] which gives a maximum dorsiflexion moment as −44 Nm and a maximum plantarflexion moment of about 37 Nm. Maximum joint torque in the inversion–eversion directions is also available from [4], where values of 33 Nm in inversion and 44 Nm in eversion were reported. Unfortunately, maximum torque for internal/external rotation is not available from the above studies. The robot used in this research was therefore designed by assuming that the maximum internal/external rotation moments are similar in magnitude to the inversion/eversion moments. In summary, the moment requirements of the ankle rehabilitation robot are set at 100 Nm for moments about the X Euler angle axis, and 40 Nm for the remaining two Euler angle axes.

Parallel mechanisms have a kinematic structure whereby the end effector is connected to a fixed base through multiple actuated links. Due to this arrangement, parallel robots have several advantages over their serial counterparts. One of these advantages is higher positioning accuracy since errors in the actuated joints no longer accumulate as in the case of serial robots. Furthermore, since the end effector is supported by multiple actuators, the load capacity of the mechanism can also be increased. As actuators of a parallel robot is located at its base rather than on its moving links, the total load moved by the manipulator is also reduced. As a result, parallel mechanisms can be used to achieve higher bandwidth in motion.

Due to its many advantages and the relatively large loads experienced at the ankle and foot, parallel mechanisms are excellent candidates for ankle rehabilitation devices. In fact, the human lower leg and foot can itself be viewed as a parallel mechanism with the foot being the end effector and the muscles spanning across the ankle being the actuating links. From the above discussion, it can be seen that there is sufficient motivation for the use of a parallel robot in this research. The major shortcomings of parallel mechanisms, however, come in the form of a reduced workspace and increased kinematic singularities [5, 6]. Fortunately, as the range of motion of the human ankle is rather limited, the smaller workspace of parallel manipulators may still be adequate provided that suitable kinematic parameters are selected for the mechanism. Singularities on the other hand pose a much greater concern and must be considered in the design of the manipulator. This research had therefore placed special attention on the workspace and singularity analyses during development of the ankle rehabilitation platform.

Existing ankle rehabilitation devices can be broadly classified as platform based or exoskeleton based and many have a parallel kinematic structure. The platform-based devices are mainly used in the rehabilitation of sprained ankle, and the typical set-up requires only the foot of the user to be secured onto the robot end effector. Exoskeleton-based devices on the other hand allow the user to don the robot and is generally used for gait rehabilitation. In this case, the base- and end-effector robot are attached to different limb segments across the ankle.

In many platform-based devices, the robot end effector is often constrained about a centre of rotation which is usually not coincident with the actual ankle centre. As a result of this, the shank of the user is unlikely to remain stationary during the operation of the device, and the rotational motion at the end effector in such platforms will not necessarily be identical to the relative rotations between the shank and the foot. Additionally, these designs also exert poorer control over the foot configuration and ankle moment since the ankle joint is not completely isolated from the remaining joints on the lower limb. For more advanced control strategies which adapt the robot behaviour with respect to the foot configuration, the above shortcoming can also lead to incorrect selection of controller gains. The above problem is avoided in some of the exoskeleton-based designs, where the human lower limb is utilised as part of the robot kinematic constraints and the shank is secured in place during operation. The downside to this, however, is that the robot kinematics is not fully known since the robot is underactuated prior to it being fitted onto the user. Consequently, the control of such robots can be more challenging than the fully constrained platform-based manipulators. Given its ability to provide more accurate estimates of ankle–foot configuration, this research has taken the latter approach and incorporated it into the design of a platform-based ankle rehabilitation robot.

The mobility or number of degree of freedom available in a spatial mechanism is given by the Grubler's mobility formula shown in (8.1) [6], where M is the mobility of the mechanism, n is the number of rigid links present in the mechanism (including the fixed base), g is the total number of active and passive joints and f_i is the degree of freedom for the ith joint.

$$M = 6(n - g - 1) + \sum_{i=1}^{i=g} f_i \tag{8.1}$$

In the set-up, the foot of the user is attached to the end effector and the shank is attached to the base of the mechanism. In the absence of any actuating links, the only kinematic constraint between the base and the end effector will be the human ankle joint. In this scenario, $n_0 = 2$ and $g_0 = 1$. Consequently, the mobility of this mechanism, M_0, is identical to that of the natural ankle joint. Clearly, actuated links must be included in the mechanism to allow control of the rehabilitation device; however, it should be noted that the mobility after the addition of actuated links must be identical to M_0 if the natural motion of the foot is to be preserved.

Since the actuated link must be connected to both the base and end effector for the formation of a parallel mechanism, the number of rigid body segments introduced by each actuated link must be one less than the number of joints added to the system (i.e. $\Delta n = \Delta g - 1$). According to (8.1), it can be seen that the mobility of the mechanism will decrease upon the addition of actuated links if the total degree of freedom of the joints on each actuated link is less than six. Based on this observation, the kinematic structure of the actuated links was chosen to be U$\underline{\text{P}}$S to maintain the mechanism mobility at that of the human ankle. In the above notation, U is used to represent a universal joint, P for a prismatic joint and S for a spherical joint. The line beneath P is used to indicate that the prismatic joint is being actuated. The joints in a U$\underline{\text{P}}$S link structure therefore has six degree of freedom in total, just enough to prevent any reduction in the mobility of the mechanism. Using this link structure, the number of actuated links also dictates the number of actuated degree of freedom in the system.

8.2 Workspace, Singularity and Force Analyses

Due to the incorporation of the human ankle as part of the parallel mechanism, its kinematic description must be established prior to any analyses on the workspace, singularities and moment capabilities of the ankle rehabilitation robot. Although foot motion is often depicted through rotations about two oblique revolute joints in series [7–9], its actual movement pattern appears to be more complicated with coupled translations and rotations. Studies had found that the orientations of the revolute joints in the biaxial model can vary significantly between individuals. Furthermore, it had also been found that such axes orientations also vary with the configuration of the foot. Based on these findings, the generality of results obtained from using a specific biaxial ankle model in the workspace and singularity analysis would be compromised. A natural choice of a kinematic model to replace the biaxial model is a spherical joint as it can cater for all possible rotational motion. However, this approach still fails to address the effects of translational motion. As the movement of the ankle can be considered primarily rotational with limited translational movement of its instantaneous axis of rotation [10], analyses which consider the ankle as a spherical joint can still be used to give an indication of the available workspace and singular regions.

8.2.1 *Analysis for 3-Link Parallel Mechanism*

As discussed previously, the addition of one U$\underline{\text{P}}$S link to the kinematic structure will add one actuated degree of freedom to the system. As the ankle joint is treated as a spherical joint, there are three rotational degree of freedom in the overall parallel mechanism. As a result, three actuated links are necessary to provide full motion control capability for this assumed mechanism. The kinematic structure of the three-link parallel robot considered in this design is shown in Fig. 8.2, together with an illustration of the variables used to parameterise the attachment points of the actuated links. It should be noted that due to the axes convention used, the kinematic structure shown in Fig. 8.2 is actually vertically inverted when compared to how the mechanism would operate in real life, where the foot of the user will be

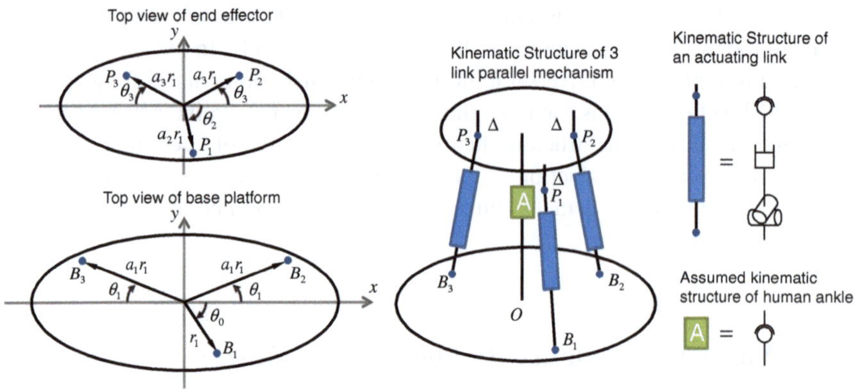

Fig. 8.2 Kinematic structure of the three-link parallel mechanism

secured on the end effector, while the shank is attached to the base platform. It is also worth noting that a symmetric distribution of actuated link attachment points about the *y*-*z* plane should be preferred due to the symmetry of the required workspace about the *Y* and *Z* Euler angles.

In Fig. 8.2, the attachment points of the actuated links on the base are denoted by B_i while their attachments on the end effector are represented by P_i. Based on the UPS link structure, point B_i is coincident with the centre of the universal joint, while point P_i is coincident with the centre of the spherical joint or equivalent on the *i*th actuated link. Point *O* had also been defined on the base platform where it acts as the origin of the robot global coordinate frame. The points B_i and *O* are constrained to lie on the same plane and their relative positions are parameterised in polar coordinates. The projections of points P_i on the end effector can similarly be represented in polar coordinates. In addition to that, the distance between P_i and the end-effector plane is also set to be constant for all *i* and is denoted by Δ. Finally, the point *A* is defined as the centre of the spherical joint used to represent the human ankle.

Using the proposed kinematic structure, the end effector can be seen to pivot about the actual ankle centre and not an external point. Consequently, when the shank is fixed on the base platform and the foot placed on the robot end effector, the robot would have completely isolated the ankle joint. Motion and moments of the end effector taken about the ankle centre will therefore, respectively, provide accurate indications of the relative orientation and moments between user's foot and shank.

8.2.1.1 Inverse Kinematics

The inverse kinematics of a parallel mechanism is the mapping that relates a particular end-effector orientation to its corresponding joint displacements in terms of lengths of the actuated links. Such a relationship can be easily established using the kinematic parameters described above. By using the subscript 0 to represent quantities relating to the zero orientation, a pose where the end-effector orientation is identical with that of the robot global frame, the link vector ($L_i \in \mathbb{R}^3$) of the ith actuated link can be written as (8.2), while its length is given by (8.3).

$$L_i = \overrightarrow{\mathrm{OA}} + R\left(\overrightarrow{\mathrm{AP}_{i,0}}\right) - \overrightarrow{\mathrm{OB}} \tag{8.2}$$

$$l_i = \sqrt{L_i^{\mathrm{T}} L_i} \tag{8.3}$$

8.2.1.2 Computation of Reachable Workspace

Results obtained from the inverse kinematics are highly relevant for the determination of the workspace available in the parallel mechanism. Assuming that the passive joints have been selected so that the limiting factor on the robot workspace is solely that of the length of the actuated prismatic joint, an end-effector orientation can only pass as a point in the robot workspace if all the actuated link lengths fall within an allowable range. This range is typically controlled by the retracted and extended lengths of the linear actuator used in the link. For the purpose of initial analysis, it is assumed that the permissible ranges for the actuator lengths are centred about their respective values at the zero orientation. More precisely, the inequality denoting the constraint on actuated link lengths can be given as (8.4), where $\Delta l_{\max}$ is the maximum stroke length of the linear actuator and $l_{i,0}$ is the length of the ith actuated link at the zero orientation.

$$l_{i,0} - 0.5\Delta l_{\max} \le l_i \le l_{i,0} + 0.5\Delta l_{\max} \tag{8.4}$$

8.2.1.3 Computation of Singularity Measure

The manipulator Jacobian is a matrix which describes the relationship between joint space and task space velocities of a robot. For parallel mechanisms where a unique set of joint space coordinates can be assigned to a given task space configuration, the manipulator Jacobian $J \in \mathbb{R}^{n_l \times 3}$ is the gradient matrix which relates the task space velocity $\dot{\Theta}$ to the joint space velocity $\dot{l} \in \mathbb{R}^{n_l}$ as shown in (8.5). Note that n_l is the total number of actuated links. It is also worth noting that the transpose of the manipulator Jacobian is used to relate the joint space forces $F \in \mathbb{R}^{n_l}$ to task space forces $\tau \in \mathbb{R}^3$, as shown in (8.6). Analysis of the manipulator Jacobian can therefore provide information on the kinematics and kinetics of a robot at a particular configuration. The manipulator Jacobian for the proposed parallel kinematic structure can be obtained from differentiation of the inverse kinematics relationship shown in (8.2). Specifically, the *i*th row of the manipulator Jacobian is given by (8.7).

$$\dot{l} = J\dot{\Theta} \tag{8.5}$$

$$\tau = J^T F \tag{8.6}$$

$$J_i = \frac{1}{l_i} L_i^{\mathrm{T}} \left[\frac{\partial R}{\partial \theta_x} P_{i,0} \quad \frac{\partial R}{\partial \theta_y} P_{i,0} \quad \frac{\partial R}{\partial \theta_z} P_{i,0} \right] \tag{8.7}$$

An important role of the manipulator Jacobian is in the identification of singular configurations of the robot. Singular configurations are poses of the robot whereby the manipulator Jacobian is rank deficient. This means that singular configurations are generally related to an infinite condition number or zero matrix determinant (if the manipulator Jacobian is a square matrix). Rank deficiency in the manipulator Jacobian will lead to the loss of controllability of the robot, where the realisation of task space forces along certain directions will not be possible regardless of the joint space forces being applied. Alternatively, singular configurations can be viewed as poses where the manipulator gains additional degree(s) of freedom in motion since the presence of a null space in the manipulator Jacobian will allow certain task space velocities to exist even though all actuators are locked (i.e. joint space velocities is uniformly zero). Clearly, singular configurations are generally undesirable and must be eliminated from the workspace of the manipulator though selection of appropriate robot kinematic parameter. Even though singularities may only occur at certain points in the robot task space, it is also generally more difficult to control the robot at configurations around these singular points. As a result, a good design should aim to improve the manipulability of the robot by reducing the condition numbers of manipulator Jacobian across all points in the task space.

8.2.1.4 Force Analysis

As the transpose of the manipulator Jacobian also acts as a linear mapping between joint space and task space forces, it can be used to identify the actuator forces required to produce a particular task space moment. This normally involves the inversion of the manipulator Jacobian (or application of the pseudo-inverse if the manipulator is redundantly actuated). Clearly, the force requirements would change with the task space coordinates of the manipulator. The maximum desired moments were therefore applied at various end-effector configurations and the largest of the resultant joint space forces was treated as the actuator force specification. The configurations considered include the neutral position, a supinated (plantarflexed, inverted and adducted) foot configuration, a pronated (dorsiflexed, everted and abducted) foot configuration, and at configurations where a rotation close to the joint motion limit is made about one of the coordinate axes, while the displacements along the remaining two are kept at zero (i.e. pure dorsiflexion/plantarflexion, pure inversion/eversion and pure abduction/adduction).

8.2.1.5 Analysis Results and Discussion

Apart from the workspace, singularity and force requirements, the resultant design must also meet certain spatial constraints to ensure that it can be used in practice. Since the robot developed in this research is used for ankle rehabilitation, the kinematic parameters of the robot must be selected in such a way that it can accommodate the placement of the foot on the end effector. With this in mind, several sets of kinematic parameters for the proposed three-link parallel mechanism had been selected and analysed. The details of these kinematic parameters are provided in Table 8.2. The actuator force requirement, robot workspace and condition numbers of the manipulator Jacobians were computed for each of these designs, and the results of these are summarised in Table 8.3.

It can be seen from these results that the manipulator workspace is rather dependent on the separation of the attachment points on the end effector, where a decrease in separation will result in an increase in workspace volume. A look at the force requirements, however, suggests that smaller separation of attachment points can potentially lead to greater force requirements at certain end-effector configurations. In terms of the robot manipulability, it can be seen that a greater difference between the separation distances of attachment points on the base and end effectors can potentially lead to reduced condition numbers in the manipulator Jacobians. Another important observation is that a region of robot configurations with ill conditioned manipulator Jacobians, or in other words, low manipulability, appears to persist within the workspace for all the parameter sets considered.

For illustrative purposes, the results for one of these mechanisms (which kinematic parameters are given in Table 8.4) are shown in Figs. 8.3, 8.4 and 8.5. Figure 8.3 shows a slice of the robot workspace when the rotation about the Z Euler axis is zero. An inspection of this plot shows that this robot configuration can produce about 32° and 36° of maximum plantarflexion and dorsiflexion, respectively. Additionally, the maximum inversion–eversion motion is around 36°. A three-dimensional view of workspace volume is also shown in Fig. 8.4, and it can

Table 8.2 Kinematic parameters of designs considered in the three-link manipulator analysis

Design ID	r_1 (m)	a_1	a_2	a_3	θ_0	θ_1	θ_2	θ_3	Δ (m)	$\overrightarrow{OA}$ (m)
A	0.2	0.9	0.4	0.45	−90°	45°	−90°	30°	0.05	$\begin{bmatrix} 0 \\ 0 \\ 0.36 \end{bmatrix}$
B	0.11		0.7	0.75	−90°			30°		
C	0.2		0.3	0.35	−90°			30°		
D	0.2		0.5	0.55	−90°			30°		
E	0.2		0.4	0.45	−60°			30°		
F	0.2		0.4	0.45	−90°			45°		

Table 8.3 Design analysis results for different three-link designs

<table>
<tr><th>Design</th><th>F_{max} (N)</th><th>Workspace</th><th>Manipulability</th></tr>
<tr><td>A</td><td>3119.1</td><td>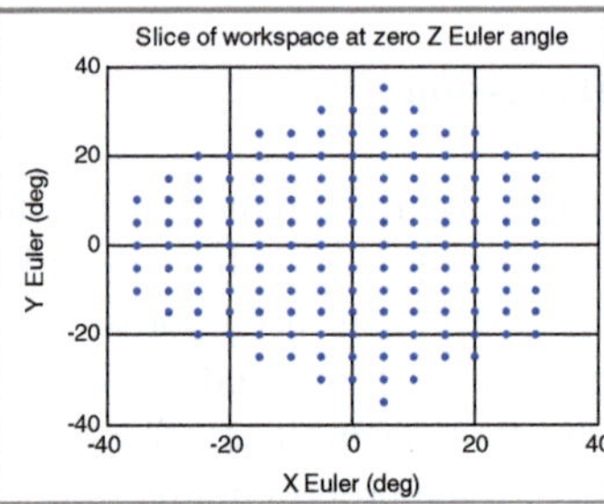
</td><td>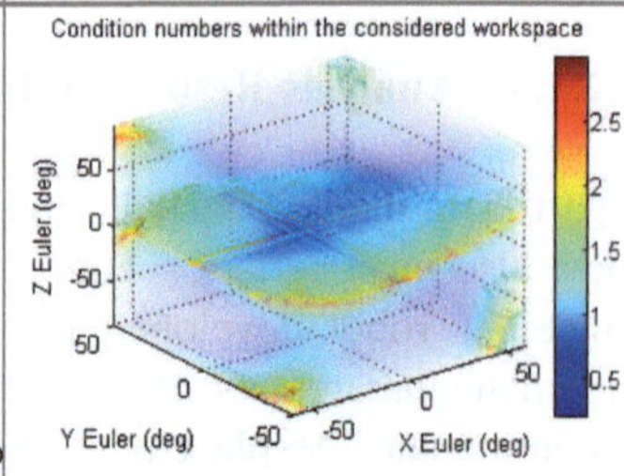
</td></tr>
<tr><td>B</td><td>6327.4</td><td>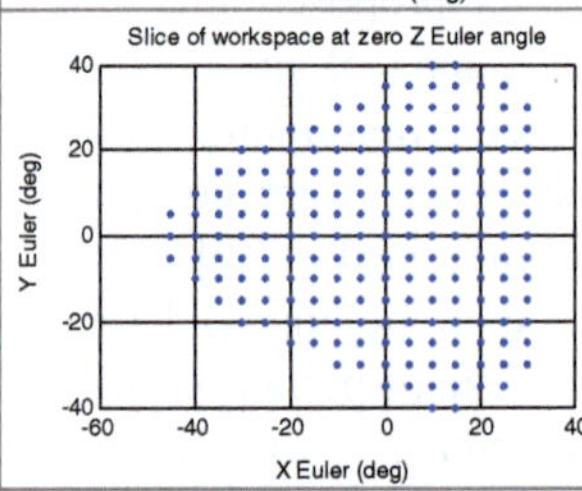
</td><td>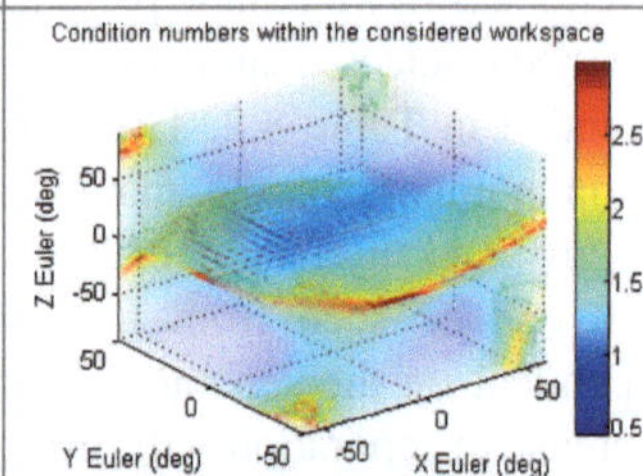
</td></tr>
<tr><td>C</td><td>4651</td><td>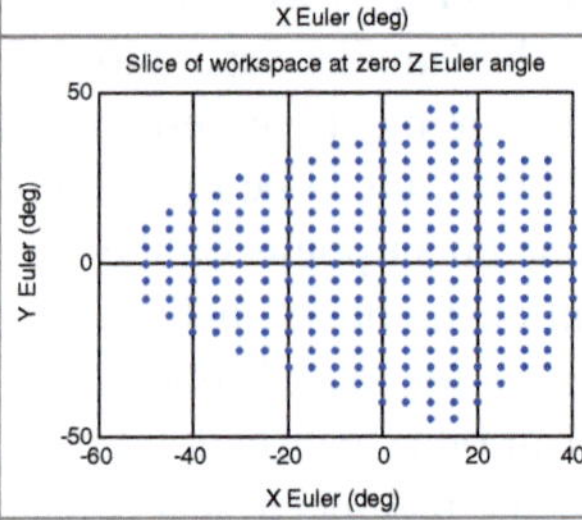
</td><td>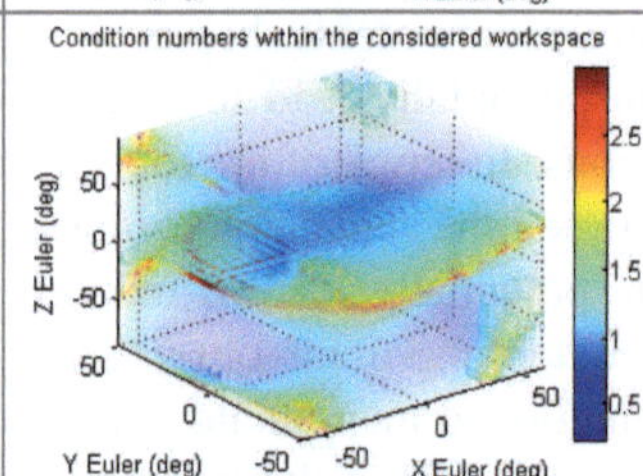
</td></tr>
<tr><td>D</td><td>4609.8</td><td>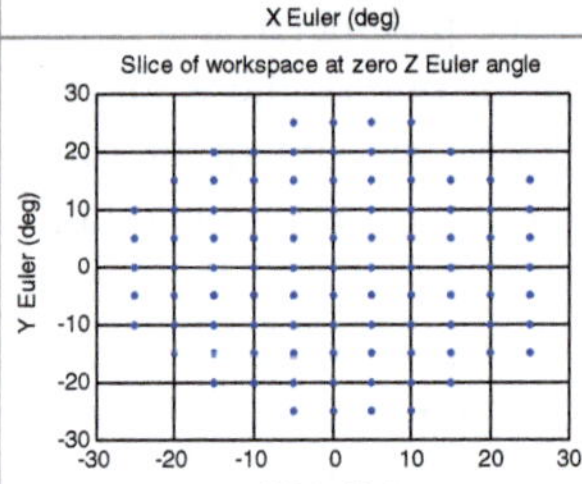
</td><td>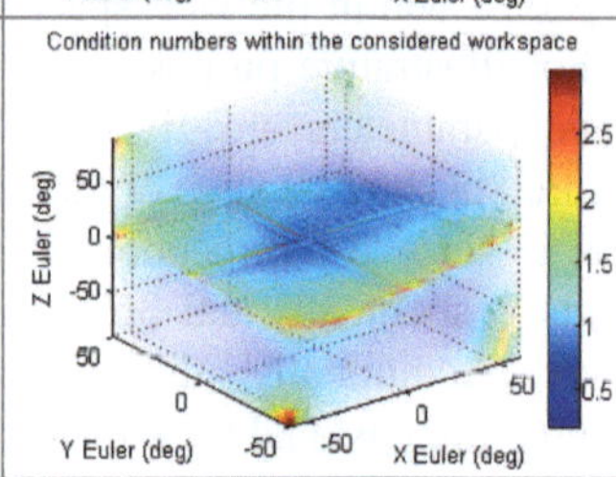
</td></tr>
<tr><td>E</td><td>3438.5</td><td>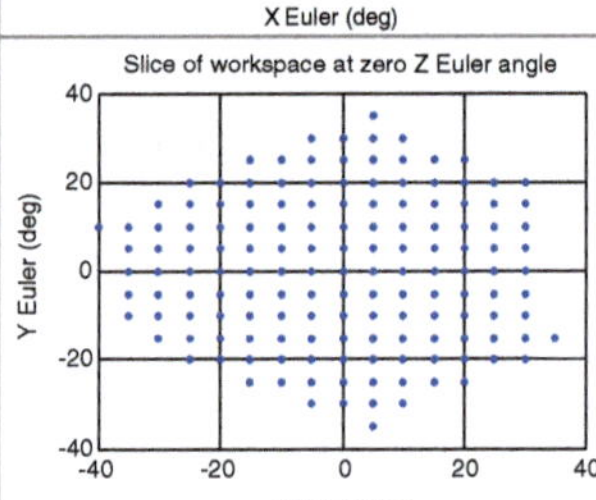
</td><td>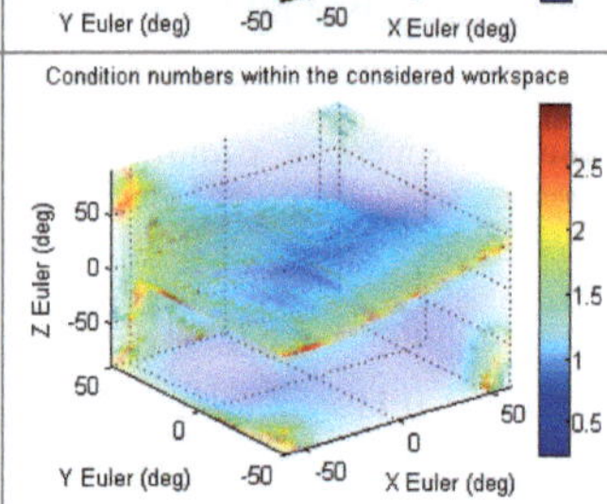
</td></tr>
</table>

(continued)

Table 8.3 (continued)

Design	F_{max} (N)	Workspace	Manipulability
F	2781.8	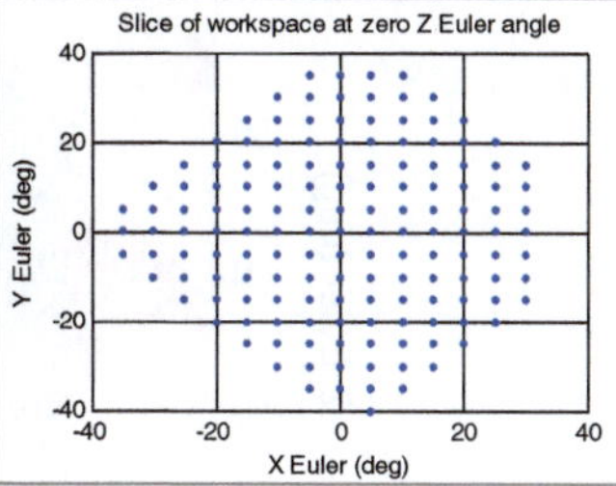	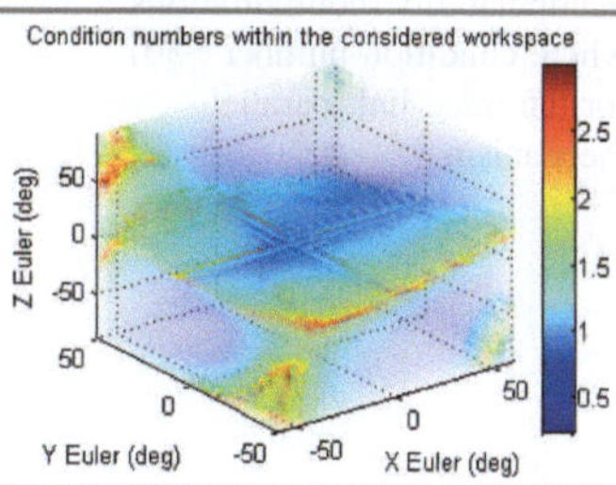

Table 8.4 Kinematic parameters for the three-link parallel mechanism

Parameter	r_1 (m)	a_1	a_2	a_3	θ_0	θ_1	θ_2	θ_3	Δ (m)	$\overrightarrow{OA}$ (m)
Value	0.2	0.9	0.4	0.45	−90°	45°	−90°	30°	0.05	$[0 \quad 0 \quad 0.36]$

be seen that the largest range of motion of the robot is by far in the yaw direction, with maximum rotations of over 90°. A better visualisation of the task space with low manipulability is given in the volumetric plot shown in Fig. 8.5. In this plot, the condition numbers of the manipulator Jacobians at different orientations are represented in a colour spectrum and plotted on the three-dimensional axes.

It can be confirmed from Fig. 8.5 that there is indeed a surface with low manipulability in the middle of the task space considered in this analysis. This surface effectively splits the workspace of the robot into two segments and prevents controlled motion from one segment to the other. This is clearly unacceptable as a full range of foot motion is desired. A remedy for this problem is the inclusion of an

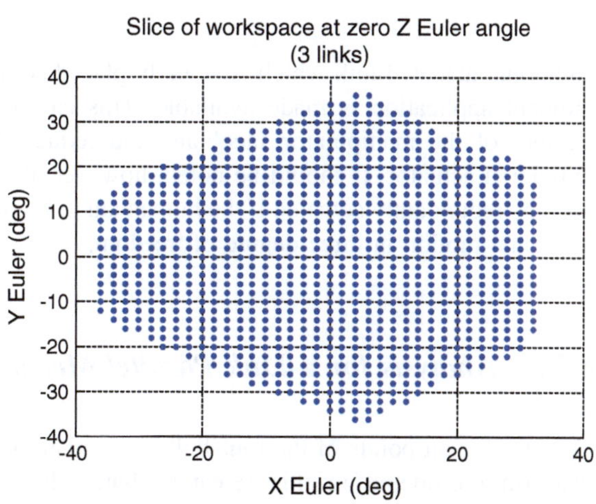

Fig. 8.3 A slice of the robot workspace at zero Z Euler angle for the three-link parallel mechanism

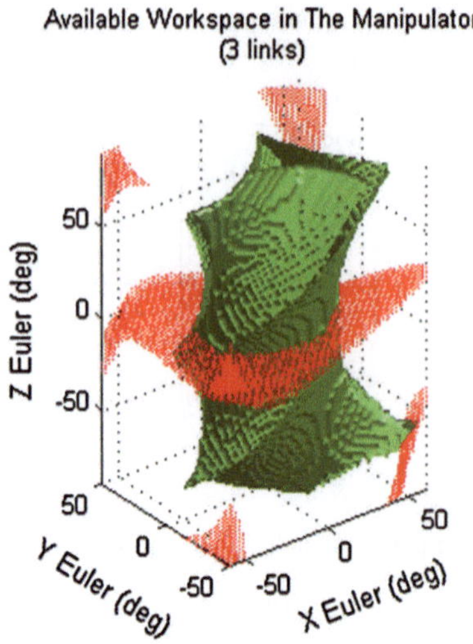

Fig. 8.4 Superposition of the workspace volume on regions of the task space with low manipulability (configurations where condition number >50) for the three-link parallel mechanism

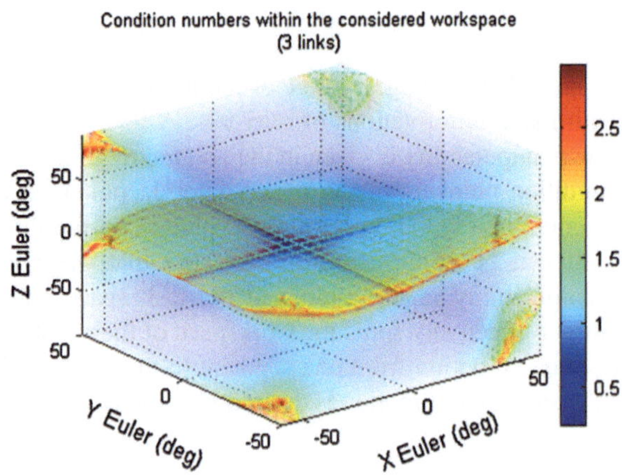

Fig. 8.5 Plot indicating the distribution of manipulator Jacobian condition numbers throughout the manipulator task space for the three-link parallel mechanism. The colour spectrum is assigned to the base 10 logarithms of the condition numbers

additional actuated link which is suitably placed so that an additional direction for moment application is made available. This can also help reduce the condition number of the manipulator Jacobians and reduce the force required from each individual actuator. It should be noted, however, that the resulting robot will then become redundantly actuated if the human ankle is considered to be only capable of rotational motion in three degree of freedom.

8.2.2 *Analysis for 4-Link Parallel Mechanism*

The attachment points of the four-link mechanism on the end effector and the base platform considered in this research shares the same parameterisation as the

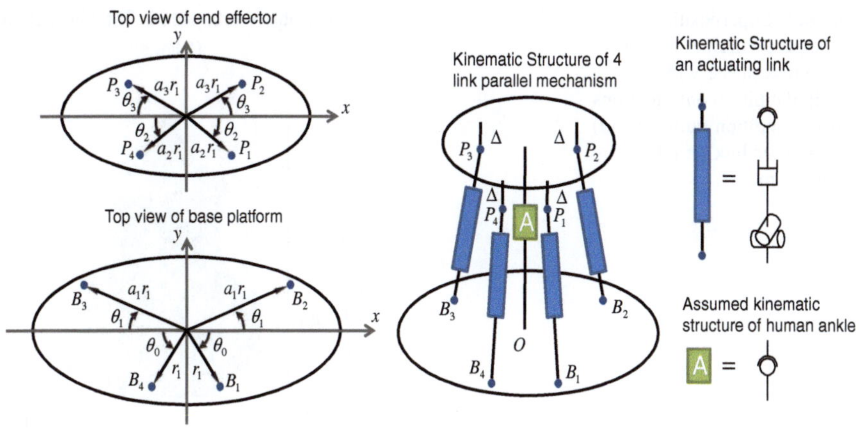

Fig. 8.6 Kinematic structure of the three-link parallel mechanism

three-link version. The kinematic structure of the mechanism can therefore be represented by Fig. 8.6.

The same workspace, singular region and actuator force analyses as above were carried out on a four-link mechanism with kinematic parameters given in Table 8.5 and the results are shown in Figs. 8.7, 8.8 and 8.9. It can be seen from these results that the manipulability of the task space has significantly improved due to the

Table 8.5 Kinematic parameters for the four-link parallel mechanism

Parameter	r_1 (m)	a_1	a_2	a_3	θ_0	θ_1	θ_2	θ_3	Δ (m)	$\overrightarrow{OA}$ (m)
Value	0.2	0.9	0.4	0.45	−45°	45°	−30°	30°	0.05	$[0 \quad 0 \quad 0.36]$

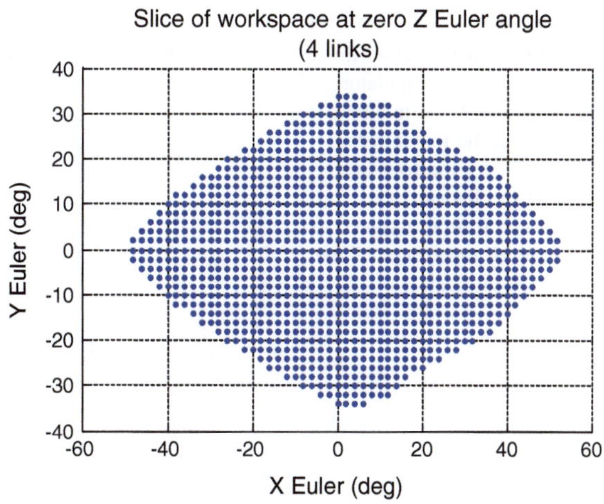

Fig. 8.7 A slice of the robot workspace at zero *Z* Euler angle for the four-link parallel mechanism

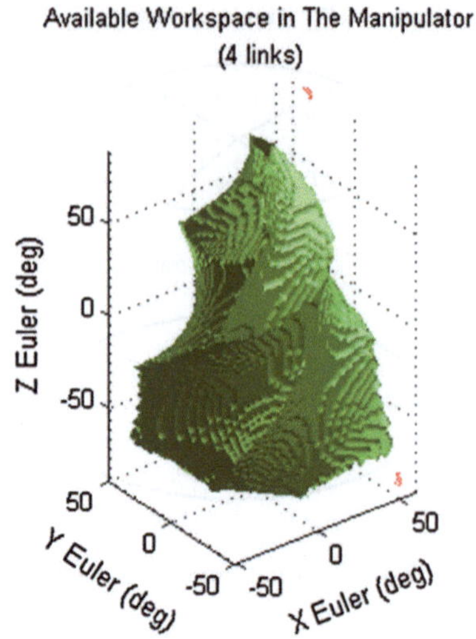

Fig. 8.8 Superposition of the workspace volume on regions of the task space with low manipulability (configurations where condition number >50) for the four-link parallel mechanism

presence of an extra actuated link, where both Figs. 8.8 and 8.9 show that the regions with the highest condition numbers are actually located outside the workspace of the robot. The new kinematic parameters of this parallel mechanism also appear to be capable of producing a larger robot workspace in the flexion directions, with maximum plantarflexion of about 52° and maximum dorsiflexion of about 48°. The motion limits about the *Y* Euler axis, however, was found to decrease slightly to 34°, but still satisfies the required range of motion. Lastly, the range of *Z* Euler rotations in the workspace is also more than adequate to accommodate the natural ankle movements. An inspection of the actuator force requirements also shows that with four actuators, the maximum actuator force exerted to achieve the prescribed task space moment is now reduced to about 1700 N from over 3000 N in the three-link mechanism.

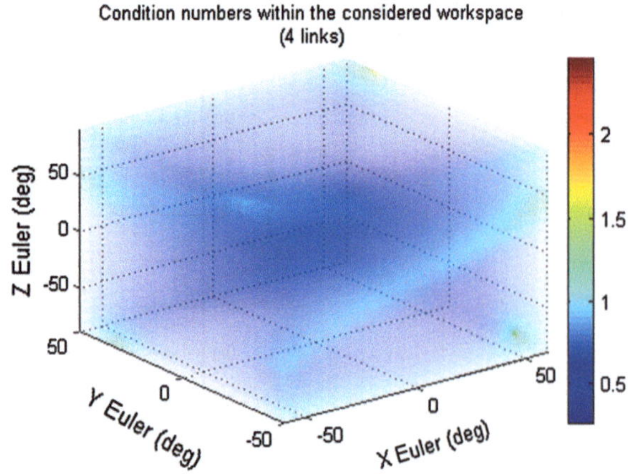

Fig. 8.9 Plot indicating the distribution of manipulator Jacobian condition numbers throughout the manipulator task space for the four-link parallel mechanism. The colour spectrum is assigned to the base 10 logarithms of the condition numbers

8.2.3 *Evaluation of 4-Link Design with Additional Constraints*

Since the four-link mechanism appears to outperform the three-link design in almost all aspects, it had been adopted in the final design of the ankle rehabilitation robot. However, it should be noted that the analyses carried out above was only completed for a single ankle centre of rotation. As discussed previously, the complex kinematics of the ankle means that this centre is likely to vary during operation of the robot. Furthermore, the previous analyses also assumed that there were no violations of passive joint limits. The actual workspace of the robot may therefore be smaller than the results shown above. Further investigation is therefore required to evaluate the true capability of the final design.

8.2.3.1 Consideration of Passive Joint Limits

The universal joint displacements were computed for different end-effector configurations to study the influence of passive joint limits on the robot workspace, and it was found that these angular displacements largely remained between ±32° throughout the entire robot workspace. This is within the permissible motion range of the universal joints used in this work (±35°) and therefore will not affect the previously determined robot workspace. The configuration of the spherical joints was also analysed, and it was found that when viewed in the local end-effector coordinates, the unit vector representing the line of action of the actuated link can deviate as much as 87° from its initial orientation. To overcome this problem, the spherical joint in the proposed mechanism is replaced with a set of three mutually intersecting revolute joints. Such a joint complex is shown in Fig. 8.10. It can be seen that the proposed joint complex will function as a spherical joint as long as axes *a* and *c* do not become parallel. This non-parallel condition therefore forms part of the passive joint constraint which must be considered in obtaining the final robot workspace. Additionally, another constraint in the passive joint displacement

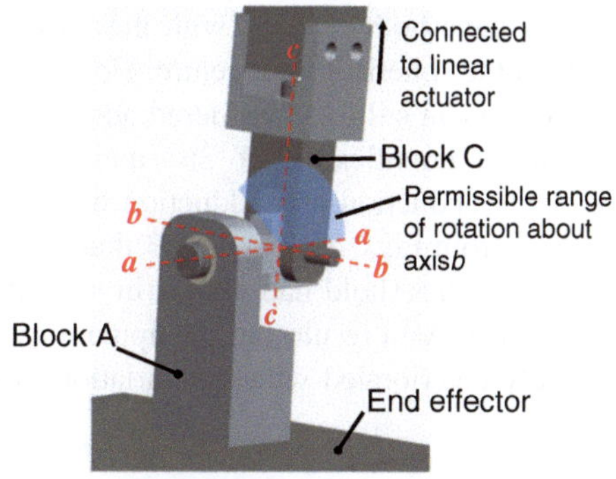

Fig. 8.10 Illustration of the joint limit on the effective spherical joint

can be obtained by imposing a non-interference condition between block A and block C. By taking into account both constraints and the geometry of the components, the permissible angle between axis a and axis c was estimated to be from 50° to 180°, as illustrated in Fig. 8.10.

8.2.3.2 Variation of Assumed Ankle Centre

In addition to the application of passive joint limits, the workspace and condition numbers for the final design were also computed for different locations of the spherical joint (i.e. $\overrightarrow{\mathrm{OA}}$) to simulate the translation of the actual ankle centre of rotation. In the final design analysis, $\overrightarrow{\mathrm{OA}}$ was varied within a 30 mm cube centred about its nominal location. Positions of the end-effector attachment points, $P_{i,0}$, were, however, held constant with respect to the global robot frame. The choice of the 30-mm cube was based on sources in the literature which estimates the range of ankle translation to be between 10 and 20 mm [10]. It should be noted that the workspace produced from this analysis will also have some safety margin against small deviations in the foot placement location on the robot end effector. The upper and lower bounds of the actuator lengths used in this analysis also differed slightly with those of the original analysis where actuator length limits are dependent on the actuator lengths at the neutral foot configuration. In the final design, the construction of the actuated links was made to be uniform across all links and they therefore share the same motion limits. Analysis of the reachable workspace had shown that this design decision had the effect of improving the maximum motion allowable in the plantarflexion direction at the expense of smaller dorsiflexion movements. Since the original dorsiflexion limit is well in excess of the natural dorsiflexion motion limit, this design change is not expected to significantly compromise the ability of the proposed robot in meeting the workspace requirements.

8.2.3.3 Analysis Results and Discussion

The results obtained from the above analysis are shown in Figs. 8.11, 8.12 and 8.13. It can be seen from these plots that the robot workspace and task space manipulability have both reduced with the introduction of passive joint limits and variations in the spherical joint centre. However, results suggest that the estimated range of motion can still be considered adequate, with a maximum plantarflexion of 44°, maximum dorsiflexion of 36° and maximum inversion–eversion of 26°. The available abduction and adduction motion remains large at about 70°. It can also be seen from Figs. 8.12 and 8.13 that the regions with condition numbers over the designated threshold had grown in size, these regions are still located outside the workspace. As a result, the manipulability of the robot within its workspace is not severely deteriorated with the variation of the spherical joint centre.

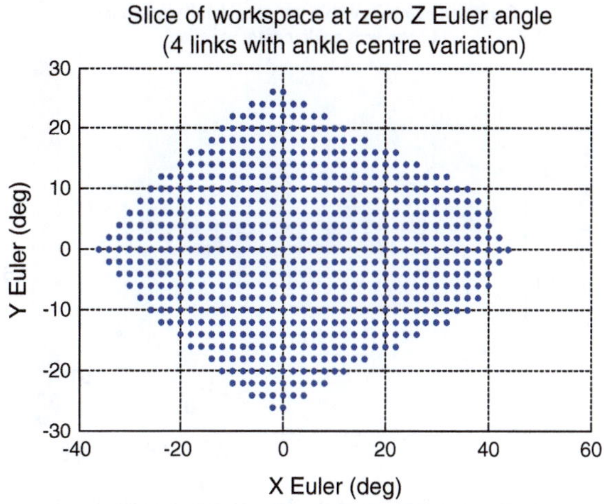

Fig. 8.11 The common robot workspace at zero *Z* Euler angle. The information shown is that for the four-link parallel mechanisms obtained by varying $\overrightarrow{OA}$ within a 30-mm cube centred about its nominal value

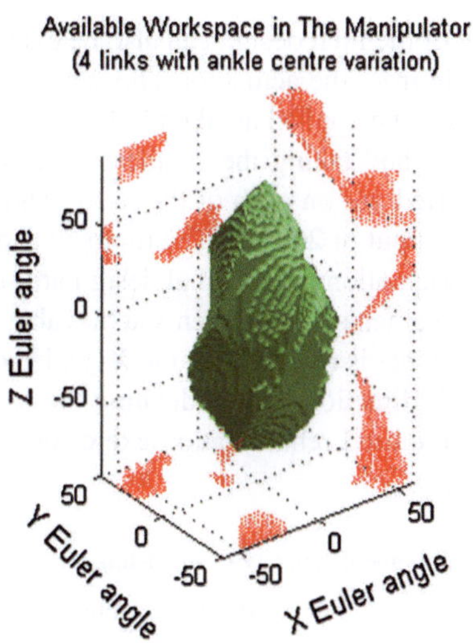

Fig. 8.12 Superposition of the common workspace volume on regions of the task space with low manipulability (configurations where largest condition number >50). The information shown is that for four-link parallel mechanisms obtained by varying $\overrightarrow{OA}$ within a 30-mm cube centred about its nominal value. Note that the common workspace shown is the intersection of all the reachable workspaces computed by varying $\overrightarrow{OA}$, while the low manipulability region shown is the union of all the low manipulability regions obtained by varying $\overrightarrow{OA}$

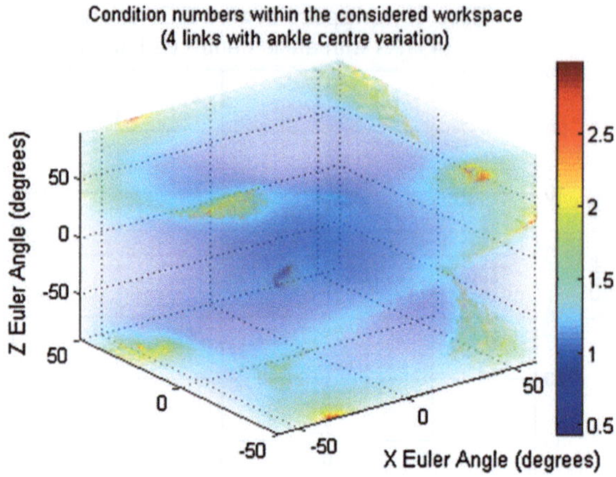

Fig. 8.13 Plot indicating the distribution of the largest manipulator Jacobian condition numbers throughout the manipulator task space. The colour spectrum is assigned to the base 10 logarithms of the condition numbers and the information shown is that for four-link parallel mechanisms obtained by varying $\overrightarrow{OA}$ within a 30-mm cube centred about its nominal value. Note that the condition numbers used to generate the plot are the largest among the results obtained from $\overrightarrow{OA}$

The moment capacity of the final design can also be evaluated by considering the maximum forces available from the actuators. This can be done by considering the maximum moments that can be applied at all end-effector orientations which belong to the common workspace and taking the smallest of these values. Note that this moment analysis was carried out on each of the *X*-, *Y*- and *Z*-directions by using a maximum actuator force output of 2000 N. The moment capacity and the maximum achievable end-effector orientations of the final design are summarised in Table 8.6. It can be seen that the movements and moments achievable by the four-link parallel mechanism are similar to what is required for the *X*- and *Y*-directions, and in excess of what is needed in the *Z*-direction, thus indicating the capability of the proposed structure to perform the required rehabilitation exercises.

Table 8.6 Motion limits and moment capacity of the 4-link parallel mechanism

Direction	Maximum motion	Moment capacity (Nm)
Plantarflexion (positive *X*)	44°	151
Dorsiflexion (negative *X*)	36°	151
Inversion (positive *Y*)	26°	38
Eversion (negative *Y*)	26°	38
External rotation/abduction (positive *Z*)	72°	68
Internal rotation/adduction (negative *Z*)	72°	68

With consideration of ankle centre variation

8.3 System Description

A prototype of the ankle rehabilitation robot had been constructed using the kinematic parameters investigated above. Brushed DC motor-driven linear actuators (Ultra Motion Bug Linear Actuator 5-B.125-DC92_24-4-P-RC4/4) had been used as the actuated prismatic joint in the prototype. The linear actuator was chosen based on the stroke length and force requirements of the mechanism, with an actuator stroke length of 0.1 m, force capacity of over 2000 N and a top speed of 0.066 m/s. In terms of sensors, linear potentiometers were built into the actuators to provide measurement of the actuator lengths. Additionally, a two axis inclinometer (Signal Quest SQ-SI2X-360DA) was also attached to the end-effector platform to allow the measurement of its pitch and roll angles. Lastly, four tension compression load cells (Omega Engineering LC201-300) were also installed at the interface between the linear actuator and the effective spherical joints to monitor the forces along the actuated links. The ankle rehabilitation robot developed in this research is shown in Fig. 8.14, both in the form of a three-dimensional model and in the form of a photograph depicting how the robot interacts with the user. In terms of controller hardware, an embedded controller (National Instruments NI-PXI 8106) had been used together with a DAQ card (National Instruments NI-PXI-6229) to carry out the signal processing and execute the real-time control functions of the prototype. The embedded controller was also connected to a PC to receive user commands and display the sensor measurements through a user interface developed using the LabView programming environment. A block diagram of the overall system is given in Fig. 8.15.

The graphical user interface (GUI) developed for the end user is also shown in Fig. 8.16. This GUI was designed to provide visual feedback regarding the foot orientation and the level of moments applied in different directions of rotation. Orientation of the actual foot is presented as the solid red block, while the desired

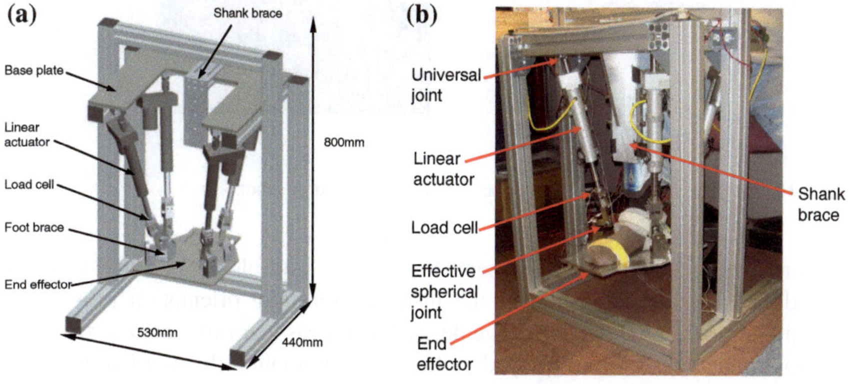

Fig. 8.14 The 3D CAD model of the developed ankle rehabilitation robot (**a**) and a photograph showing the robot with the user's lower limb attached (**b**)

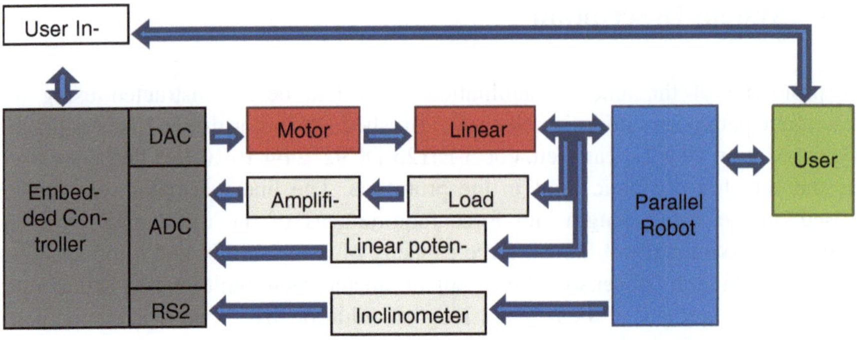

Fig. 8.15 A block diagram showing various hardware and software components of the ankle rehabilitation robot developed in this research

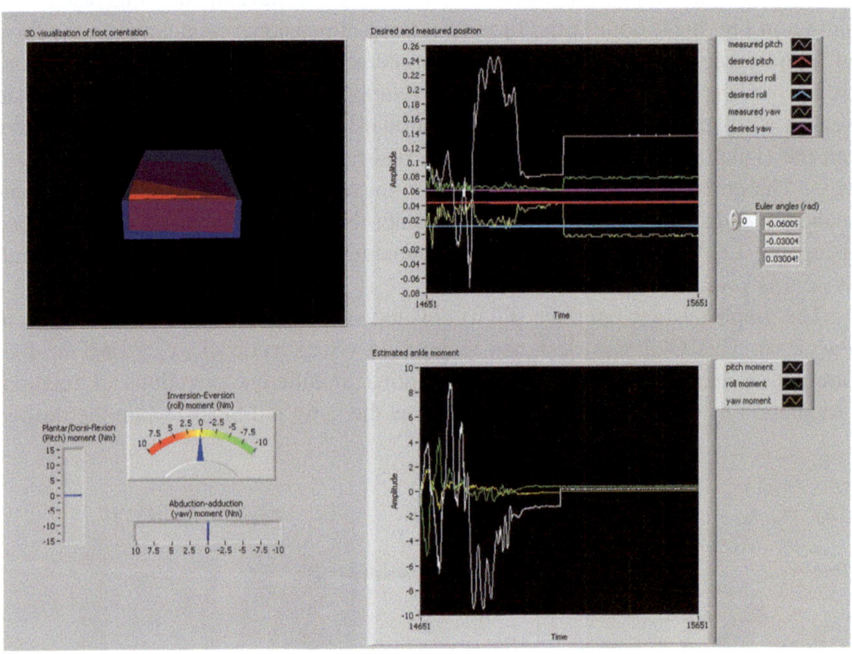

Fig. 8.16 End user GUI for the developed ankle rehabilitation robot

foot orientation is shown as the semi-transparent blue block. In addition to the three-dimensional visualisation of the instantaneous foot orientation provided in the top left plot, a time history of the desired and measured Euler angles relating to the foot orientation is also displayed in the top right graph of the user interface. The estimated instantaneous robot–user interaction moments on the other hand are presented in the bottom left area of the GUI. A separate interface is also available for the use of the therapist/technician, where it can be used to define the rehabilitation trajectory and to modify the robot control parameters to permit different types of rehabilitation exercises.

As discussed previously, the movement of the end effector will ultimately rely on the kinematic constraints of the user's ankle. As such, the effective centre of rotation of the platform is unlikely a fixed point in space. Furthermore, it is also not known precisely. However, from the perspective of the controller, the kinematics of the platform must be defined as a rotation about a known point. As a result, an assumed spherical joint centre is used. This point is the point A used in the kinematic analyses carried out in previous sections and is considered to remain constant relative to the end-effector coordinate frame. Clearly, if the actual motion of the end effector is not a perfect rotation about this assumed spherical joint centre, this point will be seen to experience translation in the global robot coordinate frame (i.e. $\overrightarrow{\mathrm{OA}}$ is not constant). The end-effector orientation estimated from kinematics based on the originally assumed $\overrightarrow{\mathrm{OA}}$ is therefore inaccurate. In fact, the forward kinematics may even fail to converge due to contradictions between the assumed and actual robot configuration. A solution to this problem proposed in this work is to incorporate sensors on the end effector to directly measure its orientation. The two axis inclinometer used in this research was therefore installed to serve this purpose. While it only provides information on two of the three rotational degree of freedom, these measurements can be used in conjunction with the four actuator link lengths to estimate the remaining yaw angle of the end effector, as well as an the correct location of $\overrightarrow{\mathrm{OA}}$.

Although most of the existing platform-based ankle rehabilitation devices utilise a six degree of freedom force torque sensor to measure the interaction torque between the foot and the robot, a different approach had been taken in this research by measuring the forces along the actuators using load cells placed along the linear actuators. The main reason for this design decision is to reduce the distance between the base of the platform and the effective centre of rotation of the user's foot, thus allowing a larger workspace for the same actuator stroke length. Additionally, it also allows monitoring of individual actuator forces to allow actuator-level force feedback control. The shortcoming associated with this approach is that the actual robot–foot interaction wrench can only be estimated by considering the measured actuator forces, robot kinematic parameters and the robot inertia properties since the sensing elements are not located at the actual robot–foot interface.

8.4 MIMO Actuator Force Control

Based on the above analyses, a gain-scheduled actuator joint force controller was proposed and implemented on the ankle rehabilitation robot. The structure of this controller is shown in Fig. 8.17, where F_c is a vector of the commanded forces and F_{meas} is a vector of forces as provided by the force sensors. K is the gain matrix

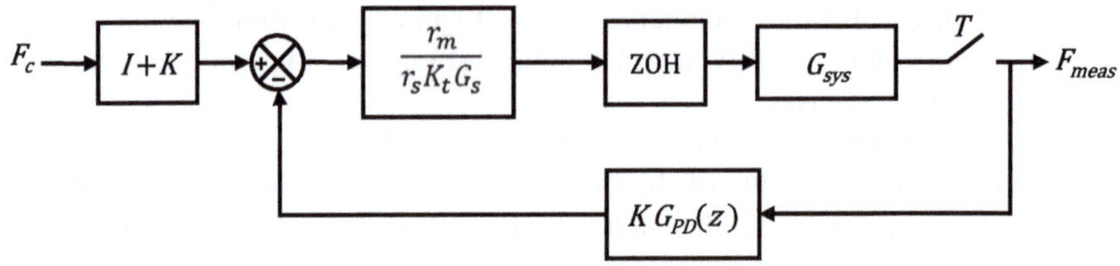

Fig. 8.17 Structure of the final actuator force control law

which is given by (8.8), where U'_m and v_0 are the output basis vectors of M'_e that can be obtained from the singular value decomposition of M'_e. Furthermore, $\mathrm{diag}(\cdot)$ is a function that forms a diagonal matrix using its argument and k_i are the controller gains applied to the ith basis vector, with $i = 0$ referring to the gain along the null space direction and $i = 1, 2, 3$ referring to gains along decoupled directions with the first, second and third largest singular values, respectively.

$$K = [\,U'_m \quad v_0\,]\mathrm{diag}([\,k_1 \quad k_2 \quad k_3 \quad k_0\,])[\,U'_m \quad v_0\,]^{\mathrm{T}} \tag{8.8}$$

Gain scheduling for the controller gains in two of the three non-null decoupled directions was done using piecewise linear functions fitted below the critical gain values. These relationships are shown as solid lines in Fig. 8.18, together with the critical gain values for comparison. The remaining non-null direction on the other hand was assigned a constant gain since the critical gain variation over the range of singular values considered is relatively small. Additionally, as the null direction is not influenced by the configuration of the manipulator, it is also assigned a constant gain which is below its gain margin.

The computational ankle model was used to obtain a more realistic operating environment for the ankle rehabilitation robot. The environmental stiffness experienced

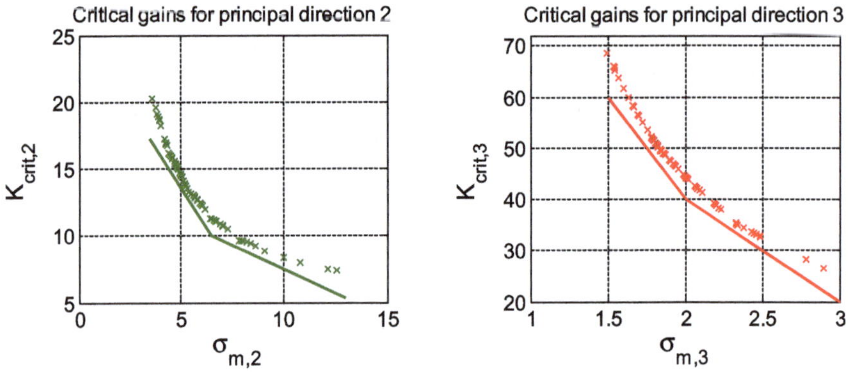

Fig. 8.18 Linear piecewise functions used for gain scheduling in different decoupled directions of M'_e

during passive ankle motion was estimated from the static torque observed at different ankle and subtalar joint displacements. These torque profiles were then numerically differentiated with respect to the ankle and subtalar displacements to produce the stiffness matrix K_{as}, which is a 2×2 matrix. This matrix was subsequently transformed into the manipulator task space to give a 3×3 stiffness matrix K_e, using a procedure which will be discussed in more detail. The environmental damping matrix B_e on the other hand was assumed to have the form shown in (8.9), with both a constant and a variable component. Here, b_e is a scalar constant which gives a base level of damping while $\gamma \ll 1$ is a proportionality constant between the damping and stiffness parameters. The variable component had been included to introduce additional damping in a proportional manner to the ankle stiffness and is mainly used to reduce the damping factor experienced at foot orientations with very high stiffness.

$$B_e = b_e I + \gamma K_e \tag{8.9}$$

A structured singular value analysis of the proposed actuator force controller was carried out to determine its stability and robustness properties. This analysis was carried out at discrete points in the task space which corresponds to different combinations of ankle and subtalar joint displacements within a certain range (±40° at 4° interval for the ankle displacement and ±30° at 3° interval for the subtalar displacement). At each of these task space coordinates, the environmental stiffness and damping matrices were obtained and used to form the nominal external environment. The environmental inertia matrix was also modified accordingly and by assuming constant principal components in the inertia tensor. The uncertainty weighting matrices used in this analysis are given in Table 8.7. The uncertainties considered represent about 5 % of the total nominal mass parameter and 10 % variations in the stiffness and damping parameters.

Stability analysis of the $A''_{z,cl}$ matrix in M_{sys} had shown that all system poles are located within the unit circle on the z-plane for the foot configurations tested, thus proving system stability and ensuring that structure singular values can be used to evaluate the robust stability of the system. The results of the structured singular value analyses are summarised in Fig. 8.19, where the computed values of $\mu(M_{sys})$ are plotted over their corresponding ankle and subtalar joint displacements. It can be seen from this figure that all the structured singular values are below unity, thus indicating that the system will remain stable as long as the environmental uncertainties remain within the prescribed bounds.

It should be noted that although the final force controller used is not exactly the same as the partial decoupling controller, they do have considerable similarities. The main feature shared by these two controllers is the application of different control gains along different decoupled directions of the M'_e matrix (recall that the

Table 8.7 Uncertainty weighting matrices used in the robust stability analysis

Uncertainty weighting	B_{wm}	B_{wb}	B_{wk}
Value/expression	$0.002R_{\Theta}$ kgm^2	$0.1I_3$	$0.1I_3$

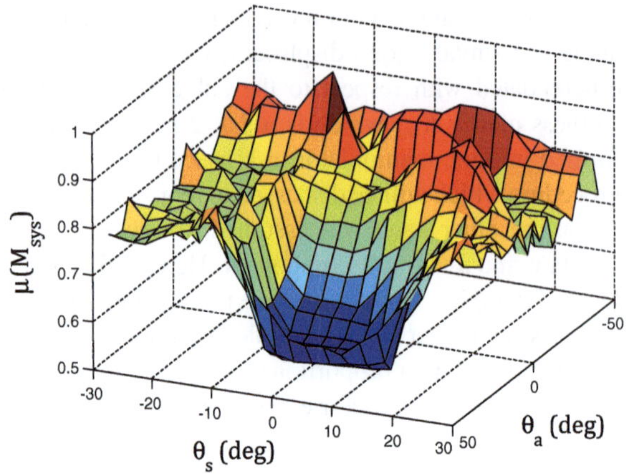

Fig. 8.19 Values of μ ($M_{\rm sys}$) computed over a range of foot orientations defined by the ankle ($\theta_{\rm a}$) and subtalar ($\theta_{\rm s}$) joint displacements

output basis vectors of M_e' can be shown to be identical to that of the coupling matrix D when the same task space mass matrix is used). Secondly, the relative magnitudes of the controller gains in the non-null decoupled directions can also be sorted in the same order for both these control laws, thus indicating that the final force control law will still achieve some level of decoupling. Furthermore, as with the partial decoupling controller, the final control law also allows independent gain selection along the null space of the manipulator Jacobian transpose (which is also the null space of M_e').

8.4.1 Simulation Results for Disturbance Rejection and Back-drivability

Simulations using the simplified state space models discussed above were carried out to evaluate the efficacy of the proposed actuator force controller. A linear state space model had been used in this simulation, where the linearisation point was taken to be the origin of the task space coordinates. This means that the manipulator Jacobian used to construct the state space model was that corresponding to this orientation. Two sets of tests were carried out to evaluate the performance improvements of the proposed controller over a force controller with uniform gains across all directions (hereafter referred to as the uniform gain controller). The first involves a test on disturbance rejection capability while the second centres on the back-drivability of the controlled manipulator. Both these simulations were carried out in the Simulink environment and continuous state space models were used to describe the plant, while the PD filter and controller were implemented as discrete time blocks. The system and parameters used are similar to those employed throughout this chapter, while the controller gain matrices used are defined according to (8.8).

8.4.1.1 Test for Disturbance Rejection

In the first test, frictional forces along the actuator rod were included as inputs to the continuous state space model to introduce disturbances into the system. A simple friction model had been used whereby the friction force F_{fric} is a saturation function of the rod velocity as shown in (8.10), with $F_{f,\max}$ being the maximum friction and η being a large constant. The simulation is run with a sinusoidal profile for the desired force and different gain matrices were applied in two separate simulations, both with the PD filter in place. The desired and actual force profiles for each actuator, along with the force errors are shown for both the proposed controller and the uniform gain controller in Fig. 8.20. In the first four plots of each column, the desired force profiles are shown as dotted lines, while actual measured forces are given as solid lines. The final plot on the other hand presents the force errors obtained from all four actuators.

$$F_{\text{fric}} = F_{f,\max}\min(\max(\eta\dot{x}_r, -1), 1) \tag{8.10}$$

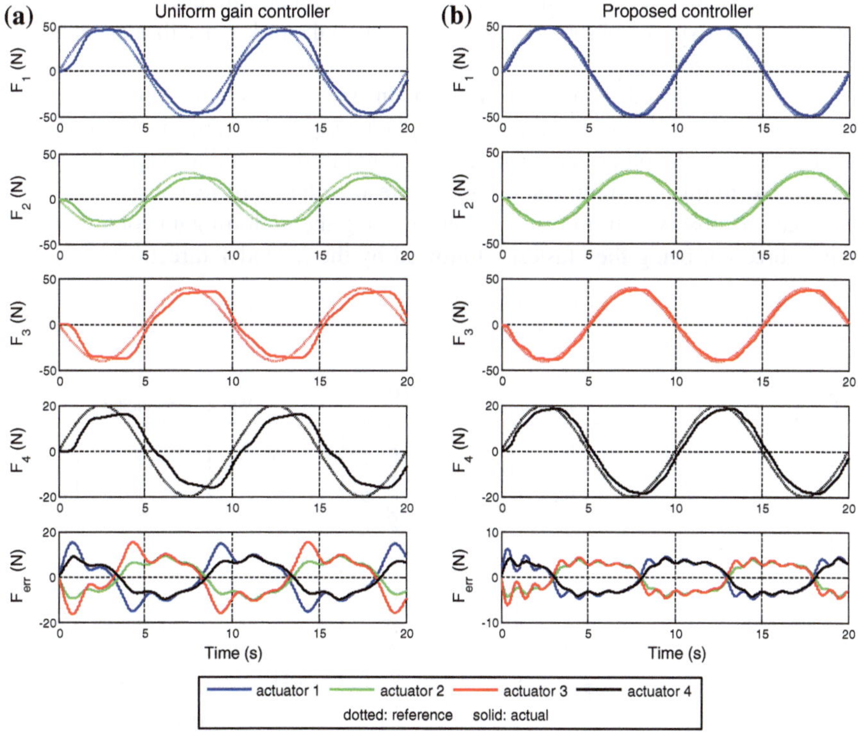

Fig. 8.20 Desired (*dotted lines*) and measured (*solid lines*) actuator force profiles, as well as force errors F_{err} for **a** the uniform gain controller and **b** the proposed controller

It is clear from the results above that the proposed controller showed much better force tracking accuracy, thus indicating its ability to better reject disturbances. This is not surprising as the gain of the uniform gain controller is limited by the least stable decoupled direction, whereas the proposed method permits the use of higher gains (and hence better disturbance rejection) in more stable directions.

8.4.1.2 Test for Back-drivability

The second test involved a study of the back-drivability of the force-controlled manipulator. In this test, the main aim was to verify that the proposed controller can partially decouple the system and result in an effective inertia which is more similar to the actual environmental inertia. This investigation therefore requires the incorporation of an external torque into the inputs of the state space system and can be easily accomplished by considering the rows of the input matrix which corresponds to the task space accelerations. The desired forces were set to be zero in this test to allow "maximum" back-drivability of the manipulator and equal levels of external torques were applied in all three task space directions. The stiffness of the environment used in this simulation was also decreased to improve the damping factor of the system and reduce oscillations to facilitate inference of acceleration from the task space displacements. Plots relating to the task space displacements are shown in Fig. 8.21.

For the proposed controller, motion in the *Z*-direction appears to have the greatest acceleration for the same applied torque. Movements in the *X*- and *Y*-directions on the other hand can be considered to have similar responsiveness to an applied torque. A significantly larger spread in terms of responsiveness, however, can be observed from results obtained using the uniform gain controller, with the *Z*-direction being the "fastest", followed by the *X*- and *Y*-directions.

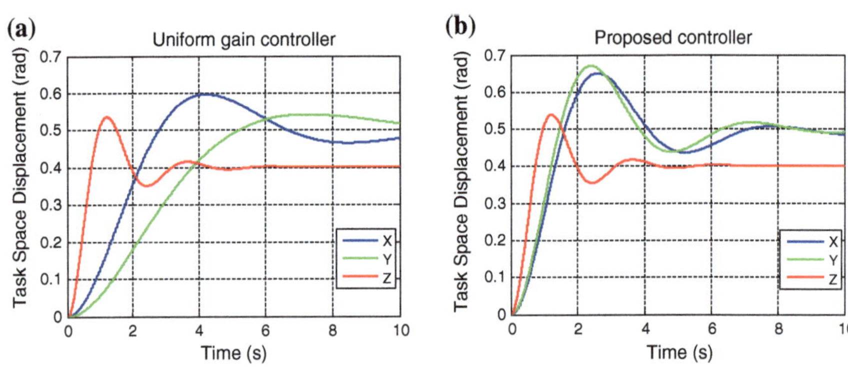

Fig. 8.21 Task space displacements of the system obtained in the back-drivability simulation with **a** the uniform gain controller and **b** the proposed controller

Table 8.8 The environmental inertia matrix and the effective inertia matrices for the force controllers considered in the back-drivability simulation

M_e	M_{eff} of final controller	M_{eff} of uniform gain controller
$\begin{bmatrix} 0.047 & 0 & 0 \\ 0 & 0.045 & 0 \\ 0 & 0 & 0.04 \end{bmatrix}$	$\begin{bmatrix} 0.2714 & 0 & 0 \\ 0 & 0.2308 & 0.0014 \\ 0 & 0.0014 & 0.0642 \end{bmatrix}$	$\begin{bmatrix} 0.6455 & 0 & 0 \\ 0 & 1.4691 & 0.0120 \\ 0 & 0.0120 & 0.0643 \end{bmatrix}$

The behaviours observed above can be better explained when considering the effective inertia matrix. Using the notations of the higher-order dynamic model, this effective mass matrix can be represented as (8.11), where K is the controller gain matrix. The effective mass matrix for both the proposed controller and the uniform gain controller, together with the original environmental inertia matrix, is given in Table 8.8. It is immediately clear from the consideration of these matrices that the effective inertia of the force-controlled system is significantly larger than that of the original environment. This is mainly due to the large effective actuator mass contributed by the high transmission ratios. However, by making a comparison between the effective inertia matrices of both the controllers, it can be concluded that the proposed control strategy is capable of producing an effective inertia matrix which is more uniform along the diagonal, with smaller off diagonal elements. Since the inertia matrix is organised in such a way that its first, second and third columns corresponds, respectively, to accelerations in X-, Y- and Z-directions, it can be seen that the responsiveness observed in Fig. 8.21 can be inversely correlated to the magnitude of elements along the diagonally dominant inertia matrix, thus confirming that the effective inertia matrix is still applicable on systems with higher-order dynamics.

$$M_{\text{eff}} = M_e + (m_{a1} + m_{a2})J^T(I+K)^{-1}J \tag{8.11}$$

8.4.2 *Experimental Results for Stability and Performance Evaluation*

Several experimental trials had been carried out on the ankle rehabilitation robot developed in this research to evaluate the effectiveness of the proposed actuator force controller. The sole participant of these experiments is an adult male (1.75 m height) and ethics approval had been granted by The University of Auckland Human Participants Ethics Committee (Ref. 2009/480). These experiments can be classified into two groups, one to highlight the effects that different force controllers have on system stability and another to evaluate and compare the force control performance of different controllers in executing tasks required by the rehabilitation exercises.

8.4.2.1 Stability Experiment

Since one of the main motivations behind the development of the proposed force controller is to improve the system stability, one of the experimental trials carried out in this work was centred on demonstrating the stability improvement brought on through the application of the proposed control scheme. This experimental trial involved the operation of the ankle rehabilitation robot under pure force control, where the force commands were selected by requiring that the vertical component of the null space forces be summed to a desired value to provide support for the user's lower limb, while all remaining non-null space forces are set to be zero. The subject was then prompted to move his foot freely in primarily the plantar/dorsiflexion direction. This experiment was done for four different actuator force controllers, which are listed and described in Table 8.9. The results of this experiment are presented in Fig. 8.22. Note that only the forces measured along one of the actuators are shown for brevity, and forces along other directions behave in a similar manner.

From the experiments, motions obtained using the first two controllers showed clear signs of instability with significant levels of oscillation. This is backed up by the actuator force measurements. Since the gains of the uniform gain controllers were selected to be the lowest gains that will result in perceptible oscillations in the robot, it can be seen that the addition of the proportional derivative term in the feedback loop does indeed improve the stability of the system and allow better performance through application of larger controller gains. Additionally, Fig. 8.22 also shows that although some of the gains applied along certain decoupled directions of the third and fourth controllers considered were larger in value than that of the second uniform gain controller, these controllers remained stable during operation. This supports the idea that there are directions which are less stable and that these directions are ultimately limiting the maximum gain that can be applied in

Table 8.9 Actuator force controllers considered in the stability experiments

Controller	Description
P control, uniform gain of 10	Measured force is fed directly into disturbance observer, the gain matrix K is obtained by selecting $k_1 = k_2 = k_3 = k_4 = 10$
PD control, uniform gain of 16	Measured force is fed into disturbance observer through a proportional derivative filter $G_{PD}(z)$, the gain matrix K is obtained by selecting $k_1 = k_2 = k_3 = k_0 = 16$
Proposed controller	Measured force is fed into disturbance observer through a proportional derivative filter $G_{PD}(z)$, the gain matrix K is obtained by observing the gain margins
Proposed controller + minimum gain of 14	Measured force is fed into disturbance observer through a proportional derivative filter $G_{PD}(z)$, the gain matrix K is obtained by setting $k_1 = k_0 = 14$, while k_2 and k_3 are obtained by observing the gain margins

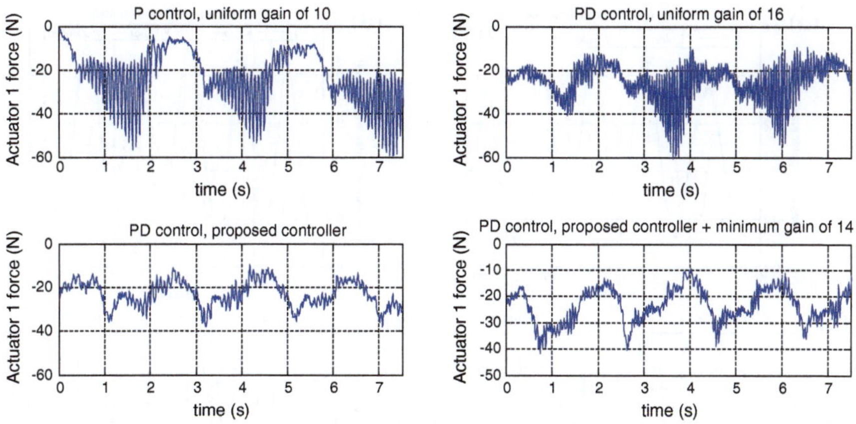

Fig. 8.22 Forces measured along actuator 1 using different actuator force controllers

a controller with uniform gains. However, when the coupling introduced by the manipulator kinematics and inertia is taken into account, it is possible to manage stability through application of different gains along different decoupled directions of M_e'. This allows higher gains in more stable directions and thus results in an improved overall performance.

8.4.2.2 Experiments for Performance Evaluation

In additional to the stability experiment, further trials were also carried out using both a uniform gain controller and the proposed controller to illustrate the performance improvements afforded through incorporation of the coupling information into the controller. These experiments were again done on the developed ankle rehabilitation robot and involve three main tasks which are considered important for implementation of ankle rehabilitation exercises. The first is the ability to maximise the back-drivability of the robot by commanding zero task space moments (such as that done in the stability experiment), the second is to move the foot passively using impedance control, while the third is explicit control of the robot–user interaction moment. All these tasks were carried out using a uniform gain actuator force controller with a gain of 5, and the proposed controller (note that the gain of 5 is also used along the output basis vector of M_e' which has the largest singular value). The results for the first two tasks described above are summarised in Figs. 8.23 and 8.24, while the root mean square values of the actuator force errors are provided in Table 8.10. Additionally, results obtained from the third task are also presented in Figs. 8.25 and 8.26.

It can be seen from the results obtained in the free and passive motion trials that utilisation of the proposed control scheme over the uniform gain controller can significantly reduce the actuator force errors, with some of the actuators

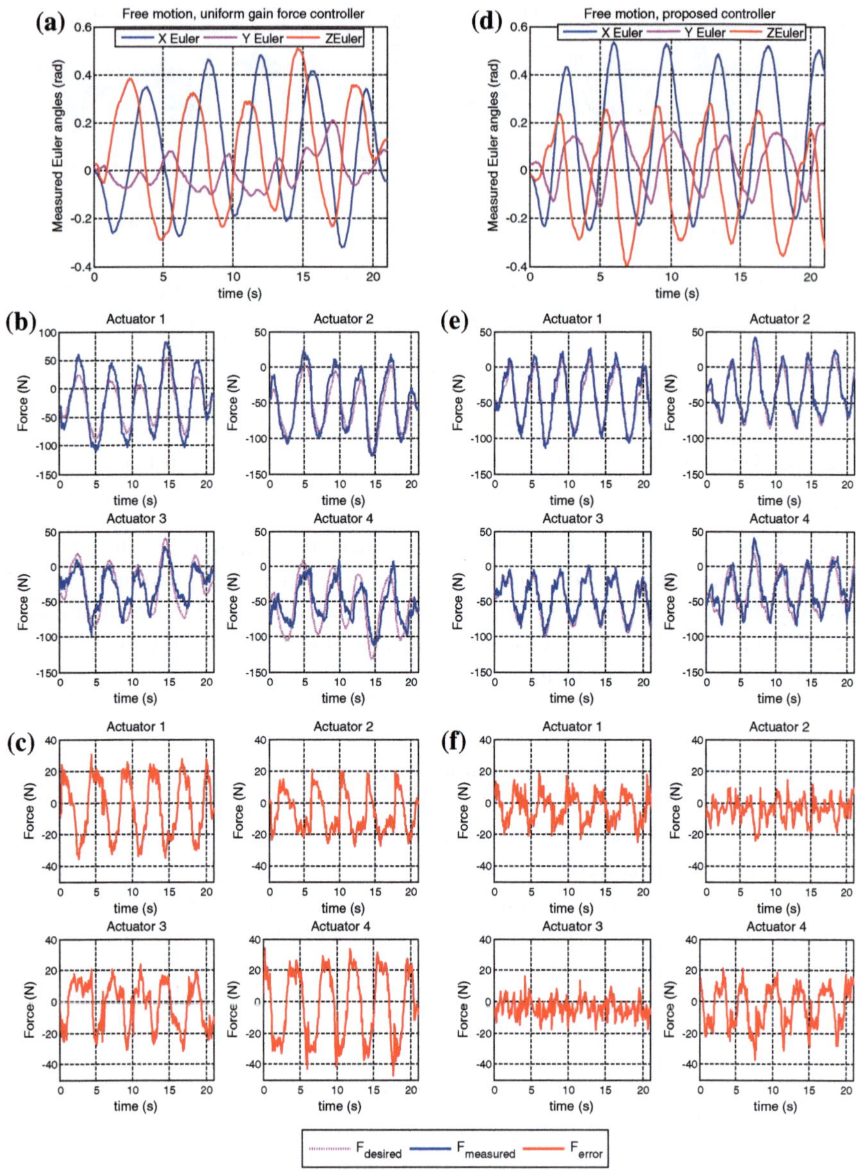

Fig. 8.23 Experimental results obtained during free motion of the user's foot on the ankle rehabilitation robot. The Euler angle trajectories for the uniform gain controller is shown in (**a**) while the associated actuator forces and force errors are given in (**b**, **c**). Similarly, the motion trajectories obtained using the proposed controller is given in (**d**) and its associated forces and force errors are shown in (**e**, **f**)

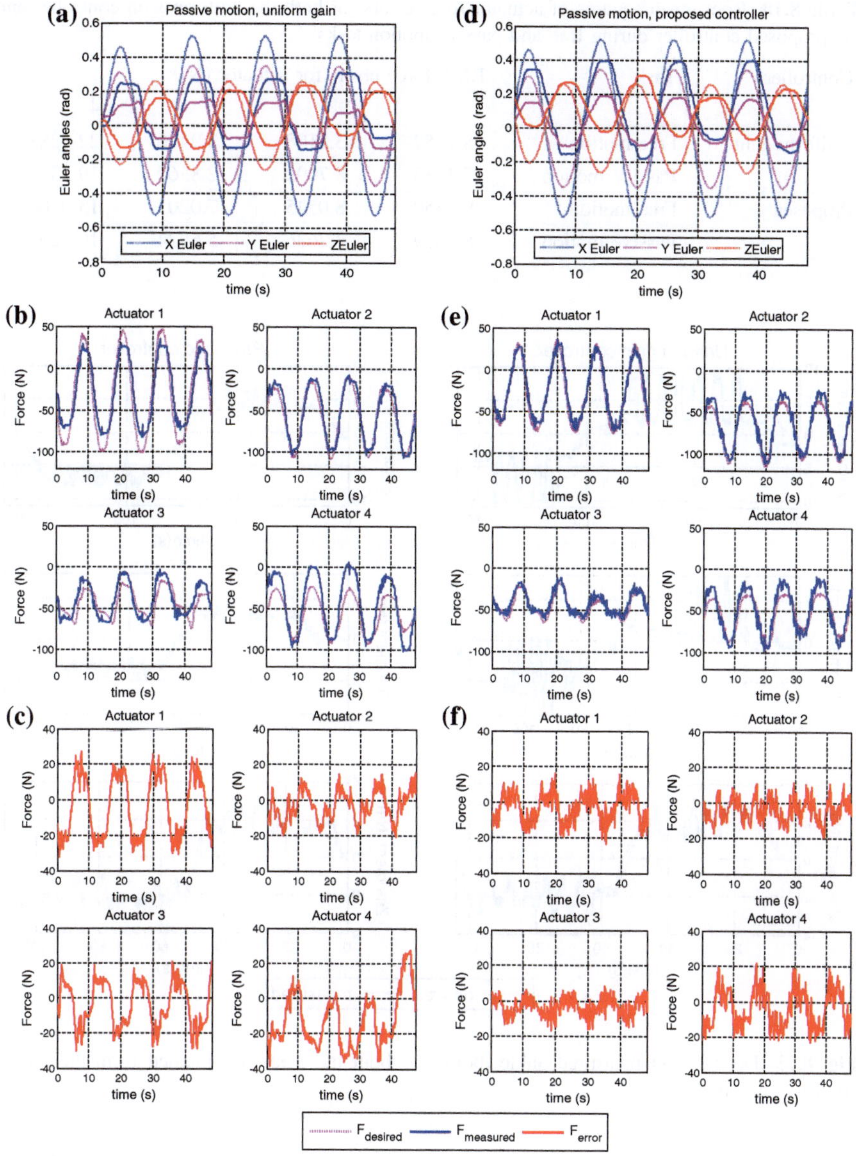

Fig. 8.24 Experimental results obtained when foot of the user is moved passively by the ankle rehabilitation robot. The Euler angle trajectories for the uniform gain controller is shown in (**a**) while the associated actuator forces and force errors are given in (**b**, **c**). Similarly, the motion trajectories obtained using the proposed controller is given in (**d**) and its associated forces and force errors are shown in (**e**, **f**)

Table 8.10 Root mean squares of actuator force errors for both the uniform gain controller and the proposed controller during free and passive motion tasks

Controller	Task	RMS force errors for actuator (N)			
		1	2	3	4
Uniform gain	Free motion	18.1557	13.8108	13.9476	22.0288
	Passive motion	17.4053	8.7092	12.8562	19.5321
Proposed	Free motion	9.2550	8.0545	7.0205	13.0206
	Passive motion	8.2829	7.2636	5.6524	10.9297

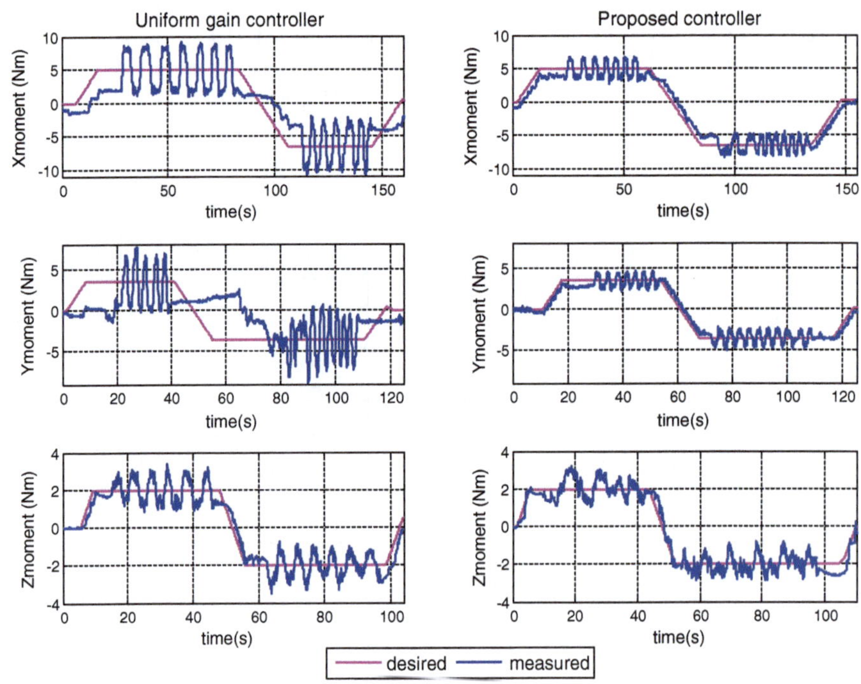

Fig. 8.25 Desired and measured ankle moments about the ankle as obtained from the torque control experiment

experiencing a force error reduction of about 50 %. Comparison of Fig. 8.23a, d also suggests that the force-proposed controller is more capable in terms of maximising the compliance of the ankle rehabilitation robot since it appears that motion recorded using the proposed controller are of larger amplitudes and velocities relative to that of the uniform gain controller. For the case of passive motion, examination of Fig. 8.24a, d indicates that the reference trajectory used in the impedance controller is tracked more closely with a smaller time delay when the proposed controller is used in place of the uniform gain controller.

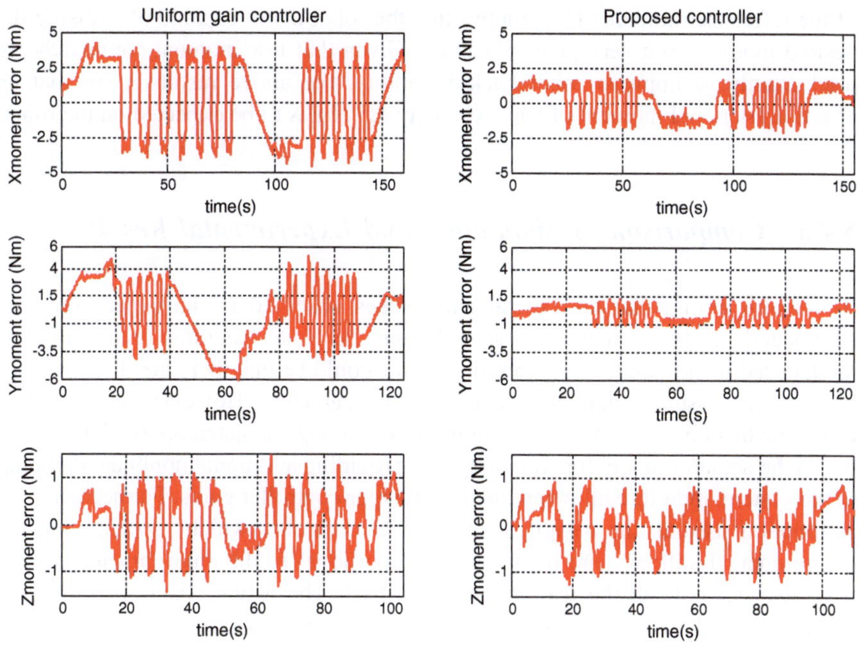

Fig. 8.26 Moment errors as obtained from the torque control experiment

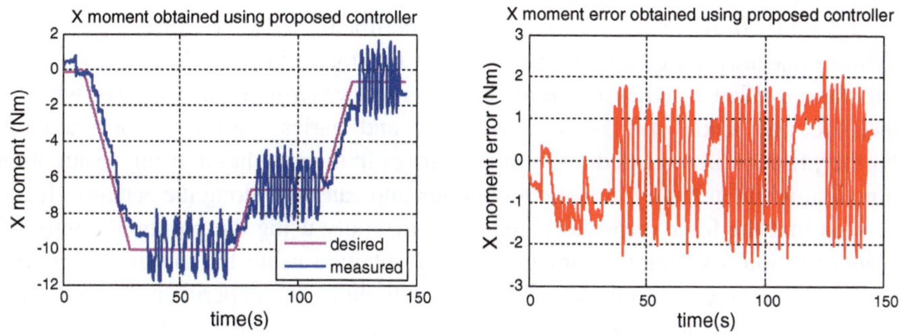

Fig. 8.27 Experimental results obtained by using the proposed controller in regulation of the *X* interaction moment about three different levels

The results of the torque control trials have suggested that the moment errors are rather large, even with the use of the proposed controller. It should be noted, however, that this error is mainly caused by frictional effects and does not vary significantly with the amplitude of the commanded torque levels. This is shown through Fig. 8.27, where the moment regulation performance of the robot in the *X*-direction was tested at three different levels. It is clear from the moment error plot that the magnitude of the errors remained relatively constant regardless of the value of the reference moment. This implies that the robot is not capable of realising the desired moment in a very precise manner. Given that low moment commands are used mainly to improve robot back-drivability, the above results mean that an effective frictional moment of approximately 1.5 Nm is to be expected on the robot.

8.4.3 Comparison of Simulation and Experimental Results

It is worth noting that the critical gain values observed in the experiments are significantly larger than those observed from the Bode diagrams (and hence the model used in simulation). The reason for this could be that there are discrepancies between the assumed and the actual system parameters. However, an additional cause for this could be that the frictional forces along the actuators (which are left out of the actuator model for simplicity) are providing additional nonlinear damping to the system, therefore allowing the use of larger controller gains. Furthermore, the assumption used in the design of the MIMO controller which specifies that the environmental stiffness and damping be proportional to the environmental inertia may also not hold in the real experimental trial. The actual changes to the gain margins caused by deviations from such an assumption will be rather difficult to explore due to the increased complexity of the problem when the transfer functions cannot be fully decoupled.

A comparison of the simulation and experimental results involving the passive motion task shows that the motion variables recorded in the simulation differed considerably from those obtained from experiments. Clearly, differences in the motion trajectories are caused mainly by the fact that a linearised model is used in simulation which assumes a constant and isotropic environmental stiffness, while in real life, the ankle stiffness is anisotropic and varies with foot configuration. Further, friction is modelled in a simple manner in the simulation using a saturation function, while in reality, it is more complex and can vary along the actuator. It can be seen that the force errors obtained experimentally using the proposed controller is indeed more oscillatory compared to that obtained using the uniform gain controller, as predicted from the simulation. Additionally, the experimental results also show an approximately 50 % reduction in force errors for certain actuators, and this trend is shared by the results obtained from simulation. This indicates that despite the simplifications, the model used in the simulation and analysis does indeed capture some of the characteristics of the real system.

8.5 Summary

This chapter presented the design of the ankle rehabilitation robot used in this research. The workspace and force requirements of the robot were established by considering the ankle characteristics and this information had been taken into account in the design process. Additionally, workspace and singularity analyses were also performed to validate the suitability of the final four-link design by factoring in the mechanical constraints imposed by the passive joints and the uncertainties in the ankle kinematics. A description of the system hardware and GUI was also presented, together with a discussion on the rationale used in sensor selection. This chapter also detailed the development of a MIMO actuator force controller for the ankle rehabilitation robot used in this research. A gain-scheduled MIMO actuator force controller was proposed in this research. Finally, experimental results have also reiterated the performance advantages brought on by the use of the proposed control scheme over a uniform gain force controller.

References

1. S. Siegler, J. Chen, C.D. Schneck, The three-dimensional kinematics and flexibility characteristics of the human ankle and subtalar joints-Part I: kinematics. J. Biomech. Eng. **110**, 364–373 (1988)
2. Y. Mrabet, http://commons.wikimedia.org/wiki/File:Human_anatomy_planes.svg
3. R.E. Kearney, P.L. Weiss, R. Morier, System identification of human ankle dynamics: intersubject variability and intrasubject reliability. Clin. Biomech. **5**, 205–217 (1990)
4. C.S. Parenteau, D.C. Viano, P.Y. Petit, Biomechanical properties of human cadaveric ankle-subtalar joints in quasi-static loading. J. Biomech. Eng. **120**, 105–111 (1998)
5. J.-P. Merlet, *Parallel robots*, 2nd edn. (Springer, Netherlands, 2006)
6. L.-W. Tsai, *Robot analysis: the mechanics of serial and parallel manipulators* (Wiley, New York, 1999)
7. J. Dul, G.E. Johnson, A kinematic model of the human ankle. J. Biomed. Eng. **7**, 137–143 (1985)
8. V.T. Inman, *The joints of the ankle* (Williams and Wilkins, Baltimore, 1976)
9. R.E. Isman, V.T. Inman, Anthropometric studies of the human foot and ankle. Biomechanics Laboratory, University of California, San Francisco and Berkeley, Technical Report 58, San Francisco, The Laboratory, May 1968
10. N. Ying, W. Kim, Determining dual Euler angles of the ankle complex in vivo using “flock of birds” electromagnetic tracking device. J. Biomech. Eng. **127**, 98–107 (2005)

Chapter 9
Adaptive Ankle Rehabilitation Robot Control Strategies

The basic formulation of the outer impedance control loop used in this research is also presented in this chapter. In this work, the basic impedance control law had been extended to yield a more advanced interaction control scheme for passive range of motion and active assistive exercises. One of these extensions involves the incorporation of an impedance parameter adjustment module in the overall interaction control scheme. This chapter explores the use of an assistance adaptation scheme to achieve the above and presents the implementation of a control module to facilitate active user participation in the rehabilitation exercises. The proposed assistance adaptation scheme is also designed to reduce the amount of resistance applied by the robot when the user is moving ahead of the reference position.

9.1 Model Integration and Elementary Robot Control

9.1.1 Dynamic Modelling of Parallel Mechanism

The dynamics of parallel mechanism can be obtained by combining the dynamics of the actuating links and the dynamics of the end effector through the mechanism's kinematic constraints. The dynamics of individual actuating links are first presented in this section, followed by that of the end effector.

The formation of the mechanism kinematic constraints first requires the definition of a set of generalised coordinates to describe the configuration of the end effector. Even though the parallel mechanism used in this research had been treated as a manipulator with pure rotational degree of freedom (DOF) in its design, the end-effector dynamics described above are still defined by assuming that the end effector is capable of general six degree of freedom motion. This had been done to ensure generality of the model, thus allowing it to be applied regardless of the type of kinematic constraints present in the environment. This is an important feature as the foot motion depicted by the commonly used biaxial ankle model is not purely rotational. The generalised coordinates used to define the end-effector configuration were selected to be the location of the end-effector centre of mass x_p and the XYZ

S.(S.Q.) Xie, *Advanced Robotics for Medical Rehabilitation*,
Springer Tracts in Advanced Robotics 108, DOI 10.1007/978-3-319-19896-5_9

Euler angles Θ used to describe the end-effector orientation. It should be noted that both these quantities are observed in the global coordinate frame and are grouped together as the generalised coordinate vector given in (9.1).

$$\xi = \begin{bmatrix} x_p \\ \Theta \end{bmatrix} \tag{9.1}$$

Having decided on the generalised coordinates, the kinematic constraints imposed by the parallel mechanism can be established by observing the collocation of the S_i points. This means that the locations of the S_i points as obtained from the task space generalised coordinates must be equivalent to those found using the actuating link coordinates. This relationship can be represented as (9.2), with u_i being a position vector describing the location of the universal joint U_i in the global frame. A mapping from the generalised coordinates $\xi \in \mathbb{R}^6$ to three of the actuating link coordinates (α_i, β_i and l_i) can therefore be obtained from (9.2). The time derivative of this relationship can then be used to obtain a Jacobian matrix $J_i \in \mathbb{R}^{3\times 6}$ which relates the derivatives of the actuating link coordinates to the generalised coordinate derivatives as shown in (9.3).

$$x_p + RP_i' = x_{s,i} + u_i \tag{9.2}$$

$$\begin{bmatrix} \dot{\alpha}_i \\ \dot{\beta}_i \\ \dot{l}_i \end{bmatrix} = J_i \dot{\xi} \tag{9.3}$$

By considering the sensor deformations as additional state variables, the expressions for the centres of mass of the actuating link segments were represented in the general form given in (9.4), with $\varsigma = a, b, f, s$. Similarly, the angular velocities of the actuating links were also written in the form as given in (9.5). Repeated differentiation of (9.4) and (9.5) then leads to the actuating link acceleration terms being represented by ξ, δ_i and their higher order time derivatives (up to the second order). With this in mind, the actuating link–end-effector interaction forces were restated as $F_{f,i} = h_i(\ddot{\xi}, \ddot{\delta}_i, \dot{\xi}, \dot{\delta}_i, \xi, \delta_i)$. It follows that the dynamic equations can be combined and viewed as (9.6), with $w_{\text{ext}} = \left[F_{\text{ext}}^{\text{T}} M_{\text{ext}}^{\text{T}}\right]^{\text{T}} \in \mathbb{R}^6$ and $\delta = [\delta_1 \delta_2 \delta_3 \delta_4]^{\text{T}} \in \mathbb{R}^4$. Additionally, $M_1 \in \mathbb{R}^{10\times 10}$ is the configuration-dependent matrix coefficient for the state acceleration variables, $N_1 \in \mathbb{R}^{10}$ is the grouping of nonlinear terms, and $A_1 \in \mathbb{R}^{10\times 6}$ is the matrix coefficient for the external wrench applied to the end effector.

$$x_{\varsigma,i} = f_{\varsigma,i}(\xi, \delta_i) \tag{9.4}$$

$$\omega_i = g_i(\xi, \dot{\xi}) \tag{9.5}$$

$$M_1(\xi)\begin{bmatrix}\ddot{\xi}\\ \ddot{\delta}\end{bmatrix}+N_1\left(\dot{\xi},\dot{\delta},\xi,\delta\right)+A_1(\xi)w_{\text{ext}}=0 \tag{9.6}$$

Even with the reparameterisation, there are still only six equations available from (9.6), while there are ten unknown accelerations. Additional equations are therefore required to obtain a definite solution to the mechanism dynamics. Appending these equations to (9.6) will then lead to the complete model of the mechanism dynamics shown in (9.7), with $F_{\text{act}}=\left[F_{\text{act},1}F_{\text{act},2}F_{\text{act},3}F_{\text{act},4}\right]^{\text{T}}$, $M\in\mathbb{R}^{10\times10}$ being the matrix coefficient of the acceleration terms, $N\in\mathbb{R}^{10}$ being the nonlinear dynamic terms, $A\in\mathbb{R}^{10\times6}$ being the matrix coefficient for the interaction wrench and $B\in\mathbb{R}^{10\times4}$ being the matrix coefficient for the actuator force vector.

$$M(\xi)\begin{bmatrix}\ddot{\xi}\\ \ddot{\delta}\end{bmatrix}+N\left(\dot{\xi},\dot{\delta},\xi,\delta\right)+A(\xi)w_{\text{ext}}=B(\xi)F_{\text{act}} \tag{9.7}$$

9.1.2 Integration of Model with Foot and Actuator Dynamics

The integration of the foot model and the mechanism model can be done by first ensuring that the interaction ports on the foot and on the end effector are collocated. If this criterion in satisfied, the wrenches acting on the interaction port of the end effector will simply be equal but opposite of that acting on the foot model. This condition can therefore be used to combine the two models. In addition to the above condition, the kinematic relationship between generalised coordinates of the ankle model and the generalised coordinates of the end effector must also be found to allow further reparameterisation of the combined dynamic equations to yield a compact state space model which can be solved exactly. Clearly, as ankle model introduces additional kinematic constraints on the end effector, the final generalised coordinate would involve the ankle and subtalar joint displacements.

It can be seen that the ankle model can be represented in the form shown in (9.8), where θ_{as} is the ankle and subtalar joint displacement, z_f is a vector of additional state variables of the ankle model (which includes ligament and muscle–tendon states), Γ is a vector of muscle activation levels, and $w_{\text{ext,f}}$ is the external wrench applied to the interaction port of the foot. Note also that the subscript *ft* is used to denote the matrix coefficients and nonlinear dynamic terms relating to the ankle model, with $M_{\text{ft}}\in\mathbb{R}^{2\times2}$, $N_{\text{ft}}\in\mathbb{R}^{2}$ and $A_{\text{ft}}\in\mathbb{R}^{2\times6}$.

$$M_{\text{ft}}(\theta_{\text{as}})\ddot{\theta}_{\text{as}}+N_{\text{ft}}\left(\theta_{\text{as}},\dot{\theta}_{\text{as}},z_f,\Gamma\right)+A_{\text{ft}}(\theta_{\text{as}})w_{\text{ext,ft}}=0 \tag{9.8}$$

The kinematic relationship between θ_{as} and ξ can be easily defined using the ankle kinematic model as long as the relative position of the end-effector centre of mass with respect to the subtalar joint centre is known at the neutral position of the ankle (by definition, this should also correspond to the end-effector orientation with zero XYZ Euler angles). This relationship was represented as (9.9) and was further differentiated with respect to time to give (9.10) and (9.11).

$$\xi = f_{\xi}(\theta_{as}) \tag{9.9}$$

$$\dot{\xi} = J_{\xi}\dot{\theta}_{as} \tag{9.10}$$

$$\ddot{\xi} = J_{\xi}\ddot{\theta}_{as} + \dot{J}_{\xi}\dot{\theta}_{as} \tag{9.11}$$

Equation (9.12) was reparameterised with θ_{as} and its time derivatives. Note that the matrix coefficient of the acceleration terms ($M' \in \mathbb{R}^{10\times 6}$) and nonlinear dynamic terms ($N' \in \mathbb{R}^{10}$) is different due to the substitution of the task space acceleration vector in (9.12).

$$M'(\theta_{as})\begin{bmatrix} \ddot{\theta}_{as} \\ \ddot{\delta} \end{bmatrix} + N'\left(\dot{\theta}_{as}, \dot{\delta}, \theta_{as}, \delta\right) + A(\theta_{as})w_{ext} = B(\theta_{as})F_{act} \tag{9.12}$$

By recognising that $w_{ext} = -w_{ext,f}$ can be rewritten as (9.13). Note that the dependencies of the nonlinear terms and matrix coefficients will be dropped hereafter for brevity. It can be seen that pre-multiplication of (9.13) by $A_{ft}^{+} = A_{ft}^{T}\left(A_{ft}A_{ft}^{T}\right)^{-1} \in \mathbb{R}^{6\times 2}$ will result in (9.14), with $v_{0,A_{ft}} \in \mathbb{R}^{6\times 4}$ being the null space matrix of A_{ft} (with the null vectors occupying the columns of $v_{0,A_{ft}}$). Equation (9.14) was then further expanded as (9.15), which showed that the actual interaction wrench can be represented by the summation of the right-hand side of (9.14) with an additional four degree of freedom vector $v_{0,A_{ft}}\rho$, with $\rho = v_{0,A_{ft}^{T}}w_{ext} \in \mathbb{R}^{4}$. Substituting this result into (9.12) then yields (9.16).

$$M_{ft}\ddot{\theta}_{as} + N_{ft} - A_{ft}w_{ext} = 0 \tag{9.13}$$

$$(I - v_{0,A_{ft}}v_{0,A_{ft}}^{T})w_{ext} = A_{ft}^{+}M_{ft}\ddot{\theta}_{as} + A_{ft}^{+}N_{ft} \tag{9.14}$$

$$\begin{aligned} w_{ext} &= A_{ft}^{+}M_{ft}\ddot{\theta}_{as} + A_{ft}^{+}N_{ft} + v_{0,A_{ft}}v_{0,A_{ft}}^{T}w_{ext} \\ &= A_{ft}^{+}M_{ft}\ddot{\theta}_{as} + A_{ft}^{+}N_{ft} + v_{0,A_{ft}}\rho \end{aligned} \tag{9.15}$$

$$M'\begin{bmatrix}\ddot{\theta}_{\text{as}}\\ \ddot{\delta}\end{bmatrix}+N'+AA_{\text{ft}}^{+}M_{\text{ft}}\ddot{\theta}_{\text{as}}+AA_{\text{ft}}^{+}N_{\text{ft}}+Av_{0,A_{\text{ft}}}\rho=BF_{\text{act}}$$
$$\Rightarrow M''\begin{bmatrix}\ddot{\theta}_{\text{as}}\\ \ddot{\delta}\end{bmatrix}+N'+AA_{ft}^{+}N_{\text{ft}}+Av_{0,A_{\text{ft}}}\rho=BF_{\text{act}} \tag{9.16}$$

Since the solution of ρ is of no interest, (9.16) was further pre-multiplied by $N_A=\left[\text{Null}\left(v_{0,A_{\text{ft}}^{\text{T}}}A^{\text{T}}\right)\right]^{\text{T}}$ to yield (9.17), where the function Null(.) returns a matrix which columns are filled by the null vectors of the function argument (i.e. $N_A\in\mathbb{R}^{6\times10}$). Inspection of (9.17) reveals that there are now six acceleration variables and six equations, which means that the acceleration variables can be solved exactly given certain actuator forces and muscle activation levels. Clearly, the state space model of the foot-manipulator system will only be complete when the state transition equations for the ligament and muscle–tendon states are included.

$$N_AM''\begin{bmatrix}\ddot{\theta}_{\text{as}}\\ \ddot{\delta}\end{bmatrix}+N_AN'+N_AAA_{\text{ft}^+}N_{\text{ft}}=N_ABF_{\text{act}} \tag{9.17}$$

Based on the actuating link coordinates, the actuator dynamics was expressed as (9.18), with $i_{\text{act,i}}$ being the actuator current, K_t being the motor torque constant, K_a being the actuator transmission ratio, J_{eff} being the effective motor inertia, b_{eff} being the effective viscous damping of the motor and $F_{\text{fric,i}}$ being the Coulomb friction experienced by the actuator. Since $\ddot{l}_i$ and $\dot{l}_i$ can ultimately be related to the accelerations and velocities of the ankle and subtalar joints, (9.18) was reorganised as (9.19). Substitution of (9.19) into (9.17) will then lead to the set of equations which describes the rigid body dynamics of the actuator, parallel mechanism and foot. This set of equations is given in (9.20), with $M_{F_{\text{act}}}\in\mathbb{R}^{4\times6}$ being a matrix which rows are consisted of $M_{F_{\text{act,i}}}\in\mathbb{R}^{1\times6}$ and $N_{F_{\text{act}}}\in\mathbb{R}^{4}$ being a vector which rows are consisted of $N_{F_{\text{act,i}}}$.

$$F_{\text{act,i}}=K_tK_ai_i-K_a^2J_{\text{eff}}\left(\ddot{l}_i-\ddot{\delta}_i\right)-K_a^2b_{\text{eff}}\left(\dot{l}_i-\dot{\delta}_i\right)-F_{\text{fric,i}} \tag{9.18}$$

$$F_{\text{act,i}}=K_tK_ai_{\text{act,i}}-M_{F_{\text{act,i}}}\begin{bmatrix}\ddot{\theta}_{\text{as}}\\ \ddot{\delta}\end{bmatrix}-N_{F_{\text{act,i}}}-F_{\text{fric,i}} \tag{9.19}$$

$$\left(N_AM''+N_ABM_{F_{\text{act}}}\right)\begin{bmatrix}\ddot{\theta}_{\text{as}}\\ \ddot{\delta}\end{bmatrix}+N_AN'+N_ABN_{F_{\text{act}}}+N_ABF_{\text{fric}}$$
$$+N_AAA_{\text{ft}}^{+}N_{\text{ft}}=K_tK_aN_ABi_{\text{act}} \tag{9.20}$$

9.1.3 Elementary Robot Control

In the context of rehabilitation robots, the force variable is the user–robot interaction force, while the motion variable is simply the movement of the joint or limb under rehabilitation. It should also be noted that the dynamic relationships described above are typically represented as a second-order mechanical system as shown in (9.21) with inertial (M_d), damping (B_d) and stiffness (K_d) parameters. Additionally, the variables f, f_d, x and x_d are, respectively, used to denote the force applied to the environment, the desired force, the actual position of the end effector and the desired end-effector position. The advantage of having the force and motion variables in relative terms is that it allows variation in the equilibrium position about which the impedance relationship is based, thus allowing the use of this control strategy for a wider range of tasks. In fact, when put in this form, pure motion control and pure force control can simply be viewed as special cases of impedance control, where pure motion control can be achieved with infinitely large impedance and pure force control with zero impedance. Due to its versatility, the interaction control scheme developed for the ankle rehabilitation robot is based on this general impedance control law.

$$f - f_d = M_d(\ddot{x}_d - \ddot{x}) + B_d(\dot{x}_d - \dot{x}) + K_d(x_d - x) \tag{9.21}$$

It is easy to see that implementation of the impedance control law can be done by issuing f as a force command to the actuator force controller. This means that an outer motion control loop is required to complete the impedance control scheme. Since the actuator force controller is defined in joint space while the impedance control law is applied in task space to allow more intuitive description of the desired manipulator behaviour, the actual input to the outer impedance loop would be the motion variables in terms of end-effector orientation and the output will be that of the torques along the task space coordinates. This torque must therefore be transformed into their corresponding actuator forces prior to it being used as force commands for the inner force control loop. In order to derive this force command, it is necessary to first consider the desired impedance relationship in task space as shown in (9.22), where τ_{ext} is the robot–user interaction torque, τ_d is the desired interaction torque, Θ is the task space coordinates in XYZ Euler angles, and Θ_d is the desired task space position. Note that the desired task space acceleration is deliberately left off the inertial component of the impedance relationship to simplify the control law. As the main focus of the impedance control law is not to achieve pure position control, this simplification is acceptable.

$$\tau_{\text{ext}} - \tau_d = -M_d\ddot{\Theta} + B_d\left(\dot{\Theta}_d - \dot{\Theta}\right) + K_d(\Theta_d - \Theta) \tag{9.22}$$

By considering the influence of the inner actuator force control law, the effective dynamics of the manipulator can be rewritten as (9.23), where M_{eff} is the effective inertia matrix and $K \in \mathbb{R}^{4\times4}$ is the gain matrix used in the inner force controller. Also, F_{distb} is used to refer to the actuator disturbance forces, C is used to represent the centripetal and Coriolis forces in the manipulator dynamics, and G is used to represent the gravitational forces in the manipulator dynamics. Finally, F_c represents the force command issued to the inner force controller. By considering (9.22) and (9.23), as well as the fact that $J^{\mathrm{T}}(J^+)^{\mathrm{T}} = I$, a suitable impedance control law can be constructed. This is shown in (9.24). The dynamics of the impedance controlled manipulator (9.25) was then obtained.

$$M_{\text{eff}}\ddot{\Theta} + C + G + \tau_{\text{ext}} = J^{\mathrm{T}}F_c - J^{\mathrm{T}}(I+K)^{-1}F_{\text{distb}} \tag{9.23}$$

$$F_c = (J^+)^{\mathrm{T}}\left[\tau_d + B_d(\dot{\Theta}_d - \dot{\Theta}) + K_d(\Theta_d - \Theta) + C + G\right] \tag{9.24}$$

$$\tau_{\text{ext}} - \tau_d = -M_{\text{eff}}\ddot{\Theta} + B_d(\dot{\Theta}_d - \dot{\Theta}) + K_d(\Theta_d - \Theta) - J^{\mathrm{T}}(I+K)^{-1}F_{\text{distb}} \tag{9.25}$$

9.1.4 *Simulation and Experimental Results*

In order to evaluate the efficacy of the proposed elementary control scheme on the ankle rehabilitation robot, the developed impedance controller, the redundancy resolution scheme and an inner actuator force controller were all applied to the integrated foot–robot model presented earlier in this chapter. The simulation was carried out to emulate the scenario where the robot is used to guide the patient's foot under impedance control along certain rehabilitation trajectory, while the user remains passive (i.e. no muscle activation). The trajectory used in the simulation was chosen to resemble pronation–supination motion of the foot and are given in (9.26), where the angles are expressed in radians and the variable t is the simulation time. The reference moment τ_d in the basic impedance control law was also set to be zero throughout the duration of the simulation.

$$[\theta_x \quad \theta_y \quad \theta_z]^{\mathrm{T}} = \left[\frac{\pi}{6}\sin\left(\frac{\pi t}{6}\right) \quad \frac{\pi}{9}\sin\left(\frac{\pi t}{6}\right) \quad -\frac{\pi}{12}\sin\left(\frac{\pi t}{6}\right)\right]^{\mathrm{T}} \tag{9.26}$$

9.1.4.1 Simulation with Rigid Biaxial Ankle Kinematics

Preliminary simulations have shown that the actuator force controller cannot be applied directly to the integrated model without causing system instability. Investigation into the problem revealed that the gains used in the proposed gain scheduling force controller were too large. Further analysis showed that the cause for this problem lied in the fact that the ankle kinematic model used was of only two DOFs. The result of this is an altered manipulator Jacobian and hence also a variation in the decoupled directions and their associated singular values. Since the gain margin along the null vector was relatively low for the three DOF manipulator model used to formulate the proposed controller, direct application of the proposed force controller to a two DOF system had resulted in an unstable system. This is because the presence of an additional vector in the null space means that some of the higher gains applied in other directions will be projected onto the null vectors instead, thus increasing the effective gains beyond the critical gain and ultimately causing system instability. A similar phenomenon can also occur for the least stable decoupled direction in the two degree of freedom model due to the mismatch of assumed and actual decoupled directions.

The above notion is supported by the fact that system stability can be restored when the force controller is redesigned by taking into account the manipulator Jacobian and inertia matrix of the two DOF system. Using constant gains along the principal directions computed from the newly formulated coupling term, it was found that higher gains can be applied along directions with smaller singular values. Results of the simulation carried out using this modified inner force controller are given in Fig. 9.1. An isotropic robot stiffness of 10 Nm/rad and a robot damping of 2 Nms/rad were used in the simulation. Additionally, a desired vertical force of −150 N was also used in the redundancy resolution scheme.

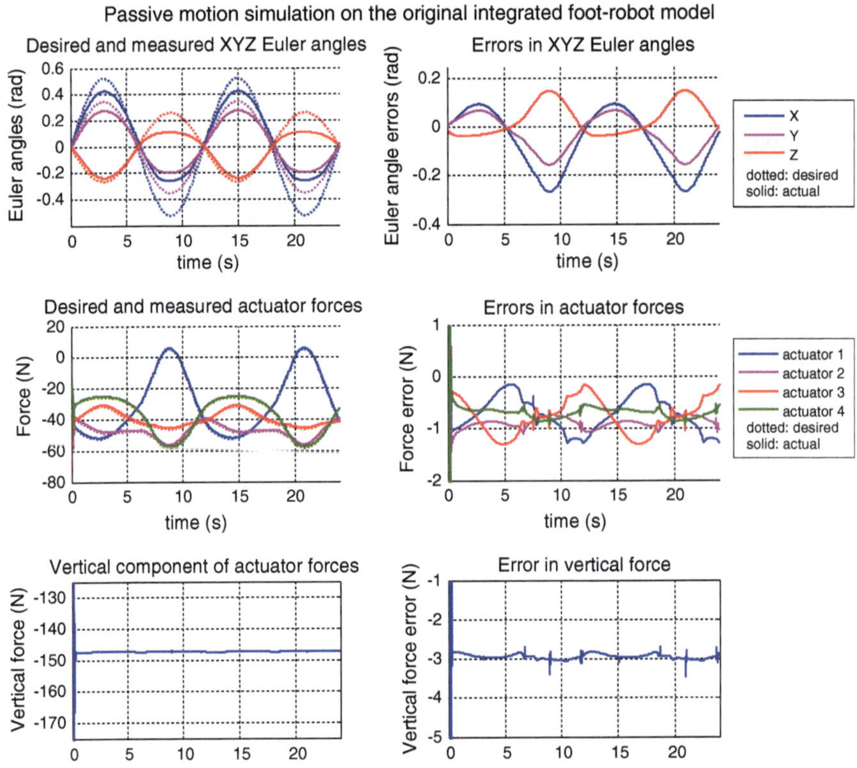

Fig. 9.1 Simulation results of a passive motion trial on the ankle rehabilitation robot. This simulation applies the proposed basic impedance controller, redundancy resolution scheme and a modified actuator force controller on the integrated foot–robot model

9.1.4.2 Simulation with Added Yaw Compliance

Based on the findings obtained from the above simulation, an important point which needs to be addressed is whether the proposed actuator force controller can be applied to the actual ankle rehabilitation robot. To represent this in the simulated system, an additional degree of freedom had been included in the ankle model through addition of an extra revolute joint at the talus. This revolute joint is fixed in the vertical (yaw) direction, and the talus was allowed to rotate about this joint. A set of linear rotational spring and damper units with reasonably large stiffness and damping ($k_z = 5\,\text{Nm/rad}$, $b_z = 2\,\text{Nms/rad}$) were also added along this joint. These parameters had been chosen manually to prevent large angular deflections about this axis while maintaining a well-damped system. It should be noted that due to added complexities in the kinematic structure of the integrated foot–robot system, there exists discrepancies between the inertia matrices to obtain the gain margins and the actual inertia matrices of the integrated system. Consequently, the gains of the proposed controller were reduced (to approximately 75 % of their original values) to ensure stability. The relative magnitudes of these gains, however, still followed the same trend as that used in the proposed controller. The results of this simulation are summarised in Fig. 9.2.

The results obtained from the simulation trials show a comparable level of force tracking capability in both systems. This, however, does not translate to a similar position following capability, with errors in the yaw compliant model much larger than that of the original foot–robot model. By noting that the same impedance controller has been used and that the force tracking capability in both systems are similar, the difference in the position errors must be caused by the addition of the yaw axis compliance. This is also believed to be partly the cause of the initial oscillations observed in the second simulation trial. Despite these differences, it is clear from both simulations that larger position errors can be found in the negative X-direction, an observation that is in line with greater ankle stiffness in the dorsiflexion direction. The simulation results also show that the redundancy resolution scheme is working well, with the total vertical force regulated to about 3 N of the desired set point in the absence of friction along the actuators.

9.1.4.3 Experimental Results

In addition to the simulations, the basic impedance controller was also tested experimentally using the actual ankle rehabilitation robot with a healthy test subject. The subject is an adult male (1.75 m height), and ethics approval had been granted by The University of Auckland Human Participants Ethics Committee (Ref. 2009/480). The foot of the user is attached onto the robot end-effector platform using Velcro strips, while the shank of the subject is attached through a shin guard to the shank brace on the ankle rehabilitation robot. The subject remained relaxed throughout the trial to minimise muscle activations, and thus, the resulting

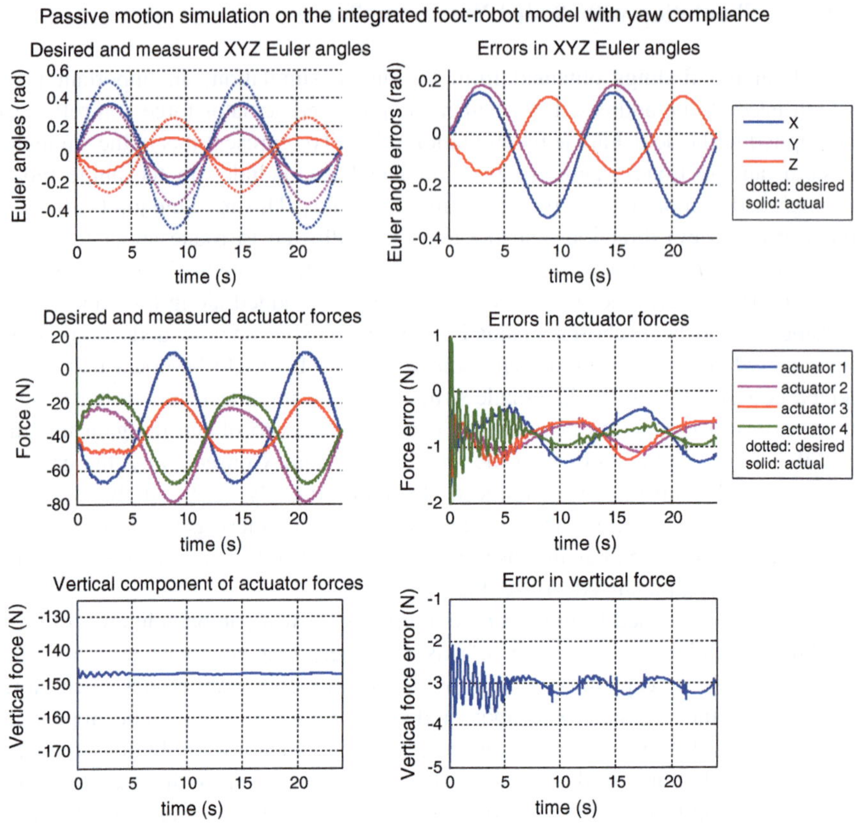

Fig. 9.2 Simulation results of a passive motion trial on the ankle rehabilitation robot. This simulation applies the proposed basic impedance controller, redundancy resolution scheme and actuator force controller on the integrated foot–robot model with added yaw compliance

motion can be considered passive. A segment of the results obtained from this experiment is shown in Fig. 9.3. Note that the inner actuator force controller used in the experiment is that of the originally proposed force controller with no gain reduction as it was found to be stable in preliminary trials on the robot, and thus, higher gains were used to improve force tracking performance.

It can be seen from the experimental results that the force tracking capability on the robot was worse than that observed in the simulation. This was expected since friction was not included in the integrated model. Focusing on the performance of the basic impedance control scheme, it can be seen that the errors in X Euler angle did follow a very similar trend to those obtained from simulations, again with much larger errors in the negative X Euler (or dorsiflexion) direction. The motion in the Y Euler angle direction, however, was rather different from those seen in simulations as there was hardly any movement in the negative *y*-direction. This can be due

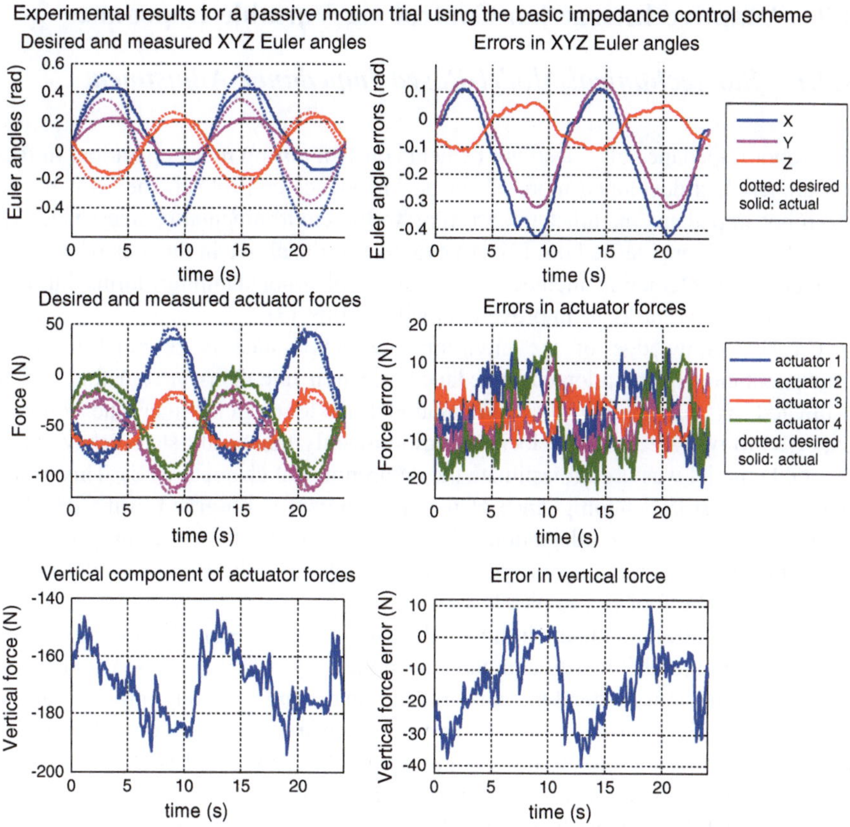

Fig. 9.3 Experimental results of a passive motion trial on the ankle rehabilitation robot. This simulation applies the proposed basic impedance controller, redundancy resolution scheme and actuator force controller on the actual ankle rehabilitation robot

to several factors, one of which is the difference between the actual ankle stiffness and the stiffness of the ankle model used in simulation. Secondly, frictions within the actuators and passive robot joints can also contribute to smaller effective moments being applied to the foot. Lastly, imperfect attachment of the shank to the robot can also lead to the robot coordinate frame not being aligned perfectly with the ideal foot coordinate frame. The results, however, suggest that the first two factors could be more dominant here due to the small amount of negative y motion observed, while if the third factor is dominant, then there should only be some form of bias/offset in the trajectory. Motion along the Z Euler angle shows that the measured motion in the z-direction is actually tracking the desired trajectory quite closely compared to the simulations. This again can be due to discrepancies between the stiffness characteristics of the ankle model and the actual foot, or it can also be due to the fact that the yaw compliance is greater than assumed in the model used for the second simulation.

9.2 Adaptive Interaction Control via Variable Impedance

9.2.1 Biomechanical Model-Based Impedance Adjustment

The robot impedance also need not be held constant during robot operation. In fact, researchers had developed more advanced impedance control schemes which vary the robot impedance parameters according to the environmental characteristics [1] or to the task being carried out [2]. An example of the above in the area of physical human–robot interaction includes the variation of robot damping during human–robot cooperative tasks to improve coupled stability [3].

Clearly, knowledge of the environmental admittance is essential to allow implementation of the adopted impedance selection rule. This information can be estimated by considering the computational ankle model. Since the robot is expected to operate in low velocity conditions, only the steady-state behaviour of the ankle model was used to estimate the environmental characteristics. This means that only the stiffness/compliance of the environment is observed in the development of this impedance adaptation scheme. Additionally, the environmental characteristics were also obtained in the absence of any muscular activation, or in other words, when the foot is completely passive.

In order to estimate the environmental stiffness, the developed ankle model was used to compute the resistive moments applied by the various force elements (ligaments and muscle–tendon units) on the ankle and subtalar joints at various points on the θ_a-θ_s plane, where θ_a and θ_s are, respectively, used to denote displacements about the ankle and subtalar joints. The ankle and subtalar moments obtained through this exercise are shown in Fig. 9.4.

The available moment–displacement data can then be numerically differentiated to obtain the stiffness matrix in the ankle and subtalar coordinates shown in (9.27),

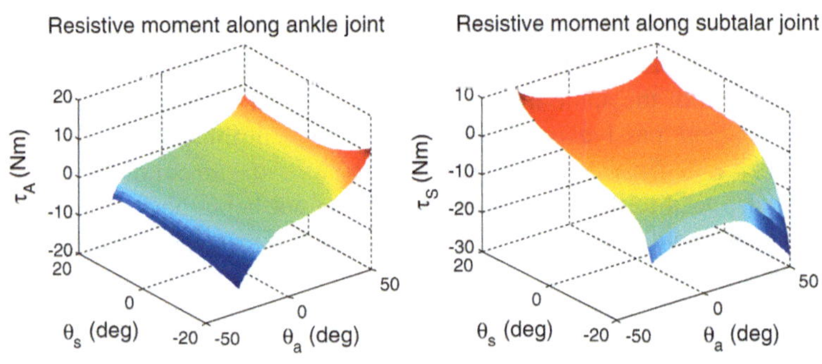

Fig. 9.4 Resistive moments contributed by the ligaments and muscle–tendon units on the ankle and subtalar joints. These moments are obtained from the computational ankle model by assuming steady-state behaviour of the force elements

where τ_A and τ_S are, respectively, the resistive moments observed along the ankle and subtalar axes. The results of these numerical differentiations are summarised in Fig. 9.5. Note that stiffness values shown are saturated at 100Nm/rad to ensure that details on the plots are not lost to accommodate the inclusion of extreme values. It is shown in Fig. 9.5 that the stiffness matrix varies quite significantly over the range of ankle and subtalar displacements considered. The results have also verified that the computed stiffness matrix is symmetric as expected.

$$K_{as} = \begin{bmatrix} k_{aa} & k_{as} \\ k_{sa} & k_{ss} \end{bmatrix} = \begin{bmatrix} \frac{\partial \tau_A}{\partial \theta_a} & \frac{\partial \tau_A}{\partial \theta_s} \\ \frac{\partial \tau_S}{\partial \theta_a} & \frac{\partial \tau_S}{\partial \theta_s} \end{bmatrix} \approx \begin{bmatrix} \frac{\Delta \tau_A}{\Delta \theta_a} & \frac{\Delta \tau_A}{\Delta \theta_s} \\ \frac{\Delta \tau_S}{\Delta \theta_a} & \frac{\Delta \tau_S}{\Delta \theta_s} \end{bmatrix} \tag{9.27}$$

Contour plots of the elements in the stiffness matrix are also given in Fig. 9.6. It can be concluded from these contour plots that there is a large region of points with relatively low stiffness near the neutral orientation. The ankle stiffness, however, increases much more rapidly as the foot is moved further away from the neutral orientation. It can also be seen that the magnitudes of off-diagonal elements in the stiffness matrix are also typically smaller than the diagonal elements, which suggests that the stiffness matrix will remain positive definite throughout the ankle's range of motion. This is confirmed by the fact that determinants of the computed stiffness matrices are all greater than zero.

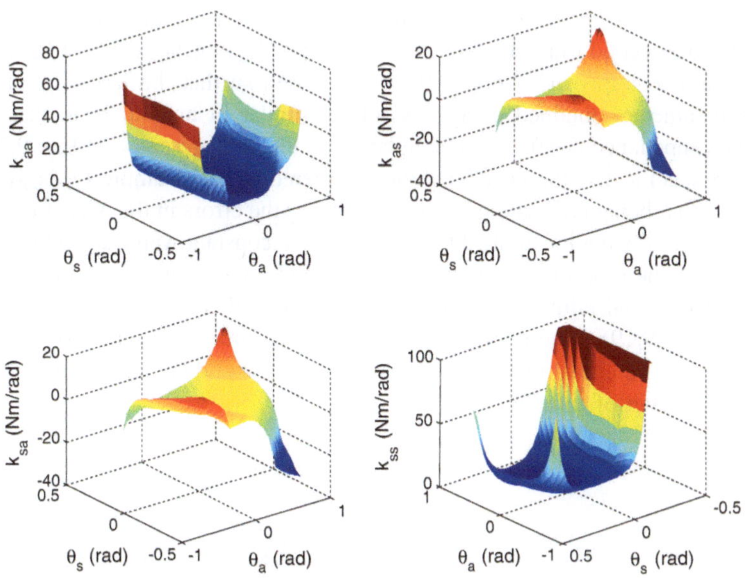

Fig. 9.5 Surface plots for different elements of the ankle stiffness matrix computed across a range of ankle and subtalar joint displacements

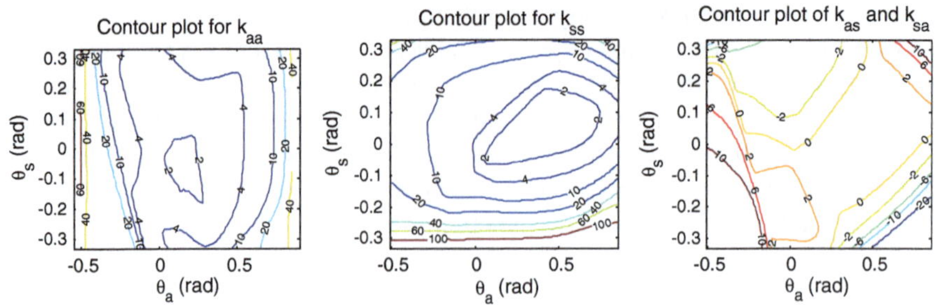

Fig. 9.6 Contour plots for different elements of the ankle stiffness matrix computed across a range of ankle and subtalar joint displacements

9.2.2 *Simulation and Experimental Results*

Simulations were carried out to verify the effectiveness of the proposed impedance adjustment rule. These simulations were done using a simplified version of the integrated foot–robot model. This simplified model leaves the force sensor and actuator dynamics out of the system to allow evaluations to be made on the fundamental concept of adapting the robot impedance according to the environmental admittance. These simulations again involved emulation of passive motion trials using the same reference trajectories as the previous chapter. Two simulation runs were carried out, a control run with the basic impedance control scheme proposed in the previous chapter, where robot stiffness and damping parameters were set to be constant (uniform stiffness and damping of 10 Nm/rad and 2 Nms/rad, respectively) and a second trial which utilised the proposed impedance adjustment rule to allow variable impedance control ($\eta = 20$, chosen so that the larger robot impedance parameters obtained using this rule is similar in magnitude to that of the constant impedance case). These simulation results are presented in Fig. 9.7.

More specifically, the cost function considered at each sample C_k is given by (9.28), with k being the sample number, Θ_e being the errors in the XYZ Euler angle coordinates, τ_k being the applied torque, and η is a constant weighting which is also the same as the proportionality constant that relates the manipulator impedance to the environmental admittance. The cost index can then be computed from this function as (9.29), where $\delta_{t,k} = t_{k+1} - t_k$ is the time between two successive samples, T_{tot} is the total time elapsed between the first and the last sample, and N is the total number of samples available.

$$C_k = \eta \Theta_{e,k}^{\mathrm{T}} \Theta_{e,k} + \tau_k^{\mathrm{T}} \tau_k \tag{9.28}$$

$$C = \frac{1}{T_{\text{tot}}} \sum_{k=1}^{k=N-1} C_k \delta_{t,k} \tag{9.29}$$

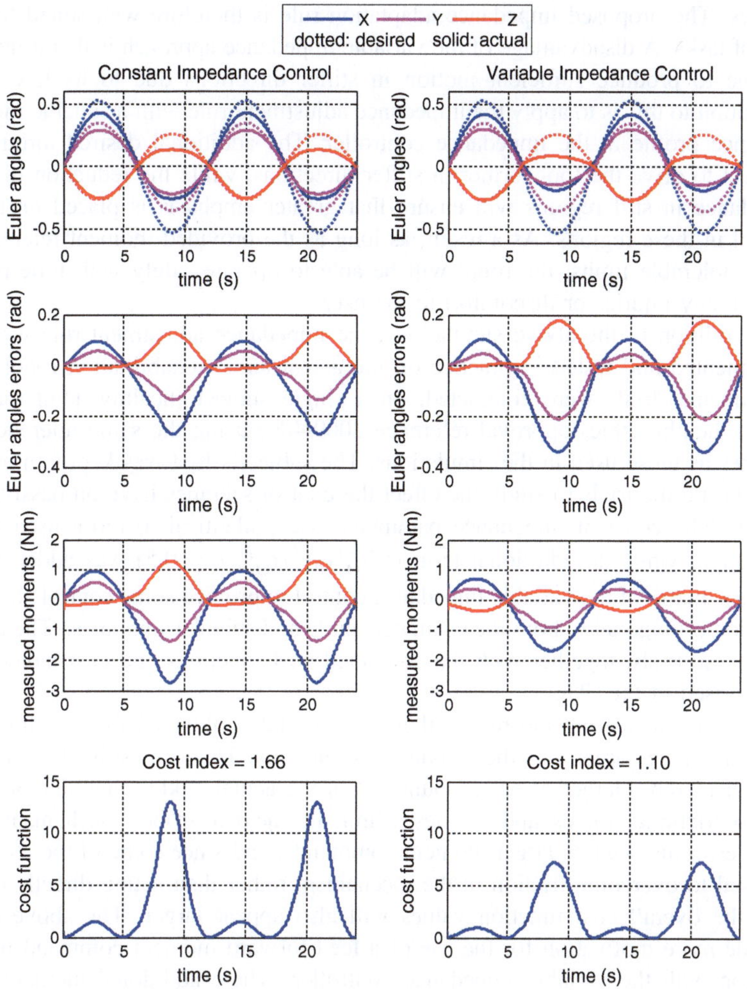

Fig. 9.7 Simulation results of passive moment trials using the constant and variable impedance control schemes

The simulation results clearly show that the variable impedance controller does indeed have a smaller cost function when compared with the constant controller. Closer inspection of the position errors and the task space moment shows that while the constant impedance case offers greater positional accuracy, it does so at the expense of significantly larger task space moments. This is particularly noticeable when the foot is moving in the pronation direction (combination of dorsiflexion, eversion and external rotation/abduction), where it is clear that the variable impedance control has considerably reduced its actuation effort compared to the constant impedance controlled system. In rehabilitation tasks, it is necessary to limit the moments applied to the user's limb or joint in order to minimise the likelihood of injuries. The proposed impedance adaptation rule is therefore well suited for this type of tasks. A disadvantage of the variable impedance approach is that it may not be able to produce sufficient motion in stiffer directions due to its low gains. A solution to this is to apply the impedance adjustment rule with a suitable moment reference profile in the impedance controller. The additional desired torque will then act to drive the foot further in stiffer directions, while the reduction of robot impedance in stiff regions will ensure that greater emphasis is placed on torque control in these regions. As a result, as long as the provided moment reference is within tolerable limits, the robot will be able to operate safely with little risk of causing any injuries or discomfort to the user.

In addition to the above simulations, the impedance adjustment rule was also implemented and tested in practice on the actual ankle rehabilitation robot. Two experimental trials were conducted, on a single subject (healthy adult male of 1.75 m height, ethics approval reference 2009/480) using the same reference trajectories as those used in the simulations. The subject's foot was kept in a relaxed state during the trials to study the effect the control schemes have on passive foot motion. The constant impedance parameters were identical to those used in the simulation, while an additional term ($\kappa H_{\Theta}^{-1} v_p v_p^{T} H_{\Theta}^{-T}$, $\kappa = 0.5$) was added to the stiffness matrix of the variable impedance control to provide some control along the direction orthogonal to both the estimated ankle and subtalar joint axes. The results from these trials, together with the computed cost functions and cost indices, are summarised in Fig. 9.8.

It can be seen from the results that the cost index obtained from both experiments are much larger than those found in simulation. This is most likely caused by the considerably larger errors encountered in the actual ankle rehabilitation robot due to frictional forces and torques within the actuator-robot mechanism. This larger error also causes larger moment commands, and since some of the moments are used to overcome friction in the mechanism rather than acting directly on the foot, the overall cost function values will also appear larger. The above issues provide more motivation for the use of a feed-forward moment command in conjunction with the variable impedance controller, where additional moment components can be added to overcome the frictional effects.

Since the ankle model was formed without using subject specific data, another source for discrepancies between simulation and experimental results comes in the form of a mismatch between stiffness characteristics of the subject's ankle and that obtained from the ankle model. The effect of this is that the robot impedance may be reduced to small values even when the actual compliance at that region is relatively high. This suggests that the stiffness or compliance characteristic should ideally be acquired online or adapted to the patient's characteristics to allow better controller performance. However, the above can be difficult to achieve, particularly as the stiffness of the ankle is not only dependent on the foot configuration but also the levels of muscle activation. This makes estimation of the instantaneous ankle stiffness challenging and is the reason for the use of a lookup table-based approach which considers only the passive foot stiffness.

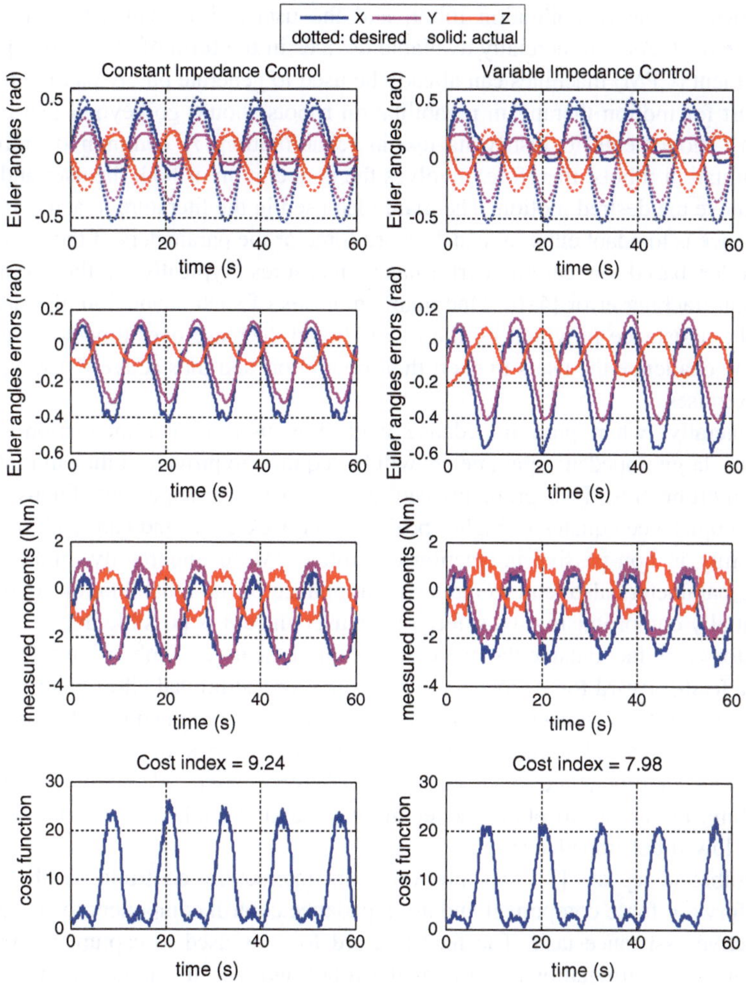

Fig. 9.8 Experimental results of passive moment trials using the constant and variable impedance control schemes

9.3 Adaptive Interaction Control via Assistance Adaptation

9.3.1 Impedance Control with Adaptive Feed-Forward Force

One of the important functionalities of rehabilitation robots is to guide the user's affected limb or joint through certain rehabilitation trajectories. For severely affected joints or limbs, the effort required to realise the motion will be completely provided by the rehabilitation robot, and the user's limb will act as a passive environment. As commercially available devices in the form of continuous passive movement (CPM) machines can already be used to generate purely passive motion, support for motion therapy in rehabilitation robots should go beyond that of pure passive movements to justify its use in rehabilitation. A common operation of rehabilitation robots, therefore, involves the cooperation of both the user and robot to achieve the desired motion. The main idea used in the literature to achieve active assistance is to adapt either a feed-forward force or the parameters of the interaction controller based on certain performance measures, typically in the form of a position tracking error [4–6]. One main emphasis of such adaptation algorithms is that the assistance provided by the robot should decrease over time so as to continually challenge the users to exert their own effort and thus actively participate in the exercises.

Generally, when pure impedance control is used in the interaction control scheme, large impedance parameters will be required to provide sufficient motion in stiff environments. Two problems can arise with this arrangement. Firstly, larger robot impedance equates to higher position feedback gains and can lead to system instability in non-passive interaction controllers. More importantly, higher impedance parameters also lead to reduced compliance of the rehabilitation robot, thus potentially compromising the safety of the user since it is possible that the desired trajectory is in fact outside the range of motion of the user's limb or joint. However, with a feed-forward force term in the controller, the additional effort contributed by this term will allow greater movements to be made and provided that the magnitude of this feed-forward term is kept at safe levels, the risk of injury will also be minimal. An advantage of a feed-forward force-based adaptation scheme is, therefore, the ability to obtain better motion tracking while still maintaining relatively low robot impedance.

Wolbrecht et al. [7] had proposed an interaction controller with both a feed-forward force component and an impedance control component to accomplish the active assistance task. The feed-forward force is used to capture information relating to the gravitational terms of the robot and user dynamics, as well as the capability of the user in producing motion at different positions. This force can, therefore, be set to be a sufficiently large value in a manner which is not directly related to the position error. The impedance component can then be chosen with small impedance parameters to permit deviations from the commanded trajectories.

The control and adaptation laws for the interaction controller given in [7] are represented by (9.30) and (9.31), respectively, where $F_r \in \mathbb{R}^m$ is the assistive force applied by the robot in the m dimensional workspace and $Y\hat{a}$ is the feed-forward component of the force. $Y \in \mathbb{R}^{m\times n}$ is the regression matrix which is obtained from the activation levels of a set of n spatially distributed Gaussian radial basis functions, and $\hat{a} \in \mathbb{R}^n$ is a vector of the weightings associated with these Gaussian functions. Additionally, $K_P \in \mathbb{R}^{m\times m}$ and $K_D \in \mathbb{R}^{m\times m}$ are the stiffness and damping matrices used in the impedance component of the control law, and x_e is the position error. Lastly, $\Gamma \in \mathbb{R}^{n\times n}$ is a symmetric positive definite matrix, and τ is the time constant of the parameter adaptation law. This control scheme had also been proven stable in the Lyapunov sense, where it was shown that the system error is bounded [7].

$$F_r = Y\hat{a} + K_P x_e + K_D \dot{x}_e \tag{9.30}$$

$$\dot{\hat{a}} = -\frac{1}{\tau} Y^{\mathrm{T}} \left(YY^{\mathrm{T}}\right)^{-1} Y\hat{a} + \Gamma^{-1} Y^{\mathrm{T}} (\dot{x}_e + \Lambda x_e) \tag{9.31}$$

An inspection of the adaptation law shows that the feed-forward assistive force is controlled by two terms, one relating to the existing parameter values and another which depends on the position tracking error. It can be seen that the matrix Γ is used to control how the position tracking error will increase the feed-forward force adaptation rate, while the time constant τ determines how quickly the feed-forward assistance reduces over time in the absence of any position tracking errors.

This adaptation law appears to be suitable for the scenario where the workspace is free of kinematic constraints or stiff regions as the adaptation law will adjust the feed-forward assistive force until the rate of decay of the force is balanced out by the position tracking error, at which stage a steady-state assistive force will be obtained. However, when uncertain kinematic constraints are present in the operating environment and engaged by the robot, such an adaptation law would continue to increase the forces applied in the constrained directions until the adaptation law reaches the steady-state assistive force. Additionally, the above control and adaptation law will also act to correct the position of the end effector regardless of whether the current position is behind or ahead of the current reference position in the desired trajectory. In assistive rehabilitation exercises, users are typically allowed to move ahead of the desired trajectory with little or no resistance. This issue has been addressed by some researchers such as in [4] where the potential function used to define the corrective forces applied to the user is defined in such a manner that resistance will not be exerted on the user when the end-effector position is further along the desired exercise path. In this work, modifications are proposed to the control and adaptation laws as shown in (9.31) to accommodate the two issues discussed above.

9.3.2 Alternative Error Dependency Functions

In order to reduce the force increase due to constraints and high stiffness in the environment, the tracking error-dependent term in the parameter adaptation law can be modified so that it does not continue to increase proportionately with the error magnitude as large tracking errors are encountered. For both methods, the adaptation law will retain a similar form as that used in (9.31). A more intuitive representation of the adaptation law in terms of the feed-forward force is shown in (9.32), where $F_{ff} = Y\hat{a}$ is the feed-forward force and k is a scalar which determines the influence of the error-dependent term. It should be noted that this form is selected so that its minimal norm solution for $\dot{\hat{a}}$ is equivalent to (9.31) when the time rate of change of the regression matrix Y is ignored and when the matrix Γ is a multiple of the identity matrix, with $\Gamma^{-1} = kI$. Using the formulation shown in (9.32), it can be seen that the relationship (9.33) holds for the adaptation law. This relationship will be referred to hereafter as the error dependency function (EDF), and two alternative EDFs were considered.

$$\begin{aligned} \dot{F}_{ff} &= -\frac{1}{\tau}F_{ff} + kYY^{\mathrm{T}}\varepsilon \\ \dot{\hat{a}} &= -\frac{1}{\tau}Y^{\mathrm{T}}\left(YY^{\mathrm{T}}\right)^{-1}Y\hat{a} + kY^{\mathrm{T}}\varepsilon \end{aligned} \tag{9.32}$$

$$\varepsilon = \dot{x}_e + \Lambda x_e \tag{9.33}$$

The first alternative EDF is rather intuitive and involves limitation of the error component used in the adaptation law by saturating the error coefficient to a certain threshold before applying it to the normalised error vector. This saturated EDF can be represented by (9.34) below, where $x_{e,\mathrm{thres}} \in \mathbb{R}$ is a positive error threshold, $x_{e0} \in \mathbb{R}^m$ is the position error normal to the direction of motion, and $x_{e1} \in \mathbb{R}^m$ is the position error along the direction of motion. The separation of error into these two components is intended to allow independent treatment of the errors between the direction where motion is possible (unconstrained) and other directions where no motion is observed (possibly constrained).

$$\varepsilon = \Lambda\left[\min\left(\|x_{e0}\|, x_{e,\mathrm{thres}}\right)\frac{x_{e0}}{\|x_{e0}\|} + \min\left(\|x_{e1}\|, x_{e,\mathrm{thres}}\right)\frac{x_{e1}}{\|x_{e1}\|}\right] + \dot{x}_e \tag{9.34}$$

The second alternative EDF investigated in this work makes use of the piecewise function as shown in Fig. 9.9 to scale the coefficient of the normalised error vector. The expression for this parabolic EDF is given in (9.35). In contrast to the saturated EDF described above which holds the error coefficient constant at large error magnitudes, this approach reduces the error coefficient as it grows beyond the error threshold. As a result, smaller feed-forward forces should be observed in directions with large position errors.

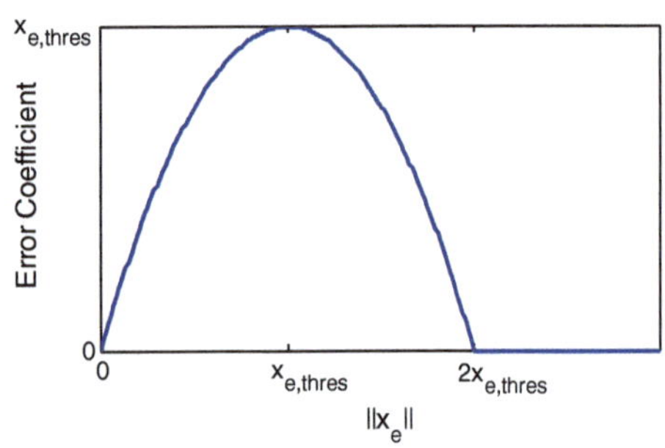

Fig. 9.9 The proposed parabolic EDF

Table 9.1 Relationship between the feed-forward adaptation rule parameters and the types of EDFs

EDF	i	A_i	ς_i
Linear	0	I	1
Saturated	1	$A_1 = \min\left(1, \frac{x_{e,\text{thres}}}{\lVert x_{e0} \rVert}\right)(I - vv^{\mathrm{T}}) + \min\left(1, \frac{x_{e,\text{thres}}}{\lVert x_{e1} \rVert}\right)vv^{\mathrm{T}}$	1
Parabolic	2	$A_2 = \max\left(0.2 - \frac{\lVert x_{e0} \rVert}{x_{e,\text{thres}}}\right)(\mathrm{I} - vv^{\mathrm{T}}) + \max\left(0.2 - \frac{\lVert x_{e1} \rVert}{x_{e,\text{thres}}}\right)vv^{\mathrm{T}}$	1

$$\varepsilon = \Lambda\left[\max\left(\frac{\lVert x_{e0} \rVert}{x_{e,\text{thres}}}(2x_{e,\text{thres}} - \lVert x_{e0} \rVert), 0\right)\frac{x_{e0}}{\lVert x_{e0} \rVert} + \max\left(\frac{\lVert x_{e1} \rVert}{x_{e,\text{thres}}}(2x_{e,\text{thres}} - \lVert x_{e1} \rVert), 0\right)\frac{x_{e1}}{\lVert x_{e1} \rVert}\right] + \dot{x}_e \tag{9.35}$$

A comparison shows that all these EDFs can be described using the same structure as shown in (9.36), where $i = 0$, 1 and 2 are used to enumerate the different EDFs discussed above. The terms used to describe the different EDFs considered in this work according to the structure given in (9.36) are summarised in Table 9.1, where the direction of motion is represented by a unit vector v.

$$\varepsilon = [\Lambda A_i \quad \varsigma_i I]\begin{bmatrix} x_\varepsilon \\ \dot{x}_\varepsilon \end{bmatrix} \tag{9.36}$$

9.3.3 *Work-Based Stiffness Adaptation*

The environment in which the robot operates is not necessarily passive as the user can actively apply forces to generate movement. The power or incremental work done by the robot can, therefore, take on both positive and negative values, where positive work indicates that the robot is providing assistance to the desired motion. In contrast, negative work indicates that the robot is impeding motion of the user. The incremental work done by the robot can, therefore, be used to identify when the motion of the patient is being resisted, and appropriate changes to the control parameters can be made to reduce this resistance during assistive exercises. In this work, it is proposed that this be achieved through modification of the desired robot stiffness matrix as in (9.37)–(9.39), where $\gamma \in \mathbb{R}$ is a state variable used to control the reduction of stiffness along the desired direction of motion given by the unit vector $\hat{v}_d \in \mathbb{R}^m$, $0 < \gamma_{\max} < 1$ is the maximum permitted value for , $\gamma, w \in \mathbb{R}$ is the amount of incremental work done by the robot, and c is a positive coefficient which governs how quickly γ changes. Additionally, $f(w)$ is a monotonic function which saturates at 0 and 1 and provides the driving force for the change in γ, with $b \in \mathbb{R}$ being a positive scaling factor for the incremental work.

$$K_P' = \left[I - \gamma \hat{v}_d \hat{v}_d^{\mathrm{T}}\right] K_P \tag{9.37}$$

$$\dot{\gamma} = c\left[-\frac{\gamma}{\gamma_{\max}} + f(w)\right] \tag{9.38}$$

$$f(w) = \max(0, \min(1, -bw)) \tag{9.39}$$

9.3.4 Reference Trajectory Modification

An additional measure that can be used to limit the forces being applied in stiff or constrained direction is to modify the reference trajectory so that the desired position is moved in the opposite direction of the position error. When used in conjunction with impedance control, this can help reduce the forces applied to the environment. However, if such an adjustment is made regardless of the magnitude of the error, the amount of forces being applied may be limited to a value which is too low to allow any useful motion. The proposed trajectory modification rule can be expressed as (9.40), where x_d' is the modified trajectory, x_d is the original reference trajectory, and Δx_d is a correction term defined using (9.41), where the regression matrix Y is the same as that used in the feed-forward force adaptation law and $\hat{\rho} \in \mathbb{R}^n$ is the parameter vector. Using the terms defined above, the adaptation law for the trajectory correction term can be expressed as (9.42), where x_e is the position error vector and $x_{e,\mathrm{th}}$ is the minimum error threshold as discussed previously. It should be noted that the pseudo-inverse is again used to obtain the minimal norm solution for the parameter time derivative in (9.42).

$$x_d' = x_d - \Delta x_d \tag{9.40}$$

$$\Delta x_d = Y\hat{\rho} \tag{9.41}$$

$$\begin{aligned} Y\hat{\rho} &= -\alpha Y\hat{\rho} + \beta\left(YY^{\mathrm{T}}\right)\max\left(0, 1 - \frac{x_{e,\mathrm{th}}}{\|x_e\|}\right)x_e \\ \dot{\hat{\rho}} &= -\alpha Y^{\mathrm{T}}\left(YY^{\mathrm{T}}\right)^{-1}\Delta x_d + \beta Y^{\mathrm{T}}\max\left(0, 1 - \frac{x_{e,\mathrm{th}}}{\|x_e\|}\right)x_e \end{aligned} \tag{9.42}$$

9.4 Simulated and Experimental Results

The adaptation laws discussed above have been tested in simulation using a two-dimensional virtual environment. The directions along which the potential functions are defined were also rotated about the controller and world reference frame. More specifically, the potential function of the environment is given by (9.43). It should be noted that u and v are the generalised coordinates of the environment. Furthermore, u_{01} and u_{02} are, respectively, the lower and upper bounds within which the potential function is constant along the u direction (a similar notation applies for the v direction). Finally, the angle Φ is used to denote the rotation which transformed the global reference frame into the principal reference frame used to define the environment. Resistive forces within the environment were obtained through partial differentiation of the potential function p_{tot} along the directions of interest.

$$p_{tot} = \sum_i p_i \tag{9.43}$$

where

$$p_1 = \frac{1}{2} k_1 [\min(0, u - u_{01})]^2$$

$$p_2 = \frac{1}{2} k_2 [\max(0, u - u_{02})]^2$$

$$p_3 = \frac{1}{2} k_3 [\min(0, v - v_{01})]^2$$

$$p_4 = \frac{1}{2} k_4 [\max(0, v - v_{02})]^2$$

$$\begin{bmatrix} u \\ v \end{bmatrix} = \begin{bmatrix} \cos\Phi & \sin\Phi \\ -\sin\Phi & \cos\Phi \end{bmatrix} \begin{bmatrix} x \\ y \end{bmatrix}$$

As some of the modifications proposed to the adaptation law are aimed at reducing the robot forces when kinematic constraints are encountered, such a constraint was also imposed on the environment during some of the simulation trials. In these trials, the kinematic constraints were given in the form of an ellipse which is centred and rotated about the global reference frame. The constraint to be satisfied is, therefore, given by (9.44), with l_a and l_b, respectively, being the minor and major radii, φ being the angle of the semi-minor axis with respect to the x-axis, while C_φ and S_φ are short for the cosine and sine of φ in that order.

$$\left[\left(\frac{C_\varphi}{l_a}\right)^2 + \left(\frac{S_\varphi}{l_b}\right)^2\right] x^2 + 2\left(\frac{1}{l_a^2} - \frac{1}{l_b^2}\right) C_\varphi S_\varphi xy + \left[\left(\frac{S_\varphi}{l_a^2}\right)^2 + \left(\frac{C_\varphi}{l_b^2}\right)^2\right] y^2 \leq 1 \tag{9.44}$$

An extensive set of simulation trials had been carried out to determine the behaviour of the control strategies discussed above under a variety of operating conditions. The potential function is plotted as a contour plot, while the resistive

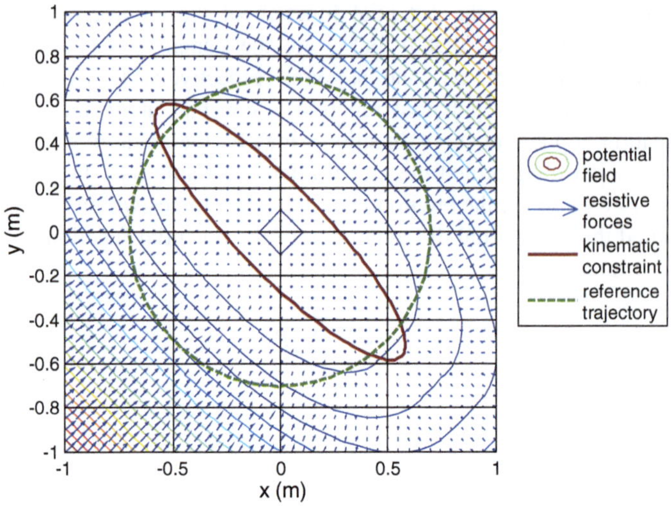

Fig. 9.10 Graphical representation of the environment used in the simulation case study

force vectors associated the potential function is given in the form of a quiver plot. The state space model used in these simulations involved a point mass moving within this environment, assisted by a propulsion force vector applied to it by the control law. The reference trajectory for the simulation trials is also given as the dashed green line in Fig. 9.10. It should be noted, however, that the initial position is located at the origin and an initial straight line reference path in the *y*-direction is used to guide the reference point from the origin to the top of the circular reference path at the start of the simulation. The trajectory has a period of 6 s and travels in the clockwise direction on the *x*–*y* plane. The simulations were run for 15 cycles of the reference trajectory.

9.4.1 Basic Feed-Forward Moment Adaptation

The experiments were used to test the different control schemes under three different scenarios. The purpose of this test was to study the robot behaviour when interacting with an abnormally stiff or constrained environment. For the purpose of this section, experiments carried out under the first scenario will be referred to as passive motion trials, and those done under the second will be termed active motion trials. Finally, constrained motion trials are used to refer to tests completed under the third scenario. The data from these experiments are presented and discussed in this section to study the assistance adaptation schemes considered above. Constant robot impedance parameters were used in all experiments, with the controller gain matrices given as follows:

$$K_P = \begin{bmatrix} 10 & 0 & 0 \\ 0 & 10 & 0 \\ 0 & 0 & 5 \end{bmatrix} \quad K_D = \begin{bmatrix} 2 & 0 & 0 \\ 0 & 2 & 0 \\ 0 & 0 & 1 \end{bmatrix}$$

Additionally, the parameters used for the feed-forward adaptation law, incremental work-based stiffness adjustment rule and the reference trajectory modification module are given in Table 9.2.

It is important to first compare the basic assistance adaptation scheme as proposed in Wolbrecht et al. [7] with a conventional impedance controller to identify the benefits and disadvantages of assistance adaptation. This was done by considering experimental results obtained from passive motion trials using a constant impedance controller and a constant impedance controller with assistance adaption. The assistance adaptation scheme used in this case was that with a linear EDF. The work-based adaptation and trajectory modification modules of the assistance adaptation controller were also deactivated in this study. The foot position and the angular errors obtained from these passive motion trials are presented in Fig. 9.11. In addition to the passive motion trials, an active motion trial was also carried out using the basic assistance adaptation scheme to allow an investigation into the behaviour of this controller when the subject is actively participating in the rehabilitation exercise. The results of this trial are given in Fig. 9.12. Lastly, constrained motion trials were also performed using both the conventional impedance controller and the basic assistance adaptation scheme, and the results are presented in Fig. 9.13.

It is clear from the passive motion trial results that the introduction of the adaptive feed-forward moment has an effect of reducing the overall motion tracking error of the foot. This is of course due to the additional effort applied by the adaptive feed-forward moments in the assistance adaptation scheme.

Results from the active motion trial shown in Fig. 9.12 indicate that the reference trajectory can be followed much more closely when the subject is actively participating in the motion. It can also be seen that the feed-forward moment used to provide additional assistance to the subject is reducing in directions with smaller position tracking errors as time progresses. This is a desired characteristic as the subject should be encouraged to produce the motion independently without relying on the rehabilitation robot. In terms of performance in constrained motion trials, the results shown in Fig. 9.13 suggest that the basic assistance adaptation scheme is applying significantly larger moments compared to the conventional impedance control scheme when the subject's foot is stiffened.

Table 9.2 Assistance adaptation scheme parameters used in the experimental trials

Control module	Feed-forward moment adaptation			Incremental work-based stiffness adjustment			Reference trajectory modification		
Parameter	τ	k	$x_{e,\text{thres}}$	$\gamma_{\max}$	c	b	α	β	$x_{e,\text{th}}$
Value	5 s	6 N/rad	0.15 rad	0.9	5 s^{-1}	25 J^{-1}	0.1 s^{-1}	0.2 s^{-1}	0.15 rad

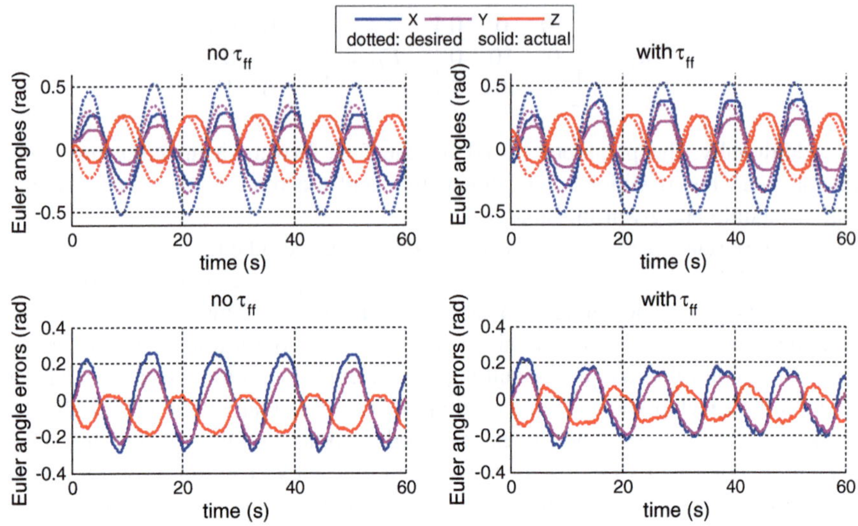

Fig. 9.11 Desired and measured foot orientation, as well as tracking errors obtained from passive motion trials using the conventional impedance controller (without feed-forward moments τ_{ff}) and the basic assistance adaptation scheme (with feed-forward moments τ_{ff})

Fig. 9.12 Desired and measured foot orientations, as well as the feed-forward torque obtained from active motion trials using the basic assistance adaptation scheme

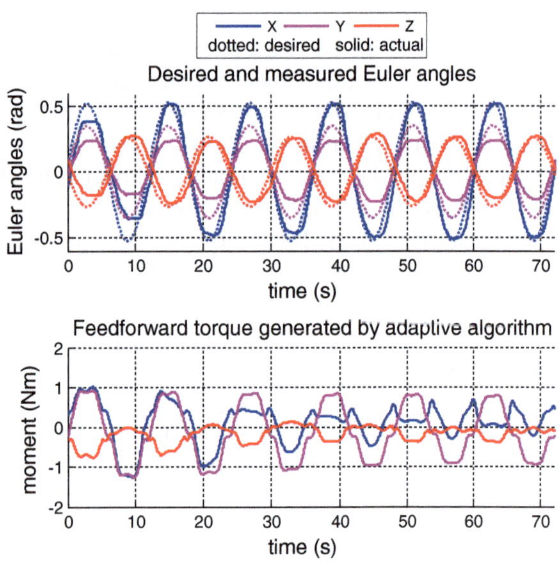

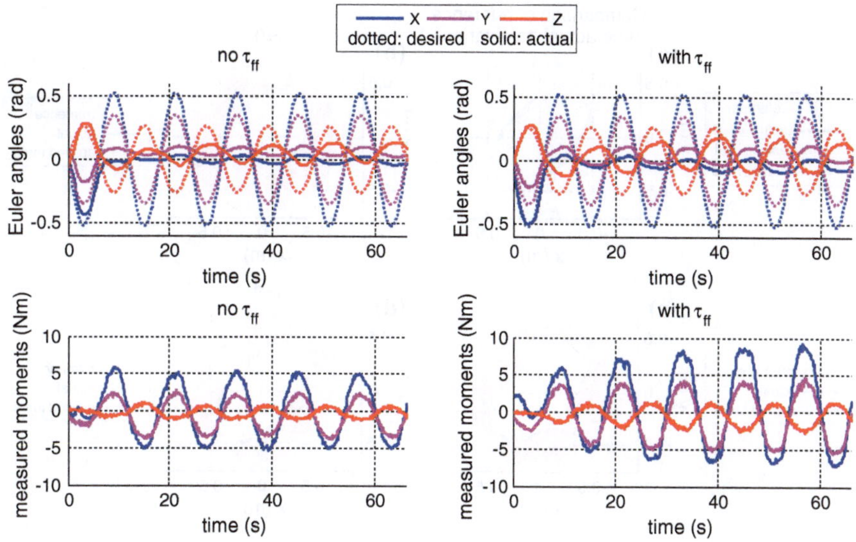

Fig. 9.13 Desired and measured foot orientation, as well as measured moments obtained from constrained motion trials using the conventional impedance controller (without feed-forward moments τ_{ff}) and the basic assistance adaptation scheme (with feed-forward moments τ_{ff})

9.4.2 Effects of Different Error Dependency Functions

Figure 9.14a shows the trajectories traced by the point mass during the last cycle in simulations involving the passive and unconstrained operating condition. It should be noted that both the work-based stiffness adjustment and trajectory modification modules are not active in these simulations. Three end point trajectories are presented, one for each type of EDF used in the adaptation law. More specifically, the blue line indicates the position recorded when the original approach based on a linear EDF (i = 0) is used in the adaptation law, while the red and green lines represent those of the saturated (i = 1) and parabolic (i = 2) approaches, respectively. The reference trajectories for all these control schemes were identical and are shown as the dotted lines. Figure 9.14b–d on the other hand shows the reference trajectory (green dotted line), the point mass trajectory (blue line) and the control force vectors applied to the point mass at the corresponding locations (red lines).

It can be seen from Fig. 9.14a that the extent of motion in the stiffer direction is greatest for the linear error dependency approach. This can be seen to be a consequence of larger forces being applied along this stiff direction. Figure 9.14c, d on the other hand reveals that limiting the contribution of error to the feed-forward force adaptation at large errors effectively reduces the forces being applied in the stiff direction, with a larger reduction in the parabolic EDF approach. As a result, the extent of motion for these two alternative approaches in the stiff direction is also smaller, although not by a large margin. Another interesting observation is that the

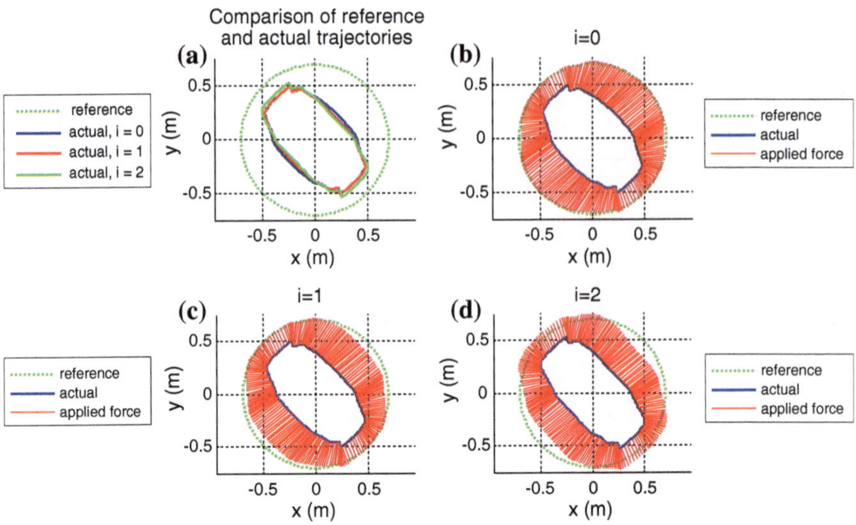

Fig. 9.14 **a** Comparison of the reference and actual trajectories obtained from simulations on unconstrained motion using different EDFs. The force vectors applied at different points along the trajectories are shown for the linear, saturated and parabolic approaches in (**b**), (**c**) and (**d**), respectively

parabolic EDF approach appears to provide the largest motion in the more compliant direction, while motion for the linear and saturated error dependency-based methods is almost identical. This is also a result of the use of a parabolic EDF in the feed-forward force adaptation law, where the feed-forward force is allowed to grow at a faster rate when the errors are small.

A similar set of plots are also shown in Fig. 9.15 for simulations involving the passive and constrained operating condition. It can be seen from these plots that the trajectory made by both the linear and saturated EDF approaches are essentially identical, while the parabolic-based adaptation approach produced larger motion in the more compliant direction. It is shown in Fig. 9.15b that rather large control forces were applied by the linear error dependency approach to the point mass, even as it was moving along the constrained surface. The magnitudes of the control forces for approaches based on the saturated (Fig. 9.15c) and parabolic (Fig. 9.15d) EDFs on the other hand are considerably smaller, with the parabolic EDF adaptation law having a more even distribution of force magnitudes along both the constrained and unconstrained direction.

While the results presented previously focused on the differences between the conventional impedance controller and the basic assistance adaptation scheme, this subsection addresses how different EDFs in the feed-forward moment adaptation law influences the overall behaviour of the rehabilitation robot. Both passive motion and constrained motion trials were considered for this purpose, and each of the linear, saturated and parabolic EDFs were tested (with the trajectory

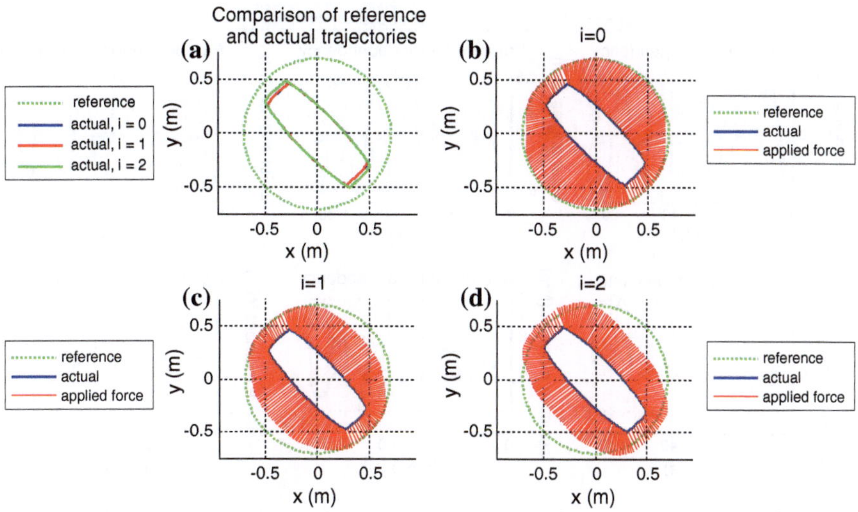

Fig. 9.15 **a** Comparison of the reference and actual trajectories obtained from simulations on constrained motion using different EDFs. The force vectors applied at different points along the trajectories are shown for the linear, saturated and parabolic EDF approaches in (**b**), (**c**) and (**d**), respectively

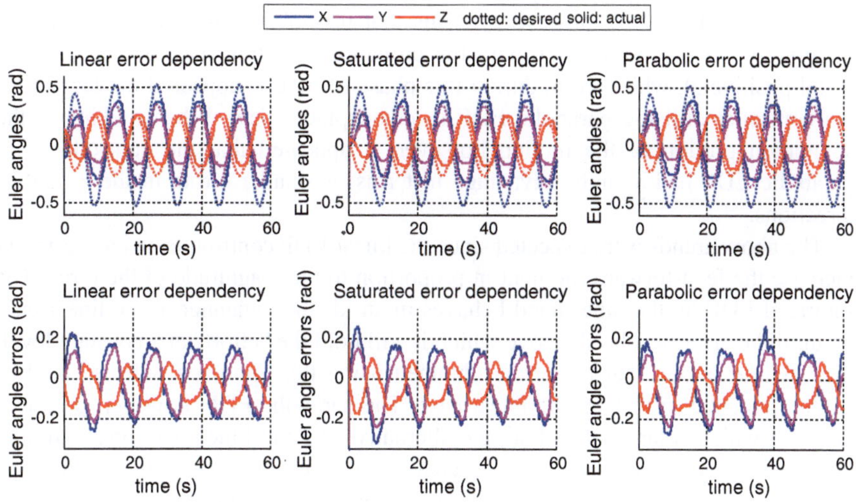

Fig. 9.16 Desired and measured foot orientations, as well as tracking errors obtained from passive motion trials using assistance adaptation schemes with different EDFs in the feed-forward moment adaptation law

modification and work-based adaptation modules disabled). The results for the passive motion trials are summarised in Fig. 9.16, while those for the constrained motion trials are shown in Fig. 9.17.

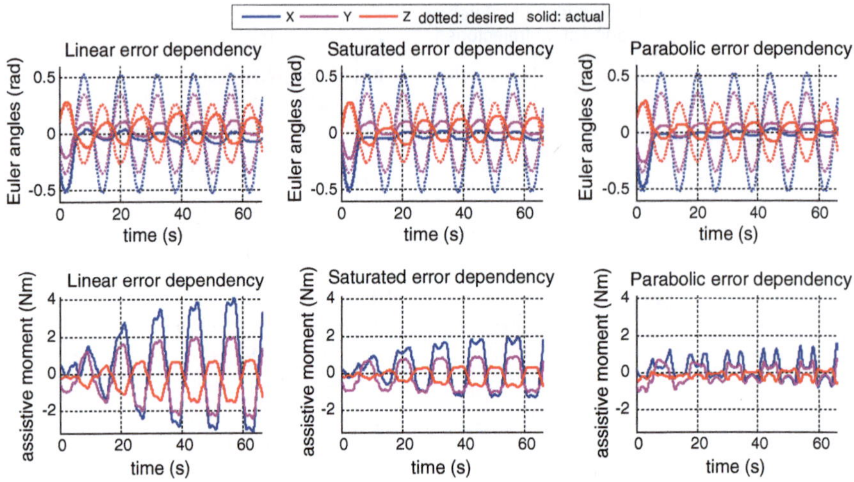

Fig. 9.17 Desired and measured foot orientations, as well as assistive moments obtained from constrained motion trials using assistance adaptation schemes with different EDFs in the feed-forward moment adaptation law

Results from the passive motion trials conducted have shown that all three EDFs appear to have very similar performances in terms of angular errors. Detailed Inspection of Fig. 9.16, however, reveals that use of the linear EDF resulted in marginally smaller position error in the pronation direction (negative x, negative y and positive z), while errors during this phase of motion appeared the largest for the controller utilising parabolic EDF in its adaptation law. When looking at the supination portion of the motion however, it appeared that the controller with parabolic EDF had a slight advantage in terms of smaller errors in the x- and y-directions.

The above trends were expected since the linear EDF contributes to an "effort" to increase the feed-forward moment in proportion to the magnitude of the error. The saturated EDF on the other hand behaves in an identical manner to the linear case up until the error threshold, above which it will hold the "effort" at a constant level; thus, it is expected that the errors obtained using this approach will be equal or slightly larger than that for the linear case. The parabolic EDF, however, produces an effort which is larger than both the alternatives up until the error threshold, and beyond that, this effort will start to decrease until it reaches zero. This provides an explanation to the observation where errors in the parabolic dependency case is larger than that of the linear dependency case during pronation, but smaller when the foot is undergoing supination motion. This is because errors in supination are smaller or near the error threshold used, while those in the pronation direction are larger than the threshold. The consequence of this is that the effort applied to increase the feed-forward moment is larger in supination for the parabolic dependency case, but smaller when the foot is moving in pronation.

9.4.3 *Effects of Incremental Work-Based Stiffness Adaptation*

Another controller module proposed in this research is the incremental work-based adjustment of the robot stiffness. The aim of this adjustment rule is to provide the robot with a means in identifying whether it is applying a force to resist the current direction of motion and subsequently allowing it to adjust its stiffness matrix so that actuator effort which acts to correct position errors along the direction of the reference velocity is minimised. This will, therefore, allow the point mass to move beyond its current reference position with smaller resistance. As discussed previously, the sign of the incremental work done by the robot can be used to identify whether resistance is being provided, with negative incremental work denoting that the robot forces are impeding motion. The goal is, therefore, to minimise the amount of negative work done by the robot. In order to study the effect of the work-based stiffness adjustment control module, the simulation results obtained under the active and unconstrained as well as active and constrained operating conditions were considered. The feed-forward force adaptation law with linear error dependency had been used to obtain these results, while the trajectory modification module was deactivated.

Figure 9.18 shows plots containing information relating to both the end point trajectory and the negative work done by the robot at a particular location. Figure 9.18a is plotted for the results obtained without any kinematic constraints,

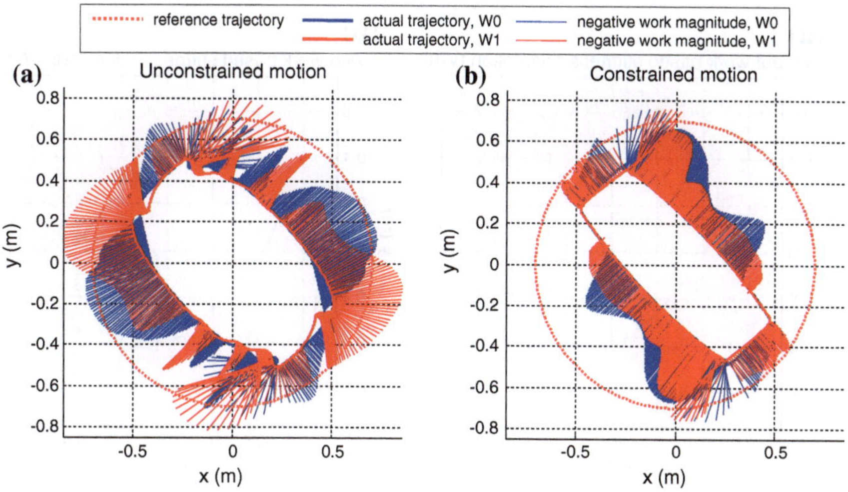

Fig. 9.18 Comparison of the motion trajectories and the magnitudes of negative work done by the controller at different trajectory points for control schemes with (*W*1) and without (*W*0) work-based adaptation for both unconstrained (**a**) and constrained (**b**) motions. Note that the lengths of the thin lines give an indication of the negative work magnitudes, with positive work having a length of zero

while Fig. 9.18b is done for those obtained when constraints are present in the environment. The red and blue lines are, respectively, used to denote quantities relating to the control scheme with and without work-based stiffness adjustment. In these plots, the negative work done by the robot at different locations are represented by lines along the normal of the end point trajectories, with the magnitude of this negative incremental work governing the lengths of these normal lines. It should also be noted that a length of zero is used where zero or positive work is recorded. Additionally, the motion of the end point was in the clockwise direction.

The advantage offered by the stiffness adjustment approach can be seen by considering Fig. 9.19, which shows the force vectors applied at various positions along the motion trajectory for the two control schemes considered under the unconstrained operating condition. One of the main points to be focused on in these plots is the spacing between these force vectors, which gives an indication of the velocity at which the end point is moving. It can be seen that this velocity towards the end of the "longer" sides of the actual motion trajectory is higher for the case when work-based adjustment module is used. This means that controller's resistance towards the active effort applied by the object is reduced, thus allowing faster motion in the direction where the active force is applied. Some other points worth noting are the spacing and magnitude of the actuator force vectors at the corner segments of the motion trajectory (where significant negative work is observed) in Fig. 9.19b.

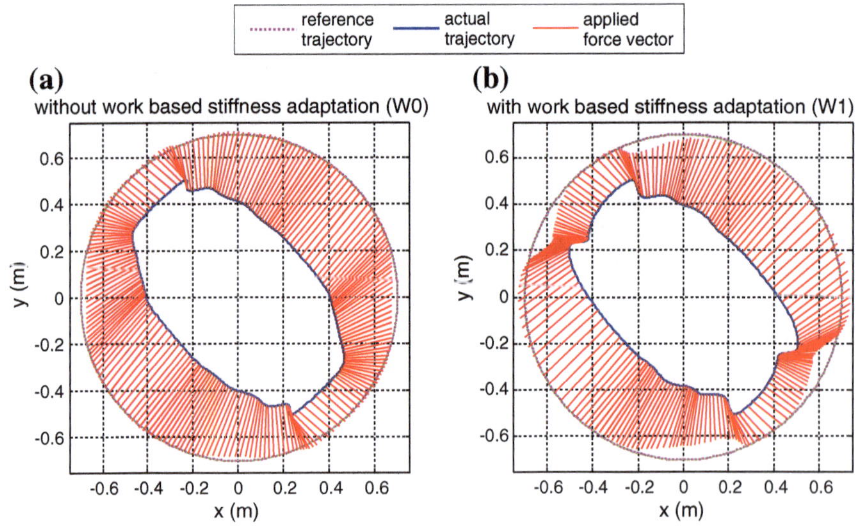

Fig. 9.19 The forces applied along the actual trajectories during unconstrained motion for the controllers without (**a**) and with (**b**) work-based stiffness adaptation. Note that force vectors are drawn at uniformly sampled time intervals

It can be seen that the negative work done by the robot does indeed increase significantly from the passive to active scenarios. This suggests that the forces applied by the robot do provide resistance to the end point motion. It is shown in Fig. 9.19 that apart from the passive unconstrained case, the use of a work-based stiffness adjustment has resulted in a reduction in the average negative work under all other operating conditions.

The dorsiflexion–plantarflexion reference trajectory is given in (9.45) as it is an easier task for the subject to drive the foot in a single direction of rotation rather than a combination of several rotational motions. The only difference between these schemes was that one had the work-based stiffness adaptation module activated, while the other had it deactivated.

$$\begin{aligned} \theta_x &= \frac{\pi}{9}\sin\left(\frac{\pi}{6}t\right) \\ \theta_y &= \theta_z = 0 \end{aligned} \tag{9.45}$$

As previously discussed in the simulation case study, negative incremental work typically indicates that the robot is impeding the motion of the user. Negative work must, therefore, be minimised in robots used to provide assistance to the user's movement. Results from the first type of active motion trials (Fig. 9.20) show that the negative incremental work done by the robot during the trials is rather similar

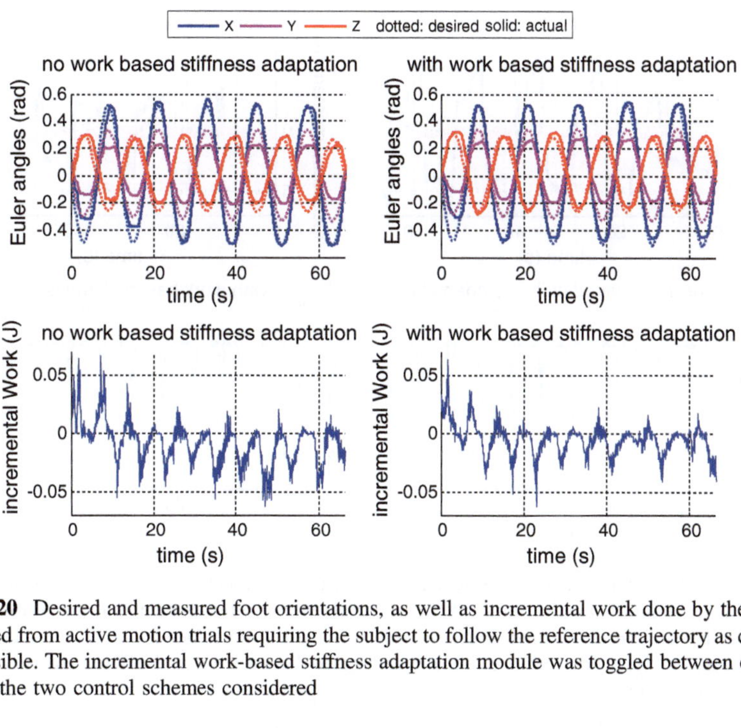

Fig. 9.20 Desired and measured foot orientations, as well as incremental work done by the robot obtained from active motion trials requiring the subject to follow the reference trajectory as closely as possible. The incremental work-based stiffness adaptation module was toggled between on and off for the two control schemes considered

between the two control schemes considered. This, therefore, makes direct comparison difficult, particularly when the difference between the two schemes is not very significant. The second type of active motion trial, however, can be used to better illustrate the contribution of the incremental work-based stiffness adaptation module. It is clear from the results of these trials (Fig. 9.21) that the controller with an active incremental work-based stiffness adaptation module provided considerably smaller resistive moments to the subject. This had led to the larger movement amplitudes and lower levels of negative work. This, therefore, suggests that the incremental work-based stiffness adaptation module is working as intended and can be incorporated into the overall assistance adaptation controller to reduce the resistive moments applied when the user is capable of moving ahead of the reference trajectory.

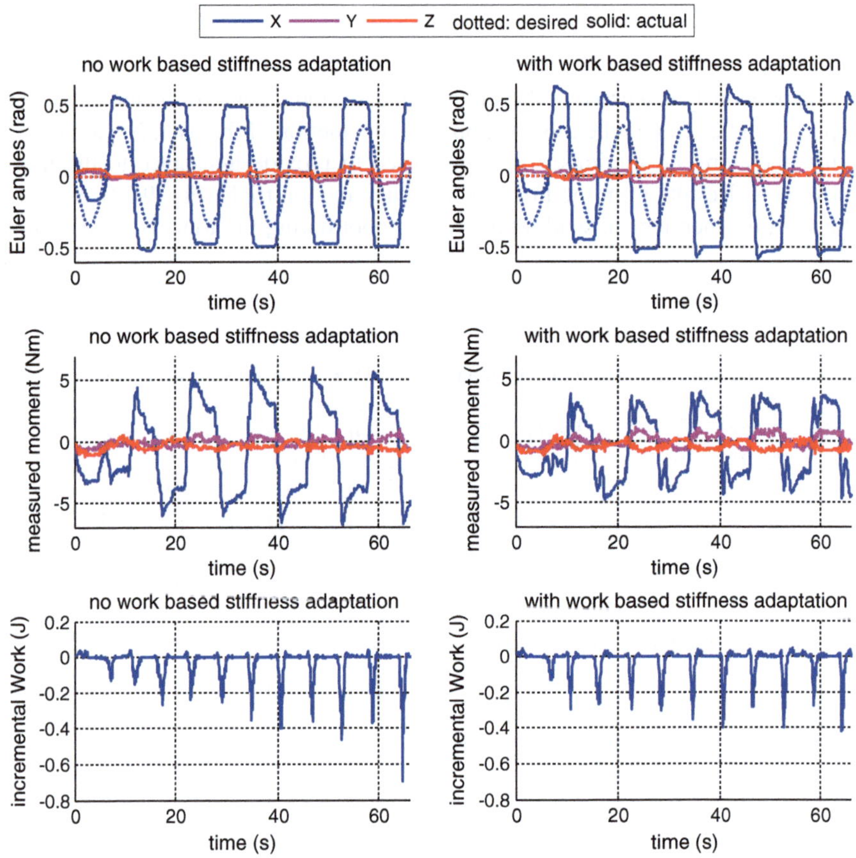

Fig. 9.21 Desired/measured foot orientations, measured moments, as well as incremental work done by the robot obtained from active motion trials where subject attempts to move the foot as much as possible in the desired direction with no regard to trajectory tracking. The incremental work-based stiffness adaptation module was toggled between on and off for the two control schemes considered

9.4.4 Effects of Reference Trajectory Modification

To study the efficacy of this trajectory modification module, simulation results carried out under both the passive unconstrained and passive constrained operating conditions were considered. While the activation of the trajectory modification module was toggled for these trials, the error dependency in the feed-forward force adaptation law was kept linear. The work-based adjustment of controller stiffness was also deactivated. The main simulation results are summarised in Fig. 9.22, with the first row of plots providing the reference (dotted lines) and actual (solid lines) trajectories obtained from the TM0W0 (blue lines) and TM1W0 (red lines) control schemes. The second and third rows then show plots of the force vectors produced

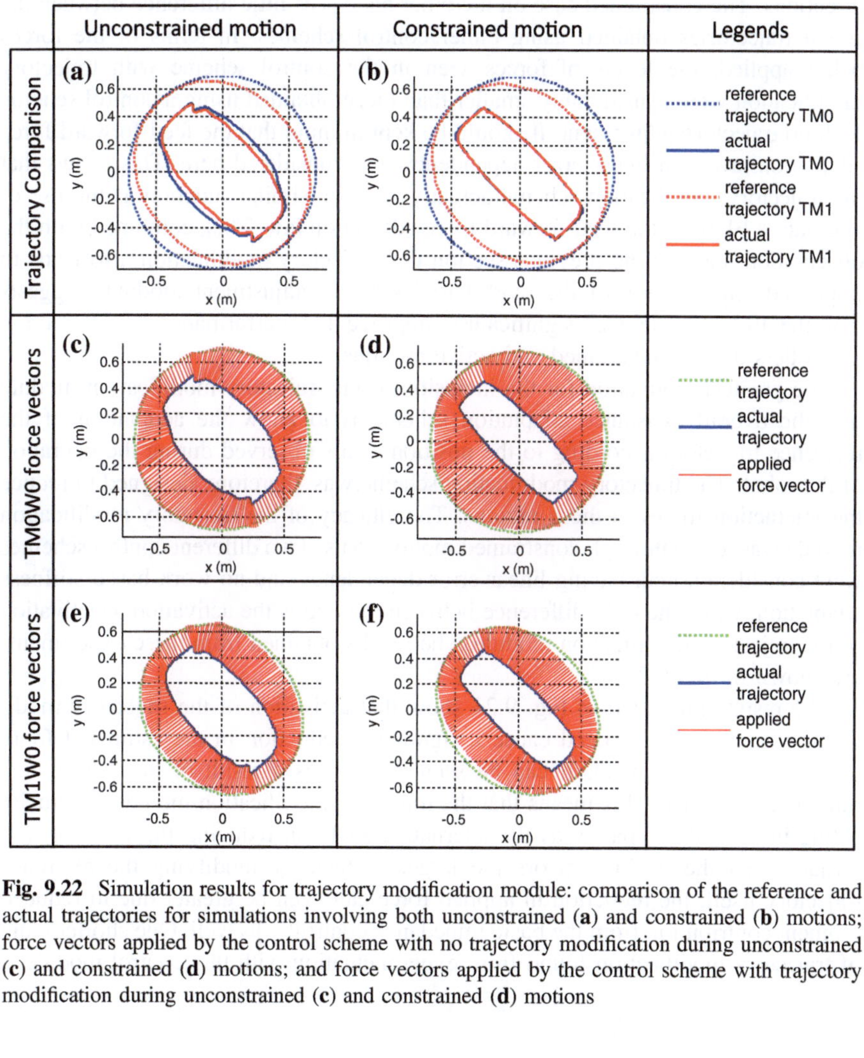

Fig. 9.22 Simulation results for trajectory modification module: comparison of the reference and actual trajectories for simulations involving both unconstrained (**a**) and constrained (**b**) motions; force vectors applied by the control scheme with no trajectory modification during unconstrained (**c**) and constrained (**d**) motions; and force vectors applied by the control scheme with trajectory modification during unconstrained (**c**) and constrained (**d**) motions

by the TM0W0 and TM1W0 control schemes, respectively. Additionally, all plots in the first column are obtained from simulations without any kinematic constraints in the environment, while those in the second column are obtained from simulations with kinematic constraints. As with the notations used in Fig. 9.22, TM1 indicates that the trajectory modification module is activated, while TM0 denotes that it is deactivated. Also, W0 is used to represent that the work-based stiffness adjustment module is deactivated.

From these results, it is shown from the first row in Fig. 9.22 that the proposed trajectory modification module does shrink the reference trajectories for both the constrained and unconstrained environments, with much greater reduction in the stiff or constrained directions. This had led to greater resemblance between the shape of the modified reference path and the actual motion trajectory. A consequence of this for the unconstrained case is lesser movement in the stiff directions. The constrained case on the other hand sees little difference between the actual trajectories obtained using either control schemes. In terms of the forces being applied, the levels of forces seen in the control scheme with trajectory modification were considerably smaller than those obtained using a control scheme with no trajectory adjustment. It should be kept in mind that the feed-forward force adaptation law with linear error dependency was considered here. This shows that the trajectory modification scheme actually serves a similar function as the use of alternative EDFs in the feed-forward force adaptation law. This, combined with the observation made in the previous section that trajectory modification also leads to improved effectiveness of the work-based stiffness adjustment module, suggests that the this module can significantly improve the performance of interaction controllers during constrained and active motions.

The greatest motivation for the inclusion of the trajectory modification module into the overall assistance adaptation scheme is to allow the adaptation of the reference trajectory according to the position errors observed during the operation of the robot. The trajectory modification scheme was, therefore, designed to reduce the interaction forces in these regions. The efficacy of the trajectory modification module was tested through constrained motion trials. Two different control schemes were considered, both having linear error dependency and no work-based stiffness adaptation, while the only difference between the two is the activation/deactivation of the trajectory modification module. The results obtained from these experiments are shown in Fig. 9.23.

The results presented in Fig. 9.23 show that activation of the trajectory modification module does indeed cause a significant reduction in the estimated foot–robot interaction moment. It can be seen that this is a result of the “shrinking” reference trajectory. This means that the trajectory modification module is actually acting in a similar capacity as the alternative EDFs in reducing the feed-forward torque when the position errors are large. In fact, by modifying the reference trajectory itself, the reduction in applied force can even be greater due to reduced moment contribution from the basic impedance controller as well. One shortcoming of trajectory modification found from experimentation with this control module is

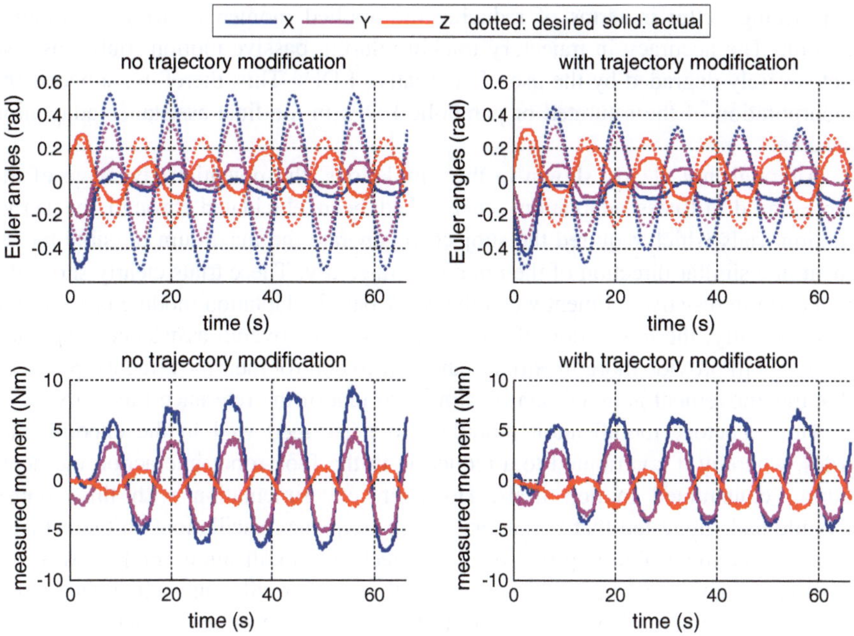

Fig. 9.23 Desired and measured foot orientations, as well as estimated interaction moments obtained from constrained motion trials using assistance adaptation schemes without and with the reference trajectory modification module

the presence of high-frequency oscillations in the actuator motors when the parameter β used in the parameter adaptation rule (10.44) is too large.

9.4.5 Summary of Experimental Results

Comparison of the basic impedance controller and the impedance controller with the existing assistance adaptation scheme [7] in place had shown that significant performance gains can be achieved through adoption of the assistance adaptation scheme, whereby the additional feed-forward assistive moment can help improve the trajectory tracking capability of the robot. Additionally, the inclusion of adaptation also means that the robot's behaviour can better adjust to suit the needs of the user in terms of assistance. At the same time, however, the experimental results had also highlighted the potential drawback of this adaptation scheme in the form of larger applied moments in stiff or constrained regions/directions. This, therefore, justifies the work in this research which attempts to modify the existing assistance adaptation scheme to address the above issue.

The experimental results on the effects of different EDFs have shown similar trends to those obtained from the simulation case studies, with the alternative EDFs performing better in terms of reducing the applied moments during constrained motion. The accuracy in trajectory tracking during passive motion trials was also not severely degraded by the use of alternative EDFs. This, therefore, supports the incorporation of the saturated or parabolic EDFs in the final assistance adaptation scheme.

Although not clearly shown in the simulations, the potential advantage of the work-based stiffness adaptation scheme had been elucidated through the active motion trials which required the subject to generate the maximum possible movement in a similar direction of the reference trajectory. These trials clearly showed a reduction in resistive moment when the work-based adaptation module is activated. Consequently, the integration of this module into the overall assistance adaptation scheme will provide more freedom to the user to control their movements, provided that this movement is in a direction similar to that of the reference trajectory.

The trajectory modification module also performed well in the experimental trials, whereby it contributed to a reduction in the foot–robot interaction moments during constrained motion trials. However, experimentation with this control module had suggested that it can cause high-frequency oscillations in the actuator motors. As the stability proof of the trajectory modification module was not attempted in this work, it is unclear whether this oscillation is inherent in the parameter adaptation law for the trajectory adjustment term or whether it is caused by un-modelled dynamics and interaction between the inner and outer control loops of the robot. Further investigation is, therefore, necessary to better understand the cause for this oscillation. Nonetheless, the problem of actuator oscillation appeared to be negligible when lower gain values are used in the adaptation rule, and given the benefits introduced by this module, a suitably tuned parameter adjustment rule can still be considered in an assistance adaptation scheme.

9.5 Overall Control Structure and Implementation of Rehabilitation Exercises

One of the main goals of this research is to develop a suitable adaptive interaction control framework to allow implementation of different ankle rehabilitation exercises on the developed ankle rehabilitation robot. The resulting interaction controller and its relation to the works presented earlier in this chapter can be summarised diagrammatically as Fig. 9.24, where the lower level controller can be considered to be made up of the inner loop MIMO actuator force controller and the elementary robot control scheme. The higher level control on the other hand consists of the ankle kinematic parameter estimator, the robot impedance adaptation module and the assistance adaptation scheme. The ankle kinematic parameter estimation algorithm is used to provide estimates for the ankle and subtalar joint displacements which are in turn used to establish the ankle compliance at a particular configuration according to a lookup table generated using the computational

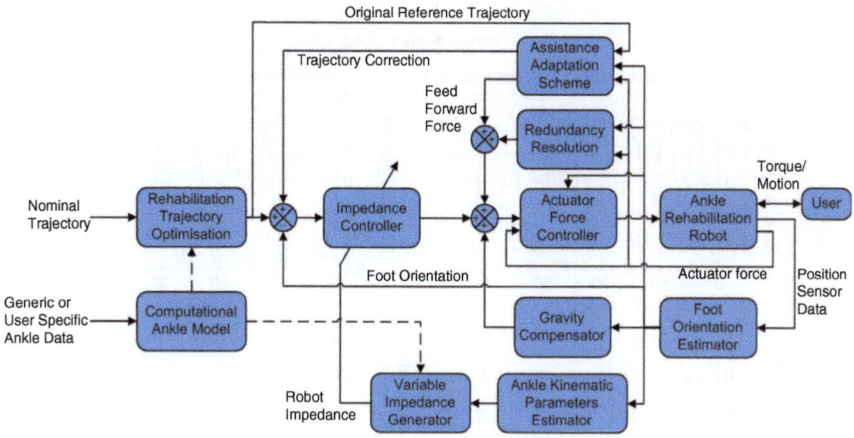

Fig. 9.24 Overview of the interaction control scheme proposed in this research

ankle model. This ankle compliance is then processed by the impedance adaptation routine to select the appropriate robot stiffness. Although not used in the experimental trials, the rehabilitation trajectory optimisation routine is also included in the diagram as it can potentially be used to generate suitable rehabilitation trajectories when desired characteristics of the rehabilitation motion such as limitations on ligament/muscle–tendon forces or ankle reaction moments are defined.

Different ankle rehabilitation exercises can be implemented using the proposed interaction controller. For instance, passive range of motion exercises can be easily implemented by using the basic impedance controller and the assistance adaptation scheme discussed in this chapter. The above control structure can also be applied directly to user-cooperative rehabilitation exercises which require active user participation in the exercises. The use of the assistance adaptation scheme means that the level of assistance provided by the robot will vary according to the capability of the user, thus allowing adaptive or assist-as-needed therapy which is widely believed to be beneficial in promoting recovery [4–7].

The developed system also has the capability to administer muscle strengthening or resistive exercises, and this can be achieved through the use of impedance control or explicit torque control. By defining a suitable robot impedance parameter and selecting a particular equilibrium position as the neutral position, the rehabilitation robot can be made to behave as a mechanical spring–damper unit which the user can work against. Using this set-up, ankle resistive exercises such as those which involve the use of elastic bands can be recreated on the rehabilitation robot. However, due to the system's ability to alter the impedance parameters and the neutral position of the developed system, a larger range of resistive exercises can be achieved. Another mode of resistive exercise that can be realised on the robot is the application of a constant resistive load to the user. This operation would require the use of pure torque control about the ankle joint, which can be accomplished on the developed system by setting the robot impedance to zero. Results obtained from

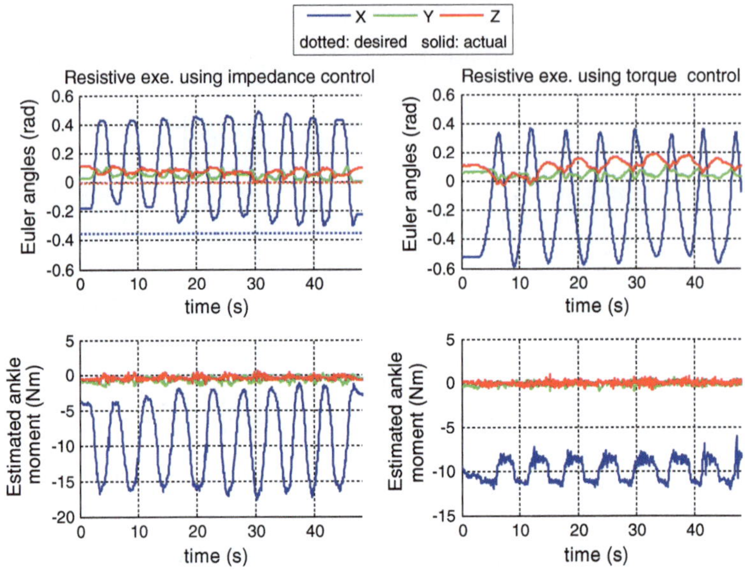

Fig. 9.25 Experimental trials showing the implementation of resistive exercises on the developed ankle rehabilitation robot through the use of impedance control and torque control

experimental trials involving the impedance-based and constant torque resistive exercises are shown in Fig. 9.25. The impedance-based resistive exercise involved the subject applying a moment at the ankle to resist the foot motion in the plantarflexion direction (positive X-direction). The torque control-based exercise on the other hand imposed a constant torque reference in the dorsiflexion direction, thus producing a resistive torque which opposed the user's plantarflexion movements.

9.6 Summary

This chapter presented the variable impedance control approach to achieve adaptive interaction control. The environment-based stiffness adaptation module is used to adapt the robot stiffness in proportion to the environmental compliance. Simulation and experiments using the proposed adaptation scheme show that the proposed robot impedance adaptation scheme does decrease the performance cost function which is computed as a weighted sum of applied moment and motion tracking error. This chapter presented the assistance adaptation scheme developed in this research to achieve adaptive interaction control. The assistance adaptation scheme is primarily used to produce a feed-forward moment which is fed into the interaction controller to provide additional assistance to the user. This scheme is based on a similar scheme proposed in Wolbrecht et al. [7], but modifications had been incorporated into the original control scheme to achieve additional control objectives.

References

1. L.J. Love, W.J. Book, Force reflecting teleoperation with adaptive impedance control. IEEE Trans. Syst. Man Cybern **34**, 159–165 (2004)
2. S. Babaci, Y. Amirat, J. Pontnau, C. Francois, Fuzzy adaptation impedance of a 6 d.o.f parallel robot. Application to peg in hole insertion. 1996, pp. 1770–1776
3. T. Tsumugiwa, R. Yokogawa, and K. Hara, Variable impedance control based on estimation of human arm stiffness for human-robot cooperative calligraphic task, in *International Conference on Robotics and Automation*, Washington DC, 2002, pp. 644–650
4. H.I. Krebs, J.J. Palazzolo, L. Dipietro, M. Ferraro, J. Krol, K. Rannekleiv, B.T. Volpe, N. Hogan, Rehabilitation robotics: performance-based progressive robot-assisted therapy. Auton. Robot. **15**, 7–20 (2003)
5. L. Marchal-Crespo, D.J. Reinkensmeyer, Review of control strategies for robotic movement training after neurologic injury. J Neuro Eng. Rehabil. **6**, 20 (2009)
6. M. Mihelj, T. Nef, R. Riener, A novel paradigm for patient-cooperative control of upper-limb rehabilitation robots. Adv. Robot. **21**, 843–867 (2007)
7. E.T. Wolbrecht, V. Chan, D.J. Reinkensmeyer, J.E. Bobrow, Optimizing compliant, model-based robotic assistance to promote neurorehabilitation. IEEE Trans. Neural Syst. Rehabil. Eng. **16**, 286–297 (2008)

Chapter 10
Conclusion and Future Work

Various aspects including the design, modelling and control of the platform-based rehabilitation robots developed in this research had been discussed in previous chapters. This book has presented an approach towards developing a neuromuscular interface, which is required for the effective interfacing between human operators and robotic devices, such as exoskeletons and prostheses. This chapter seeks to summarise the main outcomes and conclusions of this research, as well as highlight the contributions made in this work. Lastly, this chapter also provides a discussion of future directions that can be explored to extend or advance the work presented in this book.

10.1 Book Contributions

10.1.1 Human Musculoskeletal Models

10.1.1.1 Physiological Model of the Masticatory System

Previous methods have used pattern recognition techniques to identify categories of jaw movement [1, 2], but there are no developments on continuous movement prediction, even with a single degree of freedom. The physiological model of the masticatory system was therefore built from the ground up using the principles that were developed for the elbow model and is the first of its kind. The model is able to utilise the superficial mandibular muscles to predict continuous jaw motion with two DOFs, solely from the EMG signal activities of the muscles. The physiological model has a distinctive musculoskeletal component that has independent DOFs based on accessible EMG signal locations. The model can identify both vertical and lateral movement trajectories with average correlation coefficients as high as 0.74 for vertical movements. The physiological model of the masticatory system may be relevant to other multiple DOF joint systems, and it remains to be seen whether a similar approach of carefully considered model development depends on surface EMG signal accessibility and DOF identification.

S.(S.Q.) Xie, *Advanced Robotics for Medical Rehabilitation*,
Springer Tracts in Advanced Robotics 108, DOI 10.1007/978-3-319-19896-5_10

The hybrid model consists of a multiple DOF physiological model that has independent DOFs and an artificial neural network. This is the first implementation of a model that aims to maintain continuous movement prediction and movement type recognition, using only EMG signal inputs. Existing pattern recognition techniques are only able to offer discrete states or classes of movement [3, 4], while during development, physiological models were found to be significantly affected by the multiple roles a single muscle plays in movements. The effect was an average reduction of 15.6 % in the estimated position RMSE of the EMG-driven multiple DOF physiological model of the masticatory system where the performance of the physiological model by itself was compared to the performance of the physiological model and ANN combination in the hybrid model. The hybrid model therefore provides the structure and approach towards developing more sophisticated models that are capable of handling more complex movements.

The structure and function of the mandibular muscles has been thoroughly established in the available literature [5, 6]. Numerous EMG signal studies have also been conducted on the mandibular muscles to characterise them and understand their roles in mandibular movements and function [7–9]. To obtain a complete understanding of the masticatory system, these studies have involved both superficial and deep mandibular muscles [10]. The study of the superficial mandibular muscles found that the contributions of the masseters were in closing the jaw, and this can be supported by the existing literature. The study also verified that digastric activity could be identified under the chin, with the limited amount of space for bipolar electrode placement, and used to predict jaw opening. The most significant revelation of the study was the active role the anterior temporalis muscles play in lateral movements. Through ANOVA, it was shown that the temporalis muscles could be used to predict lateral movements. These findings were used to define the musculoskeletal component of the physiological model of the masticatory system, and it is only because of this study that the two DOFs of movement were identified and implemented with independent muscle actuation groups. The study therefore revealed characteristics of the mandibular muscles from a different perspective and also serves as an example that can be applied to other multiple DOF joint systems for DOF identification and musculoskeletal model development.

10.1.1.2 Analysis of Spherical Wrist Mechanisms in Shoulder Exoskeletons

In order to determine the potential issues of using a spherical wrist mechanism for the shoulder complex of an exoskeleton robot, an analysis of the 3R mechanisms used in the majority of past exoskeleton designs was carried out. This investigation highlighted major problems associated with singularity and mechanical interference of the mechanism with the user which restrict the exoskeleton's ability to operate in the shoulder workspace. These issues are caused by the exceptionally large range of motion of the human shoulder joint and are particularly challenging to solve.

Operating the mechanism at a singular configuration causes 1-DOF to be lost, making the exoskeleton unable to generate shoulder rotations about the lost axis. Furthermore, the mechanism's ability to rotate about this axis degrades as the mechanism approaches the singular configuration. Exoskeletons developed in the past that have considered singularity issues have only attempted to shift the singular configurations to regions of the workspace that are less commonly used by the shoulder and have not considered the reduction in performance near these configurations at all. For the exoskeleton designs with shifted singular configurations, analysis of mechanical interference between the exoskeleton and the user has revealed that parts of the 3R mechanism are required to operate dangerously close to the user's body in order to reach some regions of the shoulder workspace. Exoskeleton designs that have not shifted the singular configuration cannot raise the upper arm above the horizontal position at all as this will cause the 3R mechanism to collide with the user. In order to overcome both the singularity and mechanical interference problems, the use of a redundant 4R spherical wrist mechanism is proposed for use in the shoulder complex of an exoskeleton robot.

10.1.1.3 An EMG-Driven Physiological Model for the Elbow Joint

Previous interfacing methods were only able to identify discrete classes of movement after long training periods [11, 12], which limits the flexibility of an interface and restricts the versatility of the predicted movements. Some research groups have attempted to provide continuous profiles, but have resorted to enhancing the EMG signal by adding weight to the user's arm [13, 14], or employing additional sensors [15, 16]. This is unsuitable, particularly in applications with less-abled users. Other research groups have limited movement to the horizontal plane, where there are fewer forces to consider and the modelling of the system is easier, but the movements have less practical implications [17, 18]. Therefore, a physiological model that only uses the EMG signal and can identify continuous movement profiles of the elbow in the sagittal plane needed to be developed. The proposed EMG-driven physiological model for the elbow joint fills these gaps by using a unique neuromusculoskeletal structure of the elbow joint. The model consists of musculotendon, musculoskeletal and kinematic components and was able to predict the random movement of multiple subjects with a 22.4° RMSE average. This performance is comparable with previous works that focused on less complex movement trajectories [19–21]. The model's ability to handle novel movements will make it an integral element of neuromuscular interfacing approach provided that model parameters are appropriately identified and tuned.

10.1.1.4 Kinematic Parameter Estimation of Human Ankle

It had been widely reported in literature that the kinematics of human ankle is complex and can vary significantly between individuals. However, since such kinematic information can be used in the adaptation of the robot's behaviour as auxiliary variables that can be processed to adjust the robot controller parameters, this research had proposed a new online estimation algorithm based on the recursive least square filter to identify a subject-specific description of the ankle kinematics. It should be noted that while studies had been carried out to identify the kinematic parameters of a biaxial ankle kinematic model [22–24], such works had mainly utilised offline nonlinear least square methods. The proposed online estimation algorithm, driven by the need for it to be used in real-time control scheme, is therefore a new development in ankle kinematic parameter identification.

Due to its relatively simple structure, the biaxial ankle model had been identified as an ankle kinematic model that is well suited for online parameter identification. Two different online identification techniques, the extended Kalman filter (EKF) and the least mean square (LMS) method, had been considered for parameter estimation of the biaxial ankle model. A simulation-based comparison of the EKF and LMS approaches involving an ideal biaxial ankle model had shown that an EKF acting in the capacity of a recursive least square (RLS) estimator has the ability to produce the best estimation results in terms of estimation accuracy and parameter convergence. This approach had therefore been used in subsequent investigations done in this research.

As numerous studies had found the orientations of the ankle and subtalar axes in the biaxial ankle model to vary with foot orientation [25–28], the conventional biaxial ankle model with constant axis tilt angles had been extended in this research. The extension essentially allows the axis tilt angles of the biaxial model to vary with the foot configuration, and two variants of this extension had been proposed. The first version allows the axis tilt angles to vary linearly with respect to the ankle and subtalar joint displacements, while the second version varies the tilt angles according to the X and Y Euler angles used to describe the foot orientation. The feasibility of using the conventional biaxial ankle model and both the extended biaxial ankle models (with different axis tilt angle dependencies) in the RLS algorithm was also tested in a simulation study that utilised the first extended biaxial ankle model to generate the training data.

10.1.1.5 Computational Ankle Model for Controller Development

A computational ankle model in the form of a state space model had been derived in this research to facilitate the development and simulation of the robot control scheme. A three segmented rigid body model had been proposed together with the biaxial ankle kinematic constraint to reduce the computational complexity of the model, thus making it more suitable for controller simulations. Ligaments and muscle–tendon units had also been included in the model as force elements to allow monitoring of the tensions along these elements.

The developed model was validated through simulation studies involving both passive and active motions of the foot. It was found that the moment–displacement characteristic of the simulated foot along the flexion direction is largely in agreement with what is reported in literature, where larger ankle stiffness is found in the dorsiflexion direction. Simulations involving active muscular contractions also showed that activation of different muscle groups produced motion in the expected direction of motion, while also achieving movements within the typical motion limits of the human ankle. Data from an experimental trial had also been used to evaluate the validity of the developed computational model by feeding the moments computed from load cell measurements of the robot into the developed ankle model. Comparison of the simulated and actual ankle motion showed both motion trajectories to be similar in a qualitative sense for the pitch and roll directions, thus suggesting that a non-subject-specific ankle model can still be used to obtain a reasonable description of the ankle behaviour.

The computational ankle model developed in this research had been utilised in various ways to facilitate the design and implementation of the ankle rehabilitation robot. One such application is in the generation of rehabilitation trajectories. Such a problem had been studied in this research, and an optimisation-based rehabilitation trajectory generation routine which aims to minimise forces on ligaments/tendons as well as joint reaction moments had been proposed. In this context, the computational ankle model is used as a means for estimating the force and moment quantities considered in the objective function for a particular foot motion trajectory. It was found through simulation that the optimisation approach is capable of generating a trajectory with lower objective function value than the path of minimal distance between the desired start and end points. This suggests that the optimisation-based approach can potentially be used to tailor the rehabilitation trajectory according to a patient's specific condition.

In addition to trajectory generation, the developed ankle model had also been used to facilitate the development of the interaction control scheme used in this research. Apart from its obvious use in controller simulation, it had also been used to provide the ankle stiffness properties for stability analysis of the actuator force controller. Additionally, the ankle stiffness matrices derived from the model were also used to generate a lookup table for the robot impedance adaptation scheme.

10.1.2 Development of Rehabilitation Devices

10.1.2.1 A Neuromuscular Interface for the Elbow Joint

The implementation of the physiological model of the elbow joint on prototypal hardware platforms is the first step towards a physical interface between a human operator and robotic device, such as an exoskeleton or prosthesis. Such a physical interface does not exist, and there are limited existing approaches [13, 29, 30]. The neuromuscular interface uses physiological modelling principles, a modular architecture and unique communication protocols to acquire, filter and process the EMG signals. The interface was used by several subjects to successfully manipulate a single degree of freedom joint in real time, with RMSE as low as 13°, affirming the feasibility of the NI concept. The performance is comparable to that of existing exoskeletal interfaces [18, 21], and this has resulted in the filing of a provisional patent. Continued developments seek to improve the signal processing, hardware design and manufacturability, to further the commercial viability of the interface.

10.1.2.2 Optimal 4R Spherical Wrist Design for a Shoulder Exoskeleton

The proposed 4R spherical wrist mechanism is kinematically redundant, and consequently, a range of designs are possible which can achieve the entire shoulder workspace with adequate performance. In addition, the redundant 4R mechanism has infinite inverse kinematic solutions for achieving a given shoulder position. Thus, the NSGA II multi-objective optimisation algorithm was used to identify an optimal 4R design and the optimal operating configurations of the mechanism. The variables defined in the optimisation problem are used to determine the position of the base joint, the angle sizes of the three links in the 4R mechanism and the optimal operating configurations of the mechanism. The optimisation objectives are formulated with considerations for singularity, reachable workspace, interference and joint transition feasibility throughout the workspace. Analysis of performance was done for 89 uniformly distributed upper arm positions in the semi-spherical shoulder workspace. Singularity analysis was performed using the condition number of the mechanism's configuration. To measure a 4R design's singularity performance, the GCN was used to determine the average performance over the shoulder workspace and CN_{max} was used to determine the closest 4R mechanism that will operate to a singular configuration. The 4R mechanism's ability to reach the entire shoulder workspace is guaranteed. Mechanical interference between the 4R mechanism and its components or the user was carefully analysed and prevented. The movements of the 4R mechanism's joints were minimised to ensure they can transition feasibly and with minimal velocity throughout the shoulder workspace. An attempt was made to match the drift in the range of motion of the 4R mechanism joint that controls shoulder axial rotation to the drift in the range of motion of human shoulder axial rotation throughout the workspace.

10.1.2.3 5-DOF Active Upper Limb Exoskeleton System

The optimised 4R spherical wrist mechanism has been used in the design of a 5-DOF upper limb exoskeleton system. This exoskeleton is capable of performing 3-DOF spherical movements of the shoulder joint and 1-DOF movement of the elbow joint through the entire range of motion of a healthy adult's limb. Numerous considerations were made to ensure the exoskeleton design can achieve the required range of motion with adequate performance, is feasible to develop with the available resources and is user friendly. These considerations include size, weight, range of motion, velocity, torque, mechanical interference, cost, fabrication time, joint alignment, customisation for different users, options for future upgrades, ease of use, safety and noise pollution. The exoskeleton is supported by a mechanically grounded frame behind the user so that the user does not carry the weight of the exoskeleton but is instead supported by it. Length adjustments can be made to the exoskeleton structure to fit users with different arm lengths. The exoskeleton joint that controls shoulder axial rotation is implemented using a 120° curved rail encompassing the side of the upper arm which makes the exoskeleton easy to don and prevents mechanical interference issues. Each of the five joints in the exoskeleton is actuated by a compact brushless DC motor in combination with a reduction gearbox directly mounted onto the joints. Position feedback for the five exoskeleton joints is provided by rotary magnetic encoders, and force feedback is achieved using low-cost custom-built strain gauge force sensors at the hand and upper arm HRI. Numerous safety features are incorporated into the exoskeleton including mechanical stoppers to physically prevent the joints from extending beyond their standard range of motion, software to monitor the joint positions via the magnetic encoders and prevent the motor from driving the joint beyond the range of motion limits and emergency stop buttons to allow the exoskeleton user or an external user to manually stop the exoskeleton. Simulations confirm the complete exoskeleton system does not have mechanical interference issues when operating within the human workspace. A GUI has been developed for operating the exoskeleton.

10.1.2.4 Development of a Novel Ankle Rehabilitation Robot

A new parallel robot had been proposed and developed in this research for the rehabilitation of ankle sprain injuries. While there are several designs of platform-based robots used in ankle rehabilitation, the end effectors of these devices are typically constrained to rotate about a pivot which does not coincide with the human ankle's effective centre of rotation [31–35]. The design of this new robot therefore differs from most of these existing solutions in the sense that it is underactuated when the user's lower limb is not attached to the robot. This means that when in use, the user's lower limb will form part of the robot's kinematic constraint, thus ensuring that the motion performed by the robot is in line with the natural ankle–foot movements. Additionally, since movement of the shank is kept to a minimal level during operation, the robot can also estimate the relative orientation of the foot with respect to the shank with greater precision, thus allowing it to provide more repeatable rehabilitation movements and serve as a better measurement tool for evaluation of the ankle's mechanical characteristics.

The design of the device was based on workspace, singularity and force analyses which were, respectively, carried out to ascertain the motion limits of the robot, the controllability of the robot within its motion limits and the actuator forces required by the robot to produce the desired robot–foot interaction moments. By treating the ankle as a spherical joint capable of three degree of freedom rotational motion, it was found that singular regions will exist in the robot's reachable workspace if only three actuated links are used in the mechanism. More specifically, the reachable workspace will be bisected by a "surface" of orientations with ill-conditioned manipulator Jacobians, thus making the robot more difficult to control. The remedy to this issue was found through the use of a redundantly actuated mechanism by including an additional actuating link to the mechanism, which successfully eliminated these regions of large condition number in the robot's reachable workspace. In addition to the elimination of singularity in the workspace, the redundant actuation degree of freedom is also exploited in this work to allow regulation of the total vertical load applied to the ankle. To the best of the author's knowledge, this feature is not yet available in existing ankle rehabilitation devices, but can be beneficial to the treatment of ankle sprains by allowing emulation of different levels of weight bearing to suit the needs of the user.

Further analyses were also conducted to investigate the impact of uncertain ankle joint centre locations on the robot's capability to satisfy the design requirements. It was found that despite the application of conservative approaches in the workspace and singularity analyses, the desired range of motion and moment requirements are still largely satisfied by the proposed design. Additionally, it was also confirmed that this can be achieved with a good level of manipulability within the reachable workspace. The uncertainty in the ankle joint centre also presents a challenging problem for the control of the proposed ankle rehabilitation robot, particularly in the estimation of a correct foot configuration. A solution to this issue was proposed in this research through the use of redundant sensing which utilises additional pitch and roll measurements of the end effector to fully resolve the end-effector configuration of the robot.

10.1.3 Control Strategies for Robot-Assisted Rehabilitation

10.1.3.1 Smooth Trajectory Planner

In controlling the position of an exoskeleton, it is important to consider the velocities the joints move with in travelling to a target position to ensure the movement is smooth, comfortable and similar to normal human motion. It has been identified that typical human movements follow a minimum jerk trajectory where the rate of change in acceleration (jerk) is minimised throughout the trajectory. A trajectory planning algorithm based on the minimum jerk criterion has been developed for the joints in the exoskeleton. This requires an input of the target positions for the joints and the desired time for the joints to arrive at those positions. Implementation of this is fairly straightforward for the 1-DOF elbow joint since the movements of the exoskeleton joint translate directly to identical movements in the user's elbow joint. However, movements of the joints in the exoskeleton's spherical wrist shoulder mechanism have a nonlinear relationship with the movements of the user's shoulder joint. In other words, a minimum jerk trajectory of the joints in the 4R mechanism does not generate a minimum jerk trajectory for the user's shoulder.

Therefore, the minimum jerk trajectory is determined for the shoulder movement which is then converted to the respective trajectories of the 4R joints.

Due to the kinematic redundancy of the 4R mechanism, there are infinite inverse kinematic solutions as previously stated. To obtain a unique inverse kinematic solution, a set of optimal operating configurations for 89 upper arm positions in the workspace obtained during design optimisation is used. For an arbitrary target upper arm position, the optimal joint configuration is determined by interpolating the 89 known optimal configurations.

A method for combining a series of movements into a single smooth trajectory has also been developed, enabling the implementation of complex movements and task-based exercises. Changes in velocity along a trajectory path, temporarily remaining in a stationary position, reversals in movement direction and turning in shoulder movements can all be achieved by setting a sequence of target positions and the target times for reaching these positions.

10.1.3.2 Force-Based Interactive Control Strategies

Admittance and impedance control strategies have been implemented in the upper limb exoskeleton to allow it to interact and respond to movements generated by the user. A dynamic model of the system is developed with considerations for inertial, frictional and gravitational forces. Admittance control allows the user to assume control of movement such that the exoskeleton moves when pushed by the user's limb, enabling the exoskeleton to provide assistance or resistance to the user's movements. The impedance controller is used to impose a position for the user's limb with an adjustable artificial stiffness behaviour. A reduced stiffness allows user-generated forces to have a larger influence on the exoskeleton's position. Trajectory tracking can be implemented with an artificial stiffness to allow the exoskeleton to deviate from the trajectory path when a force is applied by the user's limb, thus producing an artificial compliance effect.

These types of responses to user-generated forces can be used for various types of rehabilitation applications. The difficulty level of rehabilitation exercises can be adjusted to suit users with different levels of disability by changing the amount of assistance or resistance provided by the exoskeleton.

10.1.3.3 MIMO Actuator Force Control

A prerequisite for the implementation of force-based impedance control is the availability of force/torque-controlled actuators. This, together with the need to regulate the robot vertical force in the redundancy resolution scheme, makes the development of an actuator force controller an essential aspect of this research. Due to the presence of higher order dynamics introduced by compliances in the actuator and force sensor, large force feedback gains will lead to system instability. The disturbance rejection capability of the force controller is therefore also capped by these gain limits, which are generally not uniform for coupled systems. A MIMO actuator force control had been proposed in this research to provide performance gains over independent force control along individual actuators. The proposed controller is capable of partial decoupling of the interactions between actuator forces and currents and was developed based on consideration of the stable gain limits imposed by higher order dynamics along different decoupled directions of the system.

Analyses carried out in this research had shown that motor current applied to one actuator does not exclusively affect the force output of that particular actuator due to the coupling imposed by the parallel mechanism's kinematic constraint and inertia. It was also found that allowable force feedback gain values are dependent on this coupling. These gain margins were determined to be dependent on the effective manipulator inertia along that particular decoupled direction. Based on this finding, a MIMO actuator force controller was proposed to allow improved force control performance by applying different force control gains along these decoupled directions. The major advantage that the proposed approach has over independent control of actuator forces (which uses uniform gains) is the application of larger gains along more stable decoupled directions. This can therefore improve force control performance along these decoupled directions and enhance the overall performance of the force-controlled system.

Simulation results had shown that the proposed MIMO force controller does outperform the uniform gain approach in terms of disturbance rejection. Additionally, it had also shown the proposed method to be more capable in improving the back-drivability of the mechanism by producing a more uniform (smaller condition number) effective robot inertia. Experimental results have also shown the MIMO approach to be more stable than the uniform gain approach, even when the highest gain used in the MIMO controller is larger than that of the uniform gain controller. Performance of the MIMO actuator force controller was also determined to be superior in experiments with significant reduction in force errors (approximately 50 %). However, due to the large actuator transmission ratios, a considerable level of friction still exists within the force-controlled mechanism, ultimately leading to task space moment errors in the vicinity of 1.5 Nm. This error, however, had been shown to remain relatively constant regardless of the level of desired moment. While the presence of this residual friction moment degrades the accuracy and back-drivability of the robot, it will not lead to serious safety concerns as this level of friction can be easily overcome by the user.

10.1.3.4 Adaptive Interaction Control

Interaction control is crucial for any rehabilitation robots as it takes into account both force and motion of the robot to facilitate human–robot interaction. While most of the existing ankle rehabilitation devices are capable of some basic form of interaction control, these control schemes are typically non-adaptive. This research therefore aims to enhance the safety and functionality of existing ankle rehabilitation robots through the incorporation of adaptive interaction control schemes. Adaptability was incorporated in this work through two channels, first by adjusting the robot stiffness parameters according to the environmental compliance and second by implementation of an assistance adaptation scheme to vary the assistance provided by the robot according to the user's capability.

A gain-scheduled scheme for robot stiffness adjustment had been proposed in this research. This scheme is based on the result obtained in [36] which states that the weighted sum of position error and actuating effort can be minimised by selecting the robot impedance to be proportional to the environmental admittance. Following this rule, the proposed scheme adjusts the robot stiffness by first identifying the ankle compliance with the aid of a lookup table and then scaling the compliance by a proportionality constant to yield the final robot stiffness. This lookup table is constructed using the computational ankle model, and the auxiliary variables used for the gain scheduling are those of the ankle and subtalar joint displacements estimated from the ankle kinematic model parameters provided by the online identification of the biaxial ankle model. By applying this adjustment rule, the robot was able to trade off positional accuracy for lower interaction moments, thus preventing application of large forces/moments at stiff foot configurations.

Simulation results had shown the proposed adjustment scheme to be effective, with large reductions in the cost index for the controller with stiffness adaptation. The efficacy of the stiffness adaptation had also been evaluated through experimental trials. However, although use of the adaptive controller still resulted in a lower cost index than the constant impedance controller, the relative difference was considerably smaller. This is most likely due to discrepancies between the model and actual foot stiffness, as well as to the presence of friction within the mechanism. Even so, the behaviour of the robot with stiffness adjustment showed that larger movements were allowed when the foot is moving in the more compliant supination direction, while actuator efforts were reduced in the stiffer pronation direction. This shows that the proposed stiffness adjustment scheme can still be used to produce the general desired behaviour even with mismatched model and actual foot stiffness. Additionally, the results also suggest that the proposed scheme should be used with a feed-forward moment to allow greater movements in stiff direction without resorting to the increment of the robot stiffness.

An assistance adaptation scheme was also proposed in this research. This control scheme is based on the feed-forward force adaptation strategy given in [37] but includes additional modifications designed to improve the robot's performance during constrained and active motion. The central idea of the proposed assistance adaptation scheme is to increase the assistive moments applied to the foot according to the position tracking error in a positively correlated manner up until a certain error threshold, while also reducing the assistance over time. Additionally, the incremental work done by the robot is also monitored, and the robot stiffness is adjusted in such a way that it will not act along the reference direction of motion when a negative incremental work with large magnitude is observed. The stability analysis used in [37] was also extended in this work to accommodate the changes made to the error dependency function and the inclusion of the work-based stiffness adaptation module. Lastly, the final module of the assistance adaptation scheme operates in a similar way as the feed-forward moment adaptation rule, but is instead applied to modify the reference trajectory.

A simulation case study had been carried out on a two degree of freedom point mass moving in a two-dimensional potential field. Different scenarios were simulated involving the combination of passive/active and constrained/unconstrained motions. Three error dependency functions (linear, saturated and parabolic) were tested in the adaptation of the feed-forward moment in the simulations, and it was found that while the alternative approaches (saturated and parabolic) produced slightly poorer tracking accuracy in unconstrained motion, the feed-forward forces observed from these alternative approaches during constrained motion were considerably smaller than the rule with linear error dependency. Lastly, simulations involving the trajectory modification module have shown that it is capable of maintaining a low level of feed-forward forces during constrained motion, even when a linear error dependency function is used in the feed-forward force adaptation law. Results of the simulation study therefore suggest that each of the proposed modification to the basic assistance adaptation scheme can either contribute to improved safety (by reducing forces when large position errors are observed) or reduce the resistance to constructive active motion.

Similar findings were also obtained from the consideration of experimental data involving the use of the developed ankle rehabilitation robot. In particular, the original assistance adaptation scheme used in [37] was shown to be effective in providing assistance as required to improve the tracking accuracy of the robot. However, it was also found that its use can lead to large moments in stiffer environments and that utilisation of the alternative error dependency functions in the adaptation rule can help alleviate this issue. Additionally, evaluation of the work-based stiffness adjustment module in experimental reaching movements had shown that activation of this control module did indeed reduce the level of resistance provided by the robot, both in terms of smaller negative incremental work and lower resistive moments, when the subject was moving ahead of the reference trajectory. The experimental results therefore confirmed the applicability of the proposed assistance adaptation scheme in rehabilitation.

10.2 Outlook and Future Work

10.2.1 Design Optimisation and Improvement

10.2.1.1 Improve Components of Existing System

The present exoskeleton is the first-generation prototype, and much of the exoskeleton system was developed using components that were chosen because of their low-cost or short development time rather than their suitability for an upper limb rehabilitation exoskeleton. The current exoskeleton structure is constructed almost entirely from aluminium plates which were fabricated by water jet cutting. Due to the limitations in the shapes of structural members that can be constructed using only plates, the size of these structural members is larger than is necessary. The member shapes are also not specifically designed to support the loads they are required to carry so twisting and bending of the exoskeleton structure occur. The use of better designed structural members using a stronger material can reduce the size and weight of the current exoskeleton system and improve its rigidity. In addition, the gearboxes used in the exoskeleton system are large and heavy. Four of the five current gearboxes use multi-stage reduction planetary gears which occupy a large amount of space. The size and weight of the gearbox can be reduced significantly if harmonic drives [38] are used instead. Designing a custom actuator specifically for the exoskeleton may also reduce the size and weight of the system.

10.2.1.2 Higher DOF Exoskeleton

The current exoskeleton system is capable of moving the shoulder spherically in 3-DOF and the elbow in 1-DOF flexion and extension movement. It was identified in Chap. 3 that the upper limb has 9-DOF from the shoulder to the wrist. To allow the exoskeleton to perform all possible movements of the upper limb, mechanisms for moving the remaining 5-DOF need to be added to the exoskeleton system. The most important movements to implement next are the 3-DOF spherical movements of the human wrist joint as these movements pay an important part in controlling the position of the hand. A 3R spherical wrist mechanism can be used for this joint since the range of motion of the human wrist is much smaller compared to the shoulder and it is not difficult to design the 3R mechanism to avoid singular configurations within the workspace of the wrist. The current exoskeleton has been designed with this upgrade in mind and has a forearm link that can be easily replaced with a new mechanism. Afterwards, further additions to the exoskeleton's DOF can be the 2-DOF translation movements of the shoulder joint and grasping motion for the fingers.

10.2.1.3 Human–Robot Interfaces

In the current exoskeleton system, the only interaction between the exoskeleton and its user is the mechanical force interaction at the hand and upper arm HRI. These interfaces were made using plastic parts fabricated from a 3D printer with little consideration of the user's comfort. They should have an ergonomic design and be made from a soft material that is comfortable for the user to touch. The ideal locations of the upper limb to transfer mechanical forces should also be studied. Mechanical interfaces in regions with a high pain tolerance can improve the user's safety and comfort, while attachments on stable body structures with low compliance improve load transfer between the exoskeleton and the human limb.

Apart from HRI for force transfer, other methods of interaction between the exoskeleton and its user can be used to increase the exoskeleton's capabilities. The exoskeleton can communicate with the user using haptic vibrations on the user's skin. Functional electrical stimulation can be used to electrically activate the user's muscles during rehabilitation exercises. Conversely, electrodes can be used to measure EMG signals from the user's muscles to determine the user's movement intent. The locations for these HRI will also need to be carefully considered to ensure effective interaction.

10.2.1.4 Design Optimisation and Improvement

One of the main issues compromising the performance of the developed ankle rehabilitation robot is the relatively large actuator friction. Consequently, further development of the ankle rehabilitation robot should involve a re-evaluation of the suitability of existing linear actuators, with an emphasis on decreasing the transmission ratio to reduce the effective frictional forces. However, this must be done in conjunction with the stability analysis of the force controller to ensure that reduction in effective actuator mass does not compromise system stability. An alternative solution is to modify the design of the robot in terms of the robot kinematic parameters, and this will lead to changes in singular values of the manipulator Jacobian, which will then propagate to changes in the singular values of the effective robot inertia matrix and hence will ultimately lead to modifications in gain limits of the MIMO actuator force controller. Ideally, a design optimisation problem which takes into account the workspace, singularity, force requirements, force control stability and spatial constraints can be formulated and solved to synthesise the most suitable robot kinematic parameters.

Additionally, since one of the error sources for the kinematic estimation algorithm is believed to be the unmeasured motion between the foot and shank with the ankle rehabilitation robot, improvements can also be made on the foot and shank braces to minimise unwanted motion to allow more accurate measurements of the relative orientation between the user's foot and shank and thus allow the applicability of the extended biaxial ankle model to be evaluated in greater detail.

10.2.2 Further Investigation of Human Models

10.2.2.1 Neuromuscular Interface Based on EMG

It is hoped that the utilisation of NIs will undergo continued development and extend beyond what was demonstrated for the elbow joint. During the course of the work that culminated in this book, design challenges and modelling difficulties were encountered, but also a better understanding of the nature and characteristics of the EMG signals was developed. The measurement of the signal is relatively straightforward, and it is easy to see the corresponding changes in the signal when a subject contracts their muscle. The influence of noise makes this a challenge, and subject, muscle and physiological variability (e.g. fatigue) only compound the problem of trying to identify specific muscle activation levels. It is believed that the interface will need to be adaptable to be able to accommodate such variability, and this adaptability will stem from online tuning algorithms that continuously adjust the behaviour of the model in accordance with the variability.

The advantage of the generation of a continuous movement profile that does not require training data is very appealing, but the sensitivity of the model to muscle cocontractions may trump its practical usefulness. The hybrid model is an attempt to make use of the best of both training- and tuning-based methods, and it is difficult to say how effective it is at providing a user with intuitive control, given at this stage it has only been validated offline. It is anticipated that there will be difficulties in tuning the model and identifying the most effective way to adjust parameters online to account for the amount of variability in the EMG signal. The hybrid model therefore requires further testing in real time, and the continuation should involve an investigation with multiple subjects—first with the hybrid model on its own, followed by implementation on hardware in a neuromuscular interface, as was conducted for the elbow joint. The real-time requirements of the intended end systems suggest that substantial effort and care will eventually need to go into optimising hardware specifications and processing times.

10.2.2.2 Further Investigation of Kinematic Estimation Algorithm

As discussed previously, results of the kinematic estimation algorithm are influenced by the rather large experimental errors which arise from unmeasured movements of the foot and shank during operation of the ankle rehabilitation robot. While these errors can be reduced through design improvements of the ankle rehabilitation robot, a more complete evaluation of the capability of the algorithm and the suitability of the underlying biaxial ankle kinematic model can only be done in a more controlled environment. Future work can therefore involve the use of cadaveric studies and/or optical tracking-based methods to identify the precise 6-DOF motion of the foot bones. Comparison of offline nonlinear system identification techniques and the proposed online algorithm on the more accurate measurements can then be used to establish the true efficacy of the proposed algorithm. Additionally, an online estimation algorithm which takes into account both foot orientation and translation can also be implemented and included in the future study to identify any trade-offs between simpler model and estimation accuracy.

10.2.2.3 Customisation of Computational Ankle Model

The computational model used in this research was developed based on generic information of muscles, tendons and ligaments. Although the surface geometry of the foot bones used in this research was obtained from CT scans, it is a publicly available data set and was not specific to the subject who participated in the experimental trials. The points of origin and insertion for different ligaments and tendons were also determined in accordance with anatomical resources through visual identification of bony landmarks on the available foot bone surface model. Due to the non-subject-specific nature of the computational ankle model, it cannot be expected to be able to accurately replicate the actual foot behaviour. While the "generic" computational model appeared to provide the behaviour required in the adjustment of the robot stiffness parameters in a qualitative sense, a more accurate model will be able to afford a better approximation of the ankle stiffness and thus improve the robot performance. Additionally, a subject-specific model will also be important in the generation of rehabilitation trajectory as it will be able to offer a more precise prediction of tensions along the force elements.

Further development of the ankle model presented in this research should therefore include the design of a streamlined process for incorporating patient specific data into the computational model. While it is difficult to ascertain the parameters of muscles, tendons and ligaments in an in vivo manner, information on bone surface geometry and force element attachment points should be more readily accessible through the use of medical imaging techniques. The graphical user interface developed in this research can therefore be extended to facilitate the translation of the medical imaging data into the required origin/insertion point coordinates. The axes of rotations of the biaxial ankle model can also be obtained through either inspection of foot bone geometry or parameter identification of the subject's ankle. Furthermore, the biaxial ankle model with variable axis tilt angles can also be incorporated into the computational ankle model if it were found to be applicable in the more detailed kinematic investigations.

A more meaningful evaluation of rehabilitation trajectories can also be done once a more subject-specific ankle model is established. Even though the tensions along the force elements and joint reaction moments are not directly measurable, the interaction forces between the robot and foot can be used to partially evaluate the effectiveness of the trajectory generation algorithm in an experimental study.

10.2.2.4 Disability Evaluation

Assessing disability of the upper limb is a complex task, and numerous measures of stroke severity and functional ability have been proposed in the past. These disability measures often utilise a scoring system which is performed using subjective methods. Examples include the Barthel Index (BI) for measuring a patient's performance in activities of daily life [39] and the Fugl-Meyer (FM) assessment for measuring patient recovery [40]. These assessments are performed by having the physiotherapist who gives a score to indicate how well a patient performs a movement or task. However, the information obtained from these subjective methods only provides a rough impression of the patient's disability and cannot be reliably used to compare between results [41].

An exoskeleton can make quantitative measures of patient-generated parameters such as interaction force and EMG signals during movement. This information can be used to obtain a detailed objective evaluation of individual joints and muscle groups in the patient's limb. The ability to obtain a detailed disability assessment can improve identification of the patient's problems, allow treatment intervention to be optimised according to the patient's condition, allow reliable comparison between disability assessment results and improve the quality of rehabilitation research. Objective evaluations of disability have largely been left unexplored in the past due to the lack of suitable tools; therefore, no protocols are currently available for exoskeleton-based evaluations. New guidelines will need to be developed through collaboration with physiotherapists to create a new protocol for objective evaluations that utilise the new exoskeleton tools. Objective evaluations will make rehabilitation studies more reliable which in turn will allow mankind to gain a better understanding of the human neuromuscular system and to determine the optimal rehabilitation treatment for different disability conditions.

10.2.3 Advanced Adaptive Interaction Controllers

10.2.3.1 Integration Between Human Operator and Robotic System

Further work is required to improve both the physiological model of the masticatory system and the hybrid approach and concept. Alternative multiple DOF joint systems may be targeted, such as the shoulder, which provide more accessible EMG signal electrode locations and larger underlying muscles with stronger signals. Removing EMG signal limitations would allow improvements to the modelling approach and focus on identifying the interactions between DOFs and superficial muscle groups for physiological model improvement. This would also provide another case study to test the flexibility of the neuromuscular interfacing approach and one that is more relevant to existing literature and devices.

The influence of the ANN in the hybrid model is simplistic, and while it still provides a positive effect to the model output, further work is required to improve the sophistication of its involvement in the model. The additional flexibility may allow the model to respond better and accommodate additional DOFs without much difficulty. Other pattern recognition techniques besides ANNs may also be considered as these may prove to be easier to train to allow for more flexibility when movements involve simultaneous DOFs. It is suggested that fuzzy methods may be suitable for this.

Finally, the hardware is in an early prototypal stage, and there is plenty of room for specialised improvement. This would be in the analogue filtering circuitry and processing electronics. Improving power requirements and circuitry footprints using technologies such as CMOS would also assist in reducing size and weight of the overall hardware, making it easier to embed within existing systems and much more practical to implement.

10.2.3.2 Task-Based Exercises

The human upper limb requires coordination and precise control for manipulation tasks as opposed to the lower limb which requires strength to support the body's weight. Therefore, the rehabilitation exercises for the upper limb should be designed to work on the joints' precision and control with a task-oriented approach. The ability to implement task-based exercises is an important feature of exoskeletons as these exercises are difficult to implement with conventional rehabilitation techniques that are based on hands-on methods. Exoskeletons are capable of accurately controlling multiple joints simultaneously, enabling them to produce realistic task-based exercises for the patient. The difficulty of the exercises can also be adjusted to suit different levels of disability. Task-based exercises can be incorporated into virtual games to provide a more enjoyable rehabilitation experience, thus motivating the patient to put more effort into the exercises. This will in turn accelerate the patient's rate of recovery.

In this research, the tools to implement various types of exercises have been developed in the form of the smooth trajectory planner, admittance controller and impedance controller, but specific exercises have yet to be formulated. The exercises should be developed through collaboration with physiotherapists to create highly effective exercises.

In the future, this concept can potentially be extended to teach healthy individuals more sophisticated movements such as those in sports or occupational tasks. In the entertainment sector, exoskeletons can provide a more interactive gaming experience in which the movement of the player's arm can be mimicked by the arm of a game character and the physical interactions of the game character can be felt by the player through the exoskeleton.

10.2.3.3 MIMO Actuator Force Control Design

The MIMO actuator force controller developed in this research is based on the analysis of a simplified actuator–robot–environment system. As a result, the gains selected from this approach can still be unstable for the actual system if the uncertainties assumed in the robustness analysis are in fact less than what is observed in the real system. This has been observed during simulation of the basic impedance control scheme. A more complete approach must therefore be used in the design of the MIMO force controller. This can involve the use of constrained optimisation techniques which seek to maximise the controller gains, while at the same time ensuring that robust stability is achieved when the full manipulator model is considered. The simplified approach can still be used to obtain a good starting point for the optimisation, and the controller can follow a similar structure as that proposed (i.e. parameterised by four gains acting along the principal directions of the coupling matrix) to reduce the dimensionality of the optimisation problem.

In addition to an investigation into the controller optimisation problem, different control structures along each principal direction can also be explored. In other words, alternative filters such as lead–lag controller can be used in place of the PD filter to increase the gain margin along the considered principal direction. This can be done by taking into account the frequency response along different principal directions. Last but not least, application of feed-forward friction compensators can also be explored to further improve the actuator force control performance.

10.2.3.4 Further Investigation of Adaptive Interaction Controller

Further work can also be done on the adaptive interaction control scheme proposed in this research to improve its performance. As the current environment-based stiffness adaptation scheme used in this research is reliant on the accuracy of a lookup table which is generated from consideration of the computational ankle model, its performance is dependent on the model accuracy. An alternative method which can be used to bypass the need of the ankle model is the online identification of foot stiffness. This approach can, however, be challenging due to the real-time requirements and the fact that ankle stiffness varies with respect to muscle activation. Consequently, online estimation of passive ankle stiffness will only be feasible if information on both the ankle active stiffness and the leg muscle activation levels is available. Implementation of such an estimation scheme will therefore require the robot to be capable of measuring and processing the electromyography signals of the leg muscles. Additionally, investigations into the relationship between muscle activation and ankle stiffness must be carried out.

While Lyapunov stability of the feed-forward force adaptation rule with work-based stiffness adjustment had been established in this chapter, the resulting stability conditions are overly conservative due to the consideration of worst-case scenarios. Further investigation into the stability of this proposed scheme is therefore required in order to obtain a necessary and sufficient stability condition which can be used as a better guideline to select the parameters in the adaptation rules. Additionally, as stability of the trajectory modification module has yet to be proven, efforts should also be made into identifying the associated stability criterion so that the reason behind the high-frequency oscillations observed in the experiments involving the use of this trajectory modification algorithm can be studied in more detail. Further development can also be made on the work-based stiffness adaptation scheme to obtain a smoother transition between the negative work phase (when robot stiffness is reduced along the direction of reference motion) and its complementary phase (when stiffness of the robot is returned to its nominal value) to reduce abrupt changes in the forces being applied to the foot.

Last but not least, further effort should also be placed into identifying the most suitable controller parameters for different rehabilitation exercises, and in the development of a higher level supervisory controller which automatically determines the gains required according to a given type of rehabilitation exercise and information regarding the maximum permissible moments/forces. This is important to enhance the usability of the system for healthcare professionals, who may not be familiar with the significance of different controller parameters.

10.3 Summary

This book has presented an approach towards developing a neuromuscular interface, which is required for the effective interfacing between human operators and robotic devices, such as exoskeletons and prostheses. The tools and algorithms developed throughout this book have helped to address several key limitations and requirements in realising a robot for human limb rehabilitation. Fundamental algorithms for smooth trajectory planning and force-based interactive control have been developed and can be used to implement sophisticated rehabilitation exercises. A new platform-based ankle rehabilitation robot was developed in this research with the aim of facilitating physical therapy of sprained ankles. The major works carried out are identified as as follows: development of an online identification algorithm for the biaxial ankle kinematic model; derivation of a rigid body-based computational ankle model to facilitate development of the robot interaction controller; development of a MIMO actuator force controller to realise force-based impedance control; and development of an adaptive interaction control scheme which allows the robot to adapt its behaviour to the foot configuration and user capability.

References

1. B. Fu, Classification of multi-channel EMGs for jaw motion recognition by signal processing and artificial neural networks. Master's thesis, The University of British Columbia, 2004
2. C.L. Long, Pattern recognition using surface electromyography of the anterior temporalis and masseter muscles. Master's thesis, The University of British Columbia, 2004
3. A. Smith, E.E. Brown, Myoelectric control techniques for a rehabilitation robot. Appl. Bion. Biomech. **8**(1), 21–37 (2011)
4. E. Scheme, K. Englehart, B. Hudgins, Selective classification for improved robustness of myoelectric control under nonideal conditions. IEEE Trans. Biomed. Eng. **58**(6), 1698–1705 (2011)
5. W.E. McDevitt, Functional anatomy of the masticatory system (Butterworth & Co., 1989)
6. A.G. Hannam, A.S. McMillan, Internal organization in the human jaw muscles. Crit. Rev. Oral Biol. Med. **5**(1), 55–89 (1994)
7. E. Kemsley, M. Defernez, J. Sprunt, A. Smith, Electromyographic responses to prescribed mastication. J. Electromyogr. Kinesiol. **13**(2), 197–207 (2003)
8. G.M. Tartaglia, G. Lodetti, G. Paiva, C.M.D. Felicio, C. Sforza, Surface electromyographic assessment of patients with long lasting temporomandibular joint disorder pain. J. Electromyogr. Kinesiol. **21**(4), 659–664 (2011)
9. J. Ahlgren, D.P. Lipke, Electromyographic activity in digastric muscles and opening force of mandible during static and dynamic conditions. Eur. J. Oral Sci. **85**(2), 152–154 (1977)

10. K. Hiraba, K. Hibino, K. Hiranuma, T. Negoro, EMG activities of two heads of the human lateral pterygoid muscle in relation to mandibular condyle movement and biting force. J. Neurophysiol. **83**(4), 2120–2137 (2000)
11. M. Pang, S. Guo, Z. Song, Study on the sEMG driven upper limb exoskeleton rehabilitation device in bilateral rehabilitation. J. Robot. Mechatron. **24**(4), 585–594 (2012)
12. Z.O. Khokhar, Z.. Xiao, C. Menon, Surface EMG pattern recognition for real-time control of a wrist exoskeleton. BioMed. Eng. Online **9**(41) (2010)
13. E. Cavallaro, J. Rosen, J. Perry, S. Burns, B. Hannaford, Hill-based model as a myoprocessor for a neural controlled powered exoskeleton arm—parameters optimization, in *Proceedings of the 2005 IEEE International Conference on Robotics and Automation (ICRA)*, April 2005, pp. 4514–4519
14. Q. Ding, X. Zhao, A. Xiong, J. Han, A novel motion estimate method of human joint with EMG-driven model, in *5th International Conference on Bioinformatics and Biomedical Engineering (iCBBE)*, May 2011, pp. 1–5
15. H. Kawamoto, T. Hayashi, T. Sakurai, K. Eguchi, Y. Sankai, Development of single leg version of HAL for hemiplegia, in Annual International Conference of the IEEE Engineering in Medicine and Biology Society (EMBC), Sept 2009, pp. 5038–5043
16. K. Kiguchi, S. Kariya, K. Watanabe, K. Izumi, T. Fukuda, An exoskeletal robot for human elbow motion support-sensor fusion, adaptation, and control. IEEE Trans. Syst. Man Cybern. B Cybern. **31**, 353–361 (2001)
17. D. Kistemaker, A. Van Soest, M. Bobbert, A model of open-loop control of equilibrium position and stiffness of the human elbow joint. Biol. Cybern. **96**(3), 341–350 (2007)
18. P. Artemiadis, K. Kyriakopoulos, EMG-based position and force control of a robot arm: Application to teleoperation and orthosis, in *EEE/ASME International Conference on Advanced Intelligent Mechatronics*, Sept 2007, pp. 1–6
19. A. Au, R. Kirsch, EMG-based prediction of shoulder and elbow kinematics in able-bodied and spinal cord injured indviduals. IEEE Trans. Rehabil. Eng. **8**(4), 471–480 (2000)
20. T.K. Koo, A.F. Mak, Feasibility of using EMG driven neuromusculoskeletal model for prediction of dynamic movement of the elbow. J. Electromyogr. Kinesiol. **15**(1), 12–26 (2005)
21. L. Smith, L. Hargrove, B. Lock, T. Kuiken, Determining the optimal window length for pattern recognition-based myoelectric control: balancing the competing effects of classification error and controller delay. IEEE Trans. Neural Syst. Rehabil. Eng. **19**(2), 186–192 (2011)
22. A.C. Satici, A. Erdogan, V. Patoglu, Design of a reconfigurable ankle rehabilitation robot and its use for the estimation of the ankle impedance, in *International Conference on Rehabilitation Robotics* (2009), pp. 257–264
23. A.J. van den Bogert, G.D. Smith, B.M. Nigg, In vivo determination of the anatomical axes of the ankle joint complex: an optimization approach. J. Biomech. **27**, 1477–1488 (1994)
24. G.S. Lewis, H.J. Sommer, S.J. Piazza, In vitro assessment of a motion-based optimization method for locating the talocrural and subtalar joint axes. J. Biomech. Eng. **128**, 596–603 (2006)
25. C.H. Barnett, J.R. Napier, The axis of rotation at the ankle joint in man; its influence upon the form of the talus and the mobility of the fibula. J. Anat. **86**, 1–9 (1952)
26. J.R. Engsberg, A biomechanical analysis of the talocalcaneal joint—in vitro. J. Biomech. **20**, 429–442 (1987)
27. D.M. Demarais, R.A. Bachschmidt, G.F. Harris, The instantaneous axis of rotation (IAOR) of the foot and ankle: a self-determining system with implications for rehabilitation medicine application. IEEE Trans. Neural Syst. Rehabil. Eng. **10**, 232–238 (2002)
28. N. Ying, W. Kim, Determining dual Euler angles of the ankle complex in vivo using "flock of birds" electromagnetic tracking device. J. Biomech. Eng. **127**, 98–107 (2005)
29. B. Li, EMG detection system and design. Adv. Mater. Res. **488–489**, 1011–1015 (2012)
30. I. Moon, M. Lee, M. Mun, A novel EMG-based human-computer interface for persons with disability, in *Proceedings of the IEEE International Conference on Mechatronics (ICM)*, June 2004, pp. 519–524

31. J.A. Saglia, N.G. Tsagarakis, J.S. Dai, D.G. Caldwell, Control strategies for ankle rehabilitation using a high performance ankle exerciser, in *IEEE International Conference on Robotics and Automation* (2010), pp. 2221–2227
32. J. Yoon, J. Ryu, K.-B. Lim, Reconfigurable ankle rehabilitation robot for various exercises. J. Rob. Syst. **22**, S15–S33 (2006)
33. J.A. Saglia, N.G. Tsagarakis, J.S. Dai, D.G. Caldwell, A high-performance redundantly actuated mechanism for ankle rehabilitation. Int. J. Rob. Res. **28**, 1216–1227 (2009)
34. J. Yoon, J. Ryu, A novel reconfigurable ankle/foot rehabilitation robot, in IEEE International Conference on Robotics and Automation, Barcelona, Spain (2005), pp. 2290–2295
35. G. Liu, J. Gao, H. Yue, X. Zhang, G. Lu, Design and kinematics simulation of parallel robots for ankle rehabilitation, in *IEEE International Conference on Mechatronics and Automation, Luoyang, China* (2006), pp. 1109–1113
36. N. Hogan, Impedance control: an approach to manipulation: Parts I, II and III. J. Dyn. Syst. Meas. Contr. **107**, 17–24 (1985)
37. E.T. Wolbrecht, V. Chan, D.J. Reinkensmeyer, J.E. Bobrow, Optimizing compliant, model-based robotic assistance to promote neurorehabilitation. IEEE Trans. Neural Syst. Rehabil. Eng. **16**, 286–297 (2008)
38. Harmonic Drive LLC. Available: http://harmonicdrive.net/
39. D.T. Wade, C. Collin, The Barthel ADL index: a standard measure of physical disability? Int. Disabil. Stud. **10**, 64–67 (1988)
40. D.J. Gladstone, C.J. Danells, S.E. Black, The Fugl-meyer assessment of motor recovery after stroke: a critical review of its measurement properties. Neurorehabilitation Neural Repair **16**, 232–240 (2002)
41. W.K. Anemaet, Using standardized measures to meet the challenge of stroke assessment. Top. Geriatr. Rehabil. **18**, 47–62 (2002)

Appendix A
Physiological Model of the Elbow in MATLAB/Simulink

This section contains a complete description of the implementation of the physiological model of the elbow joint in the MATLAB/Simulink environment. The highest level of the Simulink block model diagram is shown in Fig. A.1. The inputs to the model are from two MATLAB data files: data.mat, which contains the raw EMG signal data from the biceps and triceps muscles, and the motion data from the Polaris Spectra optical tracking system; and tuning.mat, which contains the tuned parameter values for a particular subject. The outputs of the Simulink model include the predicted movement from the physiological model, the actual movement measured by the tracking system and the error between the two values (used to determine RMSE). The submodel EMG Model contains the physiological model and is shown in Fig. A.2. The subsystems of the model have been grouped according to their function (in red), and their structure and purpose will be described in the remainder of this section.

A.1 Subsystem A

This subsystem performs the LEP of the raw EMG signals from the biceps and triceps muscles. The block model is shown in Fig. A.3 and it outputs the normalised activation level of both muscles.

S.(S.Q.) Xie, *Advanced Robotics for Medical Rehabilitation*,
Springer Tracts in Advanced Robotics 108, DOI 10.1007/978-3-319-19896-5

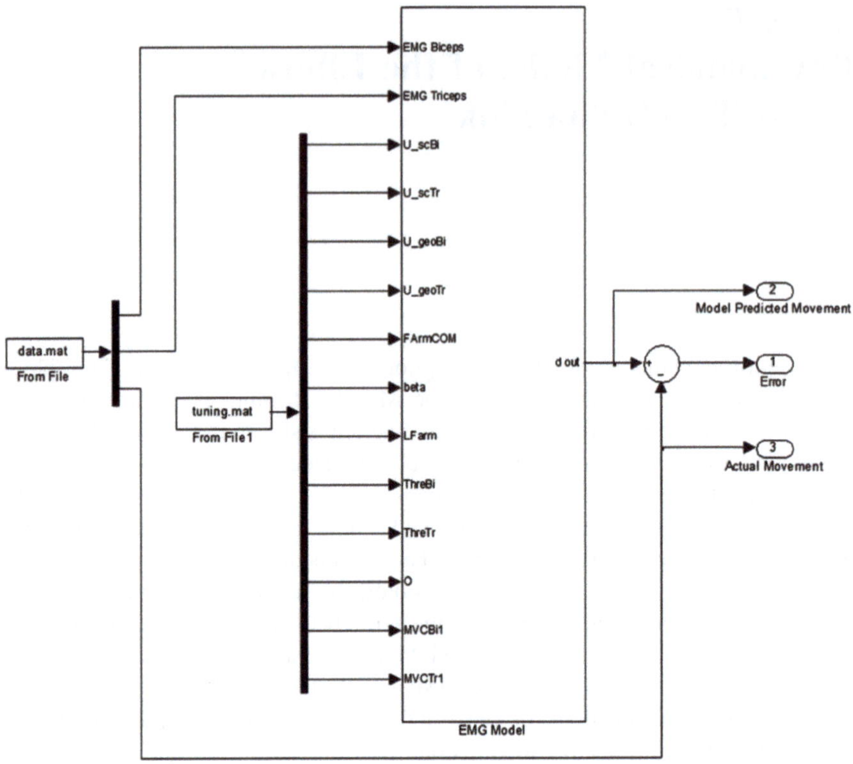

Fig. A.1 Top level view of the elbow joint Simulink model

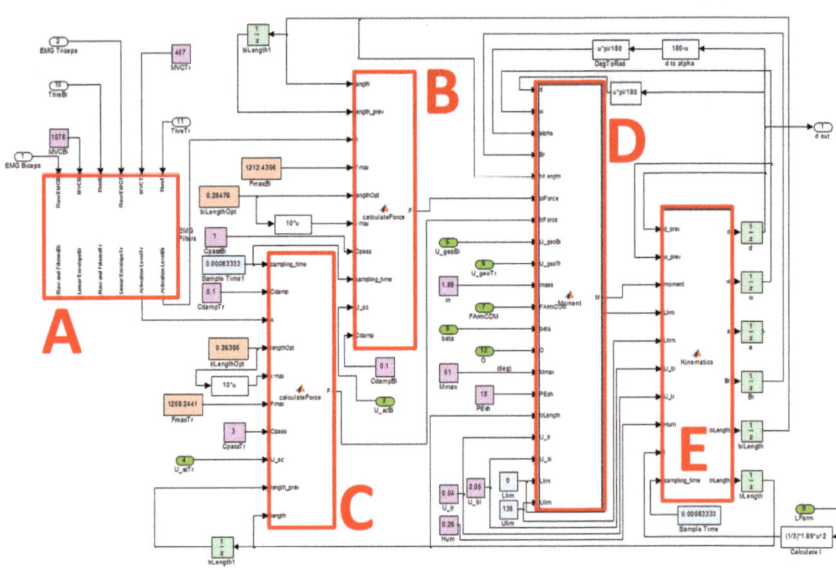

Fig. A.2 Physiological model block diagram in Simulink

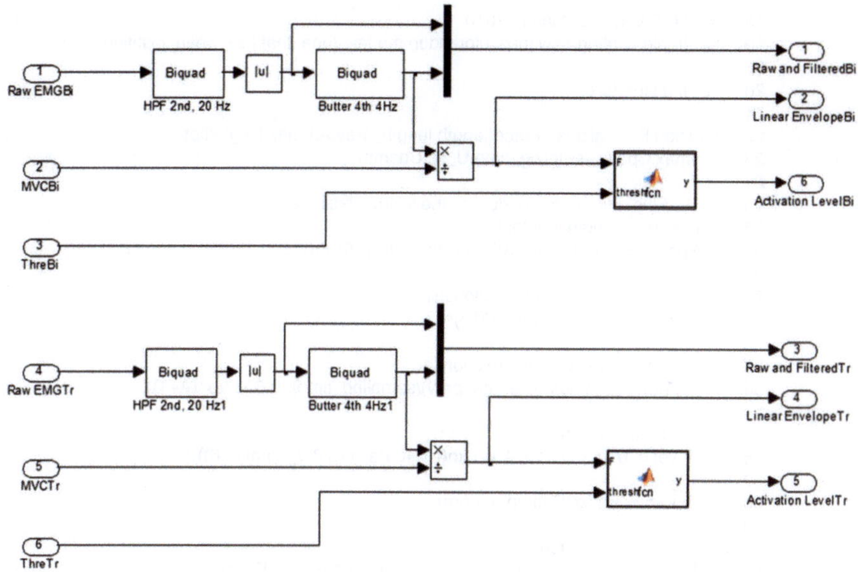

Fig. A.3 EMG signal processing subsystem

A.2 Subsystems B and C: The Musculotendon Model

These subsystems are identical with B for the biceps group and C for the triceps group. The parameters for the model are passed into the embedded MATLAB function from the Simulink model. The code for the function is shown below:

```
% This function is a generic method for calculating the force of a muscle
% given its activation level and physical properties. The function should
% be able to be used with any muscle given that the relevant properties
% have been defined. This includes the input arguments shown below. The
% output of the function is total muscle force.

    % A    activation level
    % length      current muscle length
    % lengthMax   maximum muscle length
    % lengthOpt   optimal muscle length
    % Fmax        maximum muscle force
    % Cpass       tendon stiffness
    % U_sc        muscle size

  % Author: James Pau
  % Date: 11 November 2009

```

```
% UPDATE: 23 March 2010
% Implementing new musculotendon model (one that has been justified from
% the literature)

function F = calculateForce(length,length_prev,A,Fmax,lengthOpt,...
    vmax,Cpass,sampling_time,U_sc,Cdamp)

    % Find passive force due to the tissue elasticity
    l_norm = length/lengthOpt;
    Fpass = exp(Cpass*10*(l_norm-1))/exp(5)*Fmax;

    % Find force-length relationship
    F_leng = 1 - ((l_norm-1)/0.5)^2;

    % Find force-velocity relationship
    v_norm = ((length - length_prev)/sampling_time)/(0.5*vmax*(A+1));

    % From Rosen
    F_vel = 0.1433/(0.1074 + exp(-1.409*sinh(3.2*v_norm+1.6)));

    F_visc = Fmax*Cdamp*v_norm;

    % Find total force
    F = U_sc * Fmax * A * F_leng * F_vel + Fpass + F_visc;
```

A.3 Subsystem D: Musculoskeletal Model

```
% This function calculates the moment generated at the elbow joint. The
% function is joint specific because it depends on the geometry of the
% joint and number of active muscle groups (in this case two). The input
% arguments to the function are the forces calculated using calculateForce
% and joint geometries.

% Author: James Pau
% Date: 13 November 2009

% UPDATE: 6 March 2010
%- Changed inputs to suit use in Embedded MATLAB function

% UPDATE: 8 March 2010
```

```
% - Fixed calculation of 'beta' and 'bicep' (previously was Uln, rather
% than U_bi)

% UPDATE: 17 March 2010
% - Add component to moment calculation that takes into account gravity
% - Update block inputs to support the change

% UPDATE: 10 March 2011
% - Added alternative passive joint torque calculation from Lemay and Crago

function M = Moment(d,w,alpha,Br,biLength,biForce,trForce,U_geoBi,...
U_geoTr,mass,FArmCOM,beta,O,Mmax,PEsh,trLength,U_tr,U_bi,Llim,Ulim)

% Find moment arm momentArmBi between bicep group and joint CoR
momentArmBi = U_bi * sin(Br) * U_geoBi;

a = (trLength^2+(U_bi+U_tr)^2-biLength^2)/(2*trLength*(U_bi+U_tr));

% Check that no incorrect rounding has occurred before using acos
if a < -1
a = -1;
end
tr =ACOS(a);

% Resulting moment arm
momentArmTr = U_tr * sin(tr) * U_geoTr;

% Moment due to weight of forearm
M_w = -mass*9.81*cos(alpha - pi/2)*FArmCOM;

% Calculate moments
M_bi = momentArmBi * biForce;
M_tr = -momentArmTr * trForce;

% Passive arm moment
M_damp = -beta*w;

% Total moment
M = M_bi + M_tr + M_w + M_damp + 0.25;
```

A.4 Subsystem E: Kinematic Model

Implementation of the kinematic model.

```
% This function uses the moments calculated in calculateMomentElbow and
% elbow geometry to determine the kinematics of the elbow joint. This is
% joint specific but may be adapted for other joints and if possible, a
% generic function may be developed in future.

% Author: James Pau
% Date: 13 November 2009

% UPDATE: 6 March 2010
% - Altered input parameters to suit use in embedded MATLAB fcn

% UPDATE: 17 March 2010
% - Added repulsive component to angle for reaching upper limit

% UPDATE: 10 March 2011
% - Cleaned up the code and added comments
% - Corrected the limiting function to stop erratic behaviour in velocity
% and acceleration outputs

function [d,w,a,Br,biLength,trLength] = Kinematics(d_prev,w_prev,...
moment,Llim,Ulim,U_bi,U_tr,Hum,I,sampling_time)

% Angular displacement and velocity can be determined via acceleration

% Angular acceleration = moment/moment of inertia
a = moment/I;

% Angular velocity
w = w_prev + a * sampling_time; % rad/s

% Angular displacement. Note that d_prev, and lims are in deg
d_rad = d_prev*pi/180 + sampling_time *...
(w_prev + 0.5 * sampling_time * a);

% Check that a physical limit has not been reached and
% if it has, limit the position
if d_rad _ Llim*pi/180
d_rad = Llim*pi/180;
```

```
w = 0;
a = 0;
elseif d_rad _ Ulim*pi/180
d_rad = Ulim*pi/180;
w = 0;
a = 0;
end

% Output new values
d = d_rad*180/pi; %degrees

% Geometric model update
alpha = pi - d_rad;
biLength = sqrt(U_bi^2 + Hum^2 - 2 * U_bi * Hum * cos(alpha));
temp = (U_bi^2 + biLength^2 - Hum^2)/(2*U_bi*biLength);
% Correct any rounding errors cause values to be >1
if temp > 1
temp = 1;
end
Br = acos(temp);
trLength = sqrt(biLength^2 + (U_bi+U_tr)^2 - ...
2*biLength*(U_bi+U_tr)*cos(Br));

end
```

Appendix B
Optimal 4R Mechanism Configurations

Optimal 4R mechanism configurations were obtained for reaching 89 uniformly separated upper arm positions in the workspace during the optimisation process. The 89 optimal configurations for the left shoulder are presented in this appendix (Figs. B.1, B.2 and B.3; Table B.1).

B.1 Motor Requirements

In the selection of a specific motor actuator for each of the five joints in the upper limb exoskeleton, multiple factors are considered including performance, range of motion, weight, size, back-drivability and cost. The performance requirements are torque and velocity which are approximated by considering slightly extreme scenarios of human upper limb movement.

The assumed velocity requirement for the shoulder and elbow joints is half a revolution per second or 30 rpm which is reasonably fast compared to movements

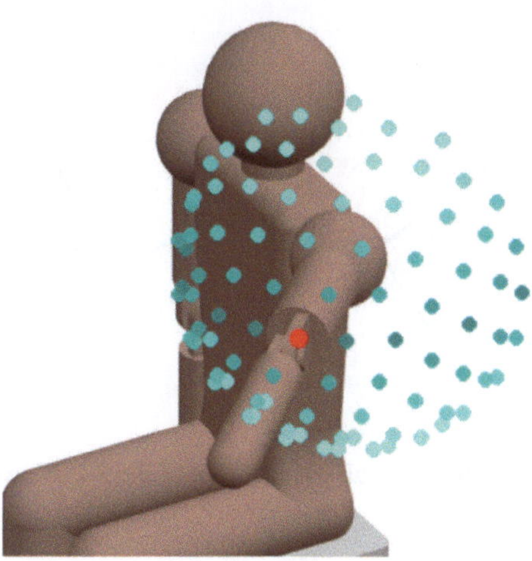

Fig. B.1 The 89 uniformly separated points in the workspace of the *left shoulder*

S.(S.Q.) Xie, *Advanced Robotics for Medical Rehabilitation*,
Springer Tracts in Advanced Robotics 108, DOI 10.1007/978-3-319-19896-5

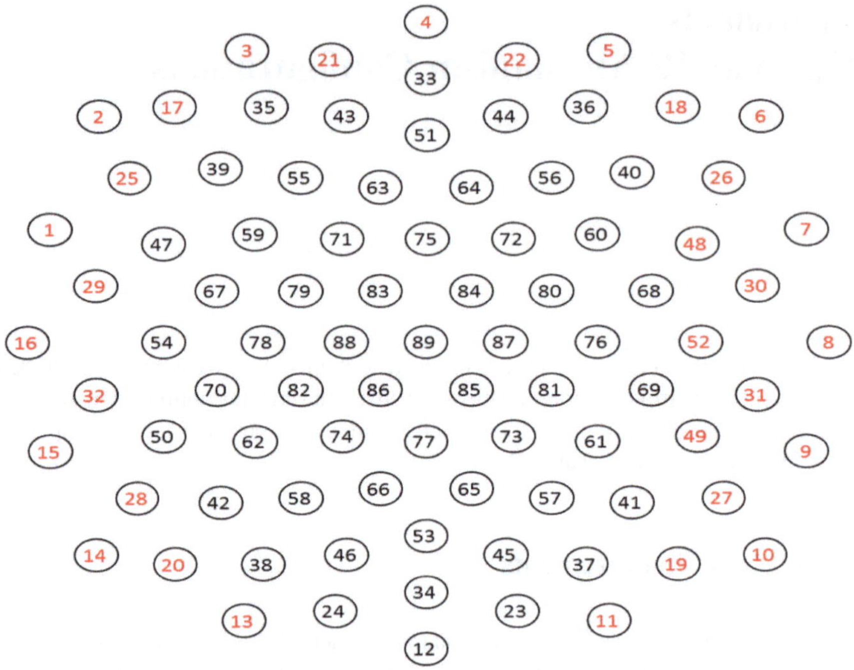

Fig. B.2 Numbers assigned to the 89 workspace points. The *red points* are not used in the GUI for operating the exoskeleton as they are considered dangerous for the user

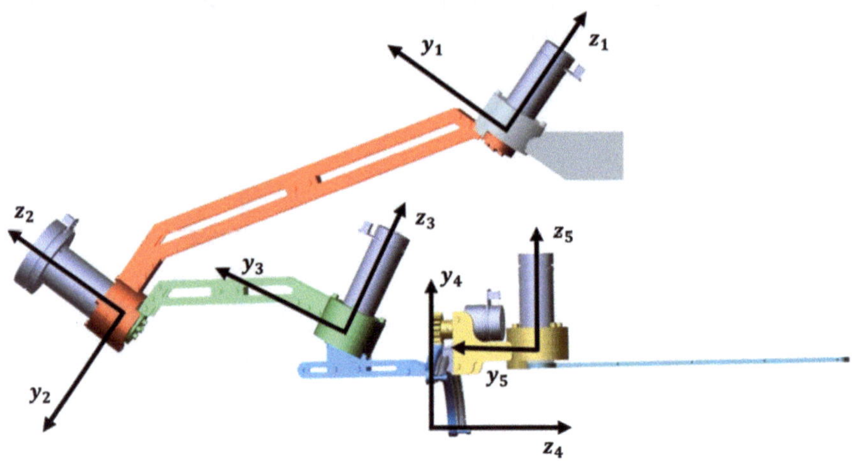

Fig. B.3 Default configuration of the 5-DOF exoskeleton

Table B.1 Optimal joint angles for reaching the 89 workspace points

Point	th1	th2	th3	Point	th1	th2	th3
1	90.3	58.2	42.1	46	159.5	107.5	95.3
2	90.0	36.4	48.8	47	110.9	53.7	56.2
3	85.0	3.0	69.7	48	178.8	−1.5	94.2
4	107.4	−26.4	74.4	49	189.5	28.3	105.9
5	116.3	−48.5	100.0	50	118.6	92.4	59.8
6	165.4	−38.0	110.9	51	127.2	−2.6	78.2
7	180.5	−24.0	117.6	52	184.2	12.8	101.0
8	199.6	−5.8	113.9	53	170.2	92.1	103.9
9	213.3	11.6	108.4	54	113.1	73.3	57.1
10	219.2	27.5	108.2	55	115.0	20.5	71.6
11	220.1	55.4	113.8	56	148.9	−7.1	87.7
12	187.4	110.3	122.8	57	179.0	63.4	111.2
13	142.3	138.3	78.5	58	147.0	101.5	82.5
14	104.1	123.4	43.0	59	118.6	41.0	66.0
15	94.2	102.1	38.3	60	164.3	4.0	89.4
16	90.4	79.6	39.4	61	179.2	44.5	105.2
17	91.2	21.1	64.5	62	134.9	90.7	71.3
18	148.5	−35.3	103.8	63	127.7	13.9	75.4
19	210.5	44.1	111.2	64	139.2	3.3	82.1
20	124.4	126.0	62.1	65	169.8	75.7	103.0
21	102.2	−7.7	72.8	66	157.3	89.6	93.4
22	125.8	−30.1	83.7	67	120.5	59.7	62.8
23	200.1	81.1	118.1	68	173.5	13.6	94.2
24	166.7	120.9	102.1	69	177.5	28.5	101.6
25	100.5	45.9	51.6	70	125.8	78.5	64.8
26	182.3	−16.9	96.6	71	129.0	30.5	72.4
27	203.9	28.0	107.6	72	150.6	11.3	85.1
28	111.6	107.3	52.5	73	168.3	59.8	101.9
29	100.2	65.9	48.9	74	147.1	83.4	83.8
30	193.8	−4.0	99.4	75	139.3	20.4	79.0
31	200.5	12.3	104.1	76	167.5	28.6	95.0
32	104.6	89.7	47.5	77	159.7	72.8	93.0
33	120.6	−15.2	75.1	78	131.0	63.6	70.1
34	177.4	102.1	112.5	79	130.0	47.1	70.6
35	101.0	11.1	70.3	80	159.8	19.9	89.5
36	146.8	−25.4	89.7	81	167.5	44.1	99.3
37	200.0	61.3	112.3	82	137.8	74.5	76.5
38	144.3	119.5	81.2	83	139.0	39.4	78.1
39	105.5	31.9	62.6	84	150.0	29.3	84.7
40	164.6	−15.0	93.1	85	159.6	54.3	91.8
41	193.5	44.7	110.9	86	148.5	65.4	84.1
42	129.5	109.0	66.7	87	157.5	38.2	91.1
43	114.6	3.5	73.1	88	140.0	55.9	77.9
44	136.5	−15.1	83.0	89	149.0	47.3	84.7
45	181.0	80.1	114.1				

Table B.2 Actuator requirements

Exoskeleton joint	Requirements	
	Velocity (rpm)	Torque (Nm)
1	30	7.7
2	30	28.2
3	20	17.1
4	20	10.4
5	30	10.2

in performing common tasks. This velocity requirement of 30 rpm is assumed for Joints 1, 2 and 5 for simplicity. The actual velocity requirements of Joints 1 and 2 in the 4R mechanism will be similar to this value for a shoulder rotation velocity of 30 rpm since the 4R mechanism is optimised to operate far away from singular configurations. Due to the smaller range of motion of Joints 3 and 4, the velocity requirement for these two joints is approximated as 20 rpm.

The torque requirement considers the weight which the joint needs to support as well as the potential torque applied by the user's limb. The torques caused by inertia, Coriolis and centrifugal effects are small since the exoskeleton operates at low accelerations and velocities and therefore are not considered in the torque requirement calculations. Firstly, the joint torque caused by the weight of the exoskeleton components and the user's upper limb is considered. Since the weight of the exoskeleton–upper limb system shifts during operation, simulation of a 3D CAD model of the exoskeleton in Creo Parametric is used to estimate the maximum torques that occur for each joint. These occur when the upper limb is lifted to a straight horizontal position. Next, the user-generated torque is approximated by applying a 25 N force at the hand position of the horizontally positioned limb. The load torque caused by the weight of motors and gearboxes chosen for distal joints are also considered in the calculation. The approximated requirements of joint velocity and torque are provided in Table B.2.

Note that the estimated torque requirement of Joint 1 is smaller than all the other joints even though it is supporting more components. This is because the axis of rotation of Joint 1 is constantly tilted resulting in a reduced component of gravitational torque acting about the joint axis. In addition, the majority of the exoskeleton mass is near the vertical plane intersecting the axis of Joint 1 during operation; therefore, the horizontal perpendicular distance to the centre of mass is small (Fig. B.4). Joint 2 has a large estimated torque requirement because the axis of rotation of Joint 2 can enter a near horizontal position during operation which maximises the load carried by the joint. Furthermore, the exoskeleton structures supported by Joint 2 tend towards one side of the joint axis (Fig. B.5). This also applies to Joint 3 which also has a relatively large torque requirement.

The torque and velocity output of a motor are inversely proportional; therefore, the actuator requirements in Table B.1 refer to the exertion of torque while operating at the specified velocity. A motor can exert a larger torque than the nominal

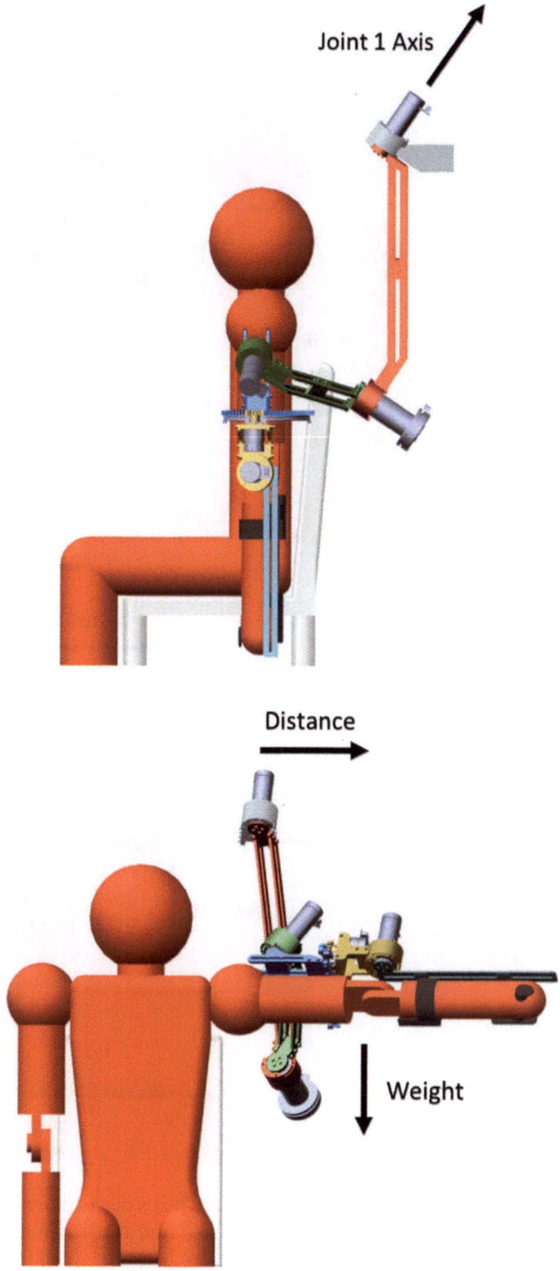

Fig. B.4 The moment acting about Joint 1 axis due to gravitational forces is relatively small due to the large angle between the Joint 1 axis and the horizontal plane and the short perpendicular distance to the weight of the system

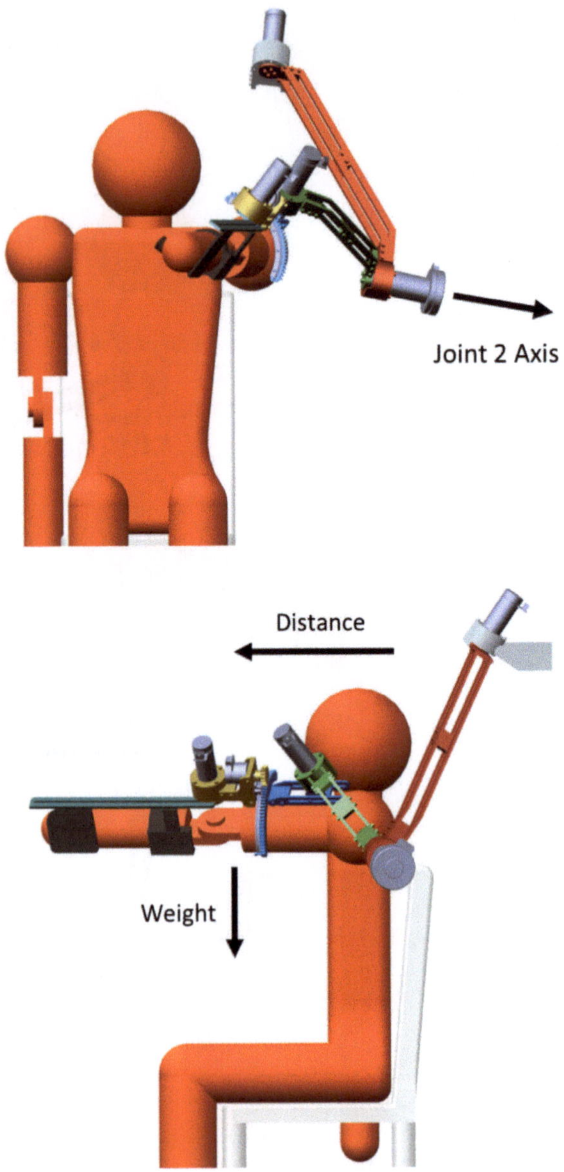

Fig. B.5 The moment acting about Joint 2 axis due to gravitational forces is relatively large due to the small angle between the Joint 2 axis and the horizontal plane and the large perpendicular distance to the weight of the system

Table B.3 Specifications of the motor–gearbox units

Joint	Motor–gearbox combination		Nominal gearbox output	
	Maxon motor	Gearbox (r:1)	Speed $\dot{\theta}_{nom}$ (rpm)	Torque τ_{nom} (Nm)
1	EC 45 Flat 50 W 24 V	156:1 planetary	33.7	9.3
2	EC 90 Flat 90 W 24 V	91:1 planetary	28.8	29.0
3	EC 45 Flat 50 W 24 V	319:1 planetary	16.5	16.9
4	EC 45 Flat 50 W 24 V	47:1 spur	111.7 (18.6[a])	3.0 (18.0[a])
5	EC 45 Flat 50 W 24 V	156:1 planetary	33.7	9.3

[a]Values after a further reduction of 6:1 by the Joint 4 rail mechanism

torque if it is running slower than the nominal velocity and can run at a higher velocity than the nominal velocity if the exerted torque is lower. The exoskeleton is not expected to operate the motors at both the required torque and velocity simultaneously. Therefore, the torque and velocity requirements are an overestimation and are only used as a guideline during motor selection. The weight and especially size of the motors are also important to ensure the motors can fit in the limited space in the exoskeleton structure.

B.2 Motor Selection

The motors chosen to actuate each of the five exoskeleton joints are Maxon 24V brushless DC motors in combination with reduction gearboxes (Maxon Motor, Switzerland). These motors are back-drivable and have a special flat design which allows them to be mounted directly at the exoskeleton joints without causing interference problems. Maxon ESCON controllers are used to drive each motor.

The motor–gearbox combinations are carefully selected for each joint (see Table B.3) to ensure the required output torque and velocity specified in Table B.2 can be achieved. Due to the high torque and low speed requirement of the exoskeleton joints, a high reduction ratio is required from the gearboxes. The gearboxes used for Joints 1, 2, 3 and 5 are planetary gearboxes with three stages of reduction for Joints 1, 2 and 5 and four stages of reduction for Joint 3. A spur gearbox with three stage reduction is used for Joint 4.

In addition, the weight and size of each motor–gearbox unit are also considered in conjunction with the structural design of the exoskeleton to ensure they can be mounted directly at the exoskeleton joints without interfering with the movements of the exoskeleton. Interference analysis is done by simulating a 3D CAD model of the exoskeleton system in Creo Parametric. In particular, extra attention was made in selecting the motor–gearbox units and designing the exoskeleton structure for Joints 3 and 4 since attaching the motor–gearbox unit onto these joints most likely causes interference. A motor–gearbox unit on Joint 3 can interfere with Link 1 (the link between Joint 1 and Joint 2) when it overlaps with Link 2 (the link between Joint 2 and Joint 3) as shown in Fig. B.6a. The structure of Links 1 and 2 is

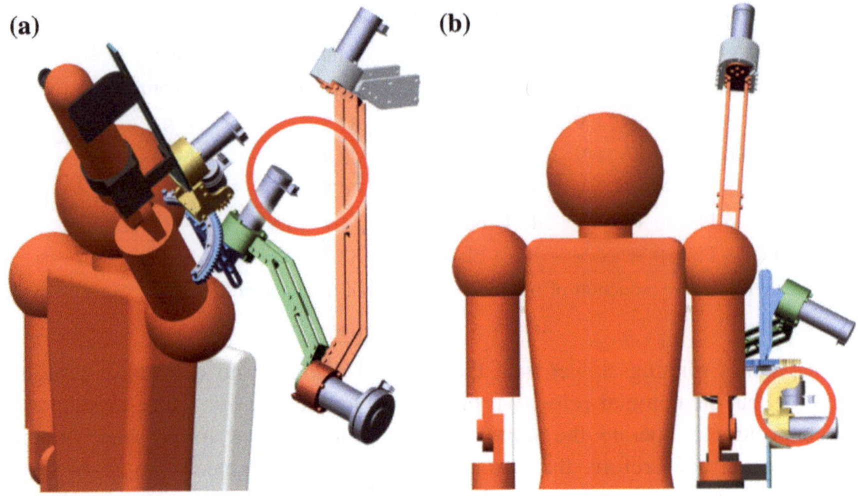

Fig. B.6 Potential occurrences of mechanical interference **a** between Joint 3 motor and Link 1 and **b** between Joint 4 motor and Joint 5

carefully designed to ensure this interference does not occur. In the case for Joint 4, there is very limited space available for the Joint 4 motor–gearbox unit since the motor–gearbox unit of Joint 5 is mounted nearby (Fig. B.6b). Therefore, a small-sized spur gearbox is selected to combine with the motor of Joint 4 instead of the larger planetary gearbox used for the other motors.

The nominal output torques and velocities of the chosen motor–gearbox units in Table B.3 are all similar or better than the approximated requirements in Table B.2. The motor–gearbox unit for Joint 3 has the largest underperformance when compared to the proposed requirements. Although a larger motor–gearbox unit would improve the performance for Joint 3, the weight of the motor–gearbox unit will increase which means the motors of Joints 1 and 2 will also need to be more powerful. Furthermore, since the motor–gearbox unit of Joint 3 can interfere with Link 1 as discussed earlier, a larger motor will require the link designs to be modified in a way which will further increase the load on Joints 1 and 2. Also, the nominal output torque and velocity are the maximum output when the joint is generating both the torque and velocity output simultaneously. This will rarely occur in the exoskeleton since its usage will often involve low velocities when a high load is applied or vice versa. The chosen motor–gearbox combination for Joint 3 is the best compromised solution after considering all the trade-offs.

B.3 Sensors

Angular position encoders pre-installed onto the motors are available, and this is a convenient option, however this cannot measure the angular displacement of the gearbox without knowing its position when the system starts up. Instead, absolute encoders are installed onto the exoskeleton joint to measure the angular displacement of the joint directly. This is achieved using AMS magnetic rotary encoders (AMS, Austria). These are high-resolution absolute encoders which measure a displacement angle relative to a pre-programmed zero position.

Force measurement is achieved using custom-made force sensors comprising of RS strain gauges attached to a specially designed aluminium load structure. This is a low-cost alternative to the otherwise very expensive commercial force sensors. Each axis of force measurement uses a pair of strain gauges, one on each side of the load structure (Fig. B.7). A force applied to the end of the load structure causes it to bend resulting in compression of one strain gauge and extension of the other. This results in an increase in electrical resistance of the strain gauge under extension and a decrease in resistance for the strain gauge under compression. The use of a pair of

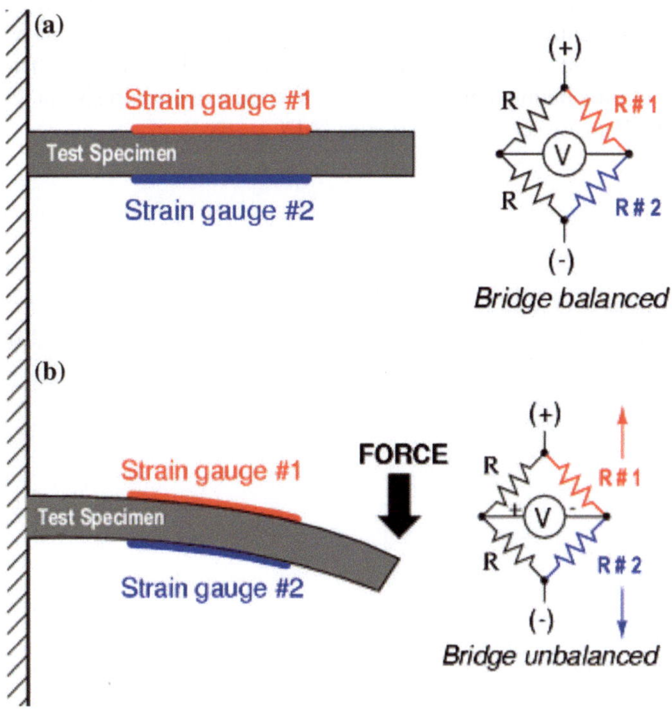

Fig. B.7 Force sensing method. **a** Load specimen with no force applied. The Wheatstone bridge is balanced and the output voltage is zero. **b** Load specimen with force applied. The Wheatstone bridge is unbalanced and the output voltage is a function of the applied force

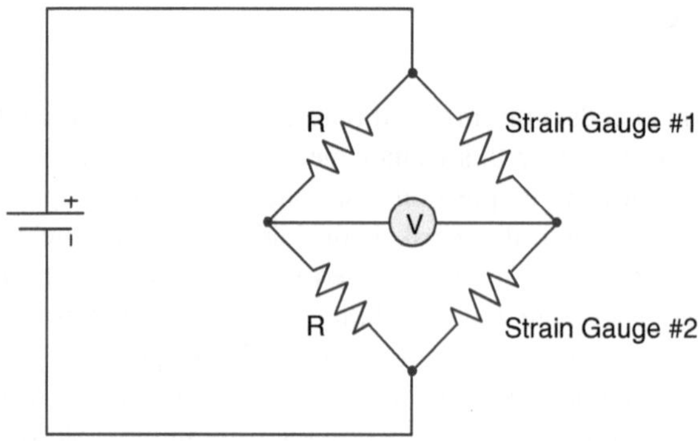

Fig. B.8 A pair of strain gauges in a Wheatstone bridge in half-bridge configuration used in the force sensor

strain gauges instead of one increases the sensitivity and compensates for changes in resistance due to temperature. The load structure is designed so that the strain gauges deform only when force is applied in the axis it is measuring and experience negligible deformation from force applied orthogonal to this axis.

The pair of strain gauges is incorporated in a Wheatstone bridge circuit in half-bridge configuration (Fig. B.8). This circuit uses the change in resistance to generate an output voltage difference. This voltage difference is then amplified using an instrumentation amplifier and is converted to a noise-resistant digital signal using an I2C analog-to-digital converter (ADC).

Appendix C
Supplementary Material on Robot Design Analysis

This appendix contains additional information on the design analysis of the ankle rehabilitation robot. This includes the test conditions used to establish the maximum actuator force requirements. Additionally, it also provides a summary of additional results on workspace, singularity and force analysis for three linked designs with different parameters.

C.1 Test Conditions for Force Analysis

The actuator force requirement was computed for different designs based on application of different moments in different end effector configurations. Table C.1 provides a summary of configuration–moment pairing considered in force analysis.

Table C.1 Configuration–moment pairings used in force analysis

End effector orientation in *XYZ* Euler angles (°)			Applied moments along the Euler angle axes (Nm)		
θ_x	θ_y	θ_z	τ_x	τ_y	τ_z
0	0	0	±100	±40	∓40
0	0	0	±100	0	0
0	0	0	0	±40	0
0	0	0	0	0	±40
40	20	−30	±100	±40	∓40
−40	−20	30	±100	±40	∓40
40	0	0	±100	0	0
0	20	0	0	±40	0
0	0	30	0	0	±40
−40	0	0	±100	0	0
0	−20	0	0	±40	0
0	0	−30	0	0	±40

S.(S.Q.) Xie, *Advanced Robotics for Medical Rehabilitation*,
Springer Tracts in Advanced Robotics 108, DOI 10.1007/978-3-319-19896-5

C.2 Simulation Parameters for MIMO Actuator Force Control

Table C.2 provides a summary of the parameters used in the analysis and simulation of the MIMO actuator force controller.

Table C.2 Parameters used in simulation and analysis of the MIMO actuator force controller

Description	Symbol	Value/expression
Motor rotational inertia	J_m	4.2×10^{-6} kg m^2
Motor viscous damping	b_m	2.6×10^{-6} Nm s/rad
Motor torque constant	K_t	0.0365 Nm/A
Belt stiffness	k_b	1×10^6 N/m
Belt viscous damping	b_b	5 N s/m
Motor pulley radius	r_m	0.004 m
Ball screw rotational inertia	J_s	1.15×10^{-6} kg m^2
Ball screw viscous damping	b_s	1×10^{-6} Nm s/rad
Ball screw pulley radius	r_s	0.02 m
Ball screw transmission ratio	G_s	$\frac{2\pi}{0.003175}$ rad/m
Actuator rod mass	m_r	0.2 kg
Actuator rod viscous damping	b_r	0.05 N s/m
Force sensor mass	m_f	0.2 kg
Force sensor stiffness	k_f	15×10^6 N/m
Force sensor damping	b_f	2500 N s/m
Derivative gain	K_d	0.002 s
Sampling time	T	0.00075 s
Environmental inertia matrix at neutral position	M_{e0}	$\begin{bmatrix} 0.047 & 0 & 0 \\ 0 & 0.045 & 0 \\ 0 & 0 & 0.04 \end{bmatrix}$ kg m^2
Environmental damping matrix	B_e	$0.1 I_{3\times3}$ Nm s/rad
		$0.1 I_{3\times3} + 0.005 K_{ankle}$ Nm s/rad
Environmental stiffness matrix	K_e	$10 \mathrm{I}_{3\times3}$ Nm/rad
		K_{ankle} Nm/rad
Gain matrix in simulation	K	$[U'_m \quad v_0]\mathrm{diag}(5 \quad 5 \quad 5 \quad 5)[U'_m \quad v_0]^T$
		$[U'_m \quad v_0]\mathrm{diag}(5 \quad 15 \quad 45 \quad 7)[U'_m \quad v_0]^T$

C.3 Simulation Parameters for Assistance Adaptation Scheme

This appendix provides the parameters used in the simulated case study to evaluate the efficacy of the different assistance adaptation scheme. Additionally, the simulation results and performance measures obtained from the passive-unconstrained, passive-constrained, active-unconstrained and active-constrained motion trials are also presented (Table C.3).

Table C.3 Parameters used in the simulation case study for the proposed assistance adaptation scheme

Description	Symbol	Value
Rotational offset of environmental coordinates from robot/global coordinates	Φ	$\frac{\pi}{4}$rad
Stiffness along negative x-axis of environment coordinates	k_1	110 N/m
Stiffness along positive x-axis of environment coordinates	k_2	110 N/m
Stiffness along negative y-axis of environment coordinates	k_3	25 N/m
Stiffness along positive y-axis of environment coordinates	k_4	25 N/m
Zero potential boundary in negative X-direction of the environment coordinates	u_{01}	−0.1 m
Zero potential boundary in positive X-direction of the environment coordinates	u_{02}	0.1 m
Zero potential boundary in negative Y-direction of the environment coordinates	u_{03}	−0.1 m
Zero potential boundary in positive Y-direction of the environment coordinates	u_{04}	0.1 m
End effector mass	m	1 kg
Environmental viscous damping	b_{env}	5 N s/m
Radius of circular reference trajectory	r_{ref}	0.7 m
Minor radius of elliptic kinematic constraint	l_a	0.2m
Major radius of elliptic kinematic constraint	l_b	0.8 m
Rotational offset of semi-minor axis from positive x-axis of global frame	φ	$\frac{\pi}{4}$rad
Stiffness of constraint boundary	k_{con}	1×10^6 N/m
Damping of constraint boundary	b_{con}	1000 N s/m

MIX
Papier aus verantwortungsvollen Quellen
Paper from responsible sources
FSC® C105338

If you have any concerns about our products,
you can contact us on
ProductSafety@springernature.com

In case Publisher is established outside the EU,
the EU authorized representative is:
Springer Nature Customer Service Center GmbH
Europaplatz 3, 69115 Heidelberg, Germany

Printed by Libri Plureos GmbH
in Hamburg, Germany